Significance of lipid
Profile assay as diagnostic
and prognostic tool

Arun Kumar

Title: *Significance of Lipid Profile Assay as a Diagnostic and Prognostic Tool.*

Author: **Arun Kumar**

ISBN-13: 978-1478325345
ISBN-10: 1478325348

Cover design and Layout: Elizabeth Log
design@imedpub.com

Publisher: **Internet Medical Publishing**
info@imedpub.com
http://imedpub.com/

First edition: 2012

Significance of lipid
Profile assay as diagnostic
and prognostic tool

Arun Kumar

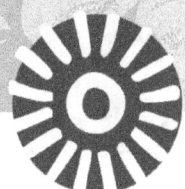

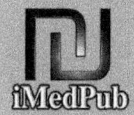

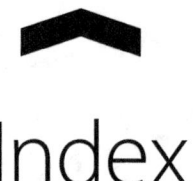

Index

V

Chapter 11
Serum TC/HDL-C, TG/HDL-C and LDL-C/HDL-C
in predicting the risk of myocardial infarction in
Normolipidemic patients in South Asia:
A case-control study   118

Chapter 12
The clinical utility of lipid profile and positive
troponin in predicting future cardiac events 128

Chapter 13
Study on lipid profile, oxidation stress and
carbonic anhydrase activity in patients with
essential hypertension   137

Chapter 14
Assessment of lipid profile in patients with
Human Immuno Deficiency Virus
(HIV/AIDS) without antiretroviral therapy   146

Chapter 15
Socio economic status, life style and behavioral
pattern of elderly normolipidemic myocardial
infarct subjects- A Case Control study from
South Asia   155

Chapter 16
Lipid parameters in predicting the risk of
myocardial infarction in elderly Normolipidemic
patients in South Asia: a multi centered
study from India, Nepal and Sri Lanka   166

Chapter 17
Cardiovascular risk factors in Elderly Normolipidemic Acute Myocardial Infarct Patients- A Case Controlled study from India 174

Chapter 18
Oxidative Stress, Endogenous Antioxidant and Ischemia-modified Albumin in Normolipidemic Acute Myocardial Infarction Patients 190

Chapter 19
Is Waist to Hip Ratio a better index than BMI in determining the risk of Myocardial Infarction in Normolipidemics? 199

Chapter 20
Thyroid Stimulating Hormone and its Correlation with Lipid Profile in the Obese Nepalese Population 205

Chapter 21
Does plasma fibrinogens and c-reactive protein predict the incidence of myocardial infraction in patients with normal lipids profile? 213

Chapter 22
Hypertriglyceridemia: A Case Report from Diagnostic Laboratory, Barasat, West Bengal, India 220

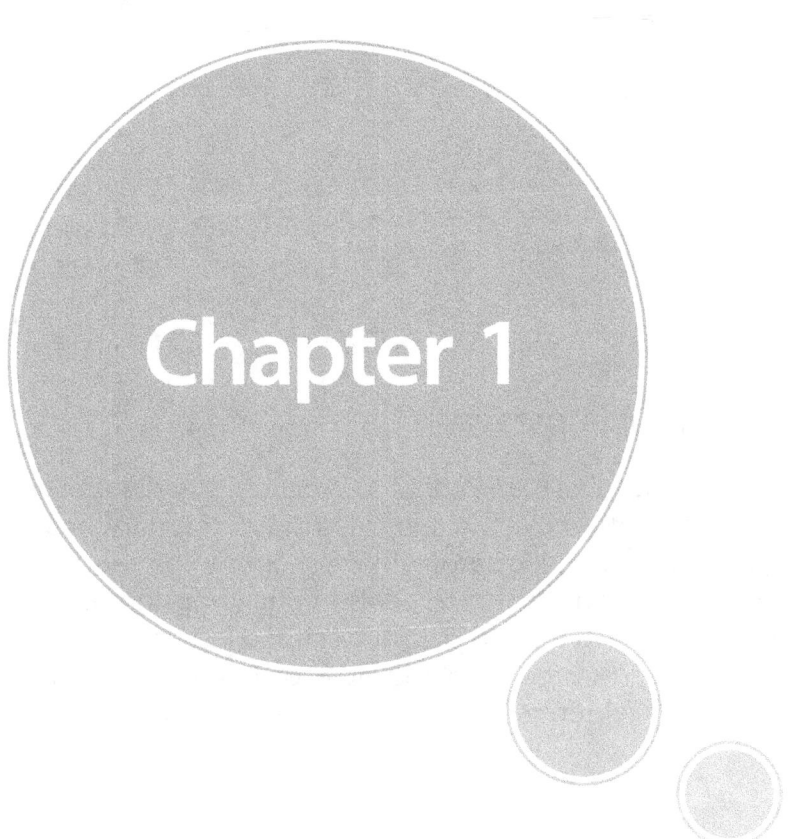

Chapter 1

Lipid Profile:
Its Importance

What does lipid profile means?

It is a group of tests that physician orders to biochemistry diagnostic laboratory in order to determine the subjects risk of coronary heart diseases. The items in the panel of profile have shown to be fantastic indicators as prognostic and diagnostic tools in analyzing the risk of subject who is likely to have a heart attack or stroke in future which can be caused due to blockage of blood flow or hardening of the arteries which in technical terms means atherosclerosis.

What are the parameters usually included when someone calls for lipid profile

Mainly it consists of measurement of Total cholesterol (TC), High density lipoprotein cholesterol (HDL-C), Low density lipoprotein cholesterol (LDL-C) and Triglycerides (TAG). Sometimes just by measuring these parameters the risk assessments cannot be fully justified so the physician calls for an extended profile. It means inclusion of some more parameters which is currently emerging biomarkers which concomitantly helps the physician in having a clear picture of the patients, how much likely they are going to be in the risk of cardiovascular disease. The parameters included in extended assay are Apolipoprotein A-I, Apolipoprotein B, High sensitivity C-reactive proteins, Lipoprotein (a), small-low density lipoprotein (sLDL), Apolipoprotein A-II, Apolipoprotein C-II, Apolipoprotein C-III and Apolipoprotein E.

Now the major concern is the ratio of total cholesterol/ HDL-C ratio, Triglycerides/ HDL-C ratio what we consider it as lipid of atherogenic potential. This risk is mainly based on the these ratios along with the variable parameters like age, sex additive to conventional risk factors like smoking, diet, exercise, sedentary life style, obesity, hypertension, diabetes. The best part is to keep your HDL-c always on the higher side (>60 mg/dl) so that you can enjoy benefit of one risk factor being subtracted.

Usually the blood sample for lipid profile assay is collected after twelve hours fasting, except water is permitted but if avoided results could be better. It is not necessary to get your lipid profile checked when you are in hospital with some ailment but it is recommended for all healthy individuals to get there blood tested for lipid profile once every five years even they do not have any risk for heart diseases. If you are known to have any remarkable risk factor and also if you are already on statins, than it is always advised to get it checked at frequent intervals say for six months interval and if your pocket does not permit than at least get your total cholesterol test done and if found drastically on the higher reference range than go for a total lipid profile assay along with the extended lipid profile and additive parameters as mentioned above to really know at how risk you are and also it would get you to check the effectiveness of your statins therapy.

Though for children and adolescents lipid testing is usually not called for routinely but it is always advised to check their profile too in case they have familial history of cardiovascular risks or death due to myocardial infarction, as the tendency for them to develop in future is always on the higher side. By seeing the children who are obese and have high blood pressure, parents of those are advised to check the lipid profile for their children. These children must get their lipid profile done when they are between two to ten years old and it is recommended by the American Academy of Pediatrics.

Soon when you get your results of lipid profile, your physician would determine at how risk you are after taking in consideration with your additive risks and then it would be considered whether you must start with lipid lowering drugs or just advised to be of low fat diet and exercise.

Our idea should be always to be on the safer side and our lipid profile should adhere to the guidelines laid down by National Cholesterol Education Program (NCEP).

As per NCEP, the following are the values of lipid profile-.

LDL-Cholesterol: <100 mg/dl (2.59 mmol/l).

Boderline high: 130-159 mg/dl (3.37-4.12 mmol/l).

High: 160-189 mg/dl (4.15-4.90 mmol/l).

Very high: > 190 mg/dl (4.90 mmol/l).

If you would find your LDL-C is ≤130 mg/dl than you are in safe zone but if increases, than you are approaching to risk. Keep a check on your diet pattern and if never go for brisk walking, you must start at least 30 min/day to burn your fat and calories.

As far as Total cholesterol is concerned.

Desirable range of Total -Cholesterol: <200 mg/dl (5.18 mmol/l).

Boderline high: 200-239 mg/dl (5.18-6.18 mmol/l).

High: ≥240 mg/dl (6.22 mmol/l).

It is always advisable to keep your HDL-Cholesterol always towards higher side because it is a negative risk factor and it is considered as good cholesterol and it is also called as a scavenger lipoprotein as it decreases the load of lipids from other circulating lipoproteins (lipids + proteins). Moreover HDL-C is associated with arylesterase activity (the enzyme which decreases the generation of free radicals and does not allow other lipoproteins to get oxidized, means much more atherogenic.

As per NCEP guidelines the risk increases when your HDL-C is well below >40 mg/dl (1.0 mmol/l) for men and for women > 50 mg/dl (1.3 mmol/l). The average risk is when it is between 40-50 mg/dl (1.0-1.3 mmol/l) for men and 50-59 mg/dl (1.3-1.5 mmol/l) for women. And as your HDL-C tends to be on higher side you are much safe and your levels should be >60 mg/dl for both genders (1.55 mmol/l).

As far as Triglycerides (TG) are concerned the desirable range should be <150 mg/dl(1.70 mmol/l), borderline high is from 150-159 mg/dl(1.7-2.2 mmol/l), high is from 200-499 mg/dl(2.3-5.6 mmol/l) and very high when found >500mg/dl(5.6 mmol/l).

Now when the physician gets aware of your lipid profile status, the first step in the treatment is to advice the patient to change his life style specifically targeting their dietary pattern, consisting of low cholesterol and also motivate them to go for mild to moderate exercise. If it is observed that these two parameters are not adequate enough to lower the cholesterol than the next step is to begin with drug therapy. These days several class of drugs are being marketed mainly to lower the cholesterol, mainly statins. First to begin with a low dosage and drastically adjust the dose depending on the lipid profile values and the dose is adjusted.

For knowledge for the commoners, the lipid profile consists of TC, LDL-C, VLDL-C, HDL-C, TG. All these lipoproteins are classified based on the content and composition of cholesterol, protein and triglycerides. LDL contains highest cholesterol concentration, VLDL contains highest TG and HDL contains the highest amount of protein. Usually as mentioned earlier HDL is always been an beneficial for its scavenging properties. The VLDL is derived by Friedwald's equation of TG/5 as it contains maximum TG.

Since TG is considered to be dangerous due to its atherogenic nature, their ability to initiate or fasten the process of atherogenesis, which causes the deposition of atheromas, lipid and calcium in the arterial lumen, so the risk of heart disease and stroke is directly related to VLDL concentrations. In technical term all cholesterol coming from Non-HDL-c fragment are considered to be atherogenic, they can cause narrowing of blood vessels and blockages.

Sometimes we must be aware when exactly the sample for lipid profile needs to be collected, because it might cause pre-analytical errors in results if the standard operating procedure is not followed. As far my studies are concerned, this test can be done any time of the day without fasting, as I worked in Acute Myocardial Infarct subjects who were admitted to Intensive Coronary Care Unit, so I never allowed any subjects who were already stressed out to go for fasting and my results were almost similar to those who went for fasting for twelve hours before undergoing lipid profile assay. Ideally, if this test is done with 12-hours fasting (no food and drink, except water) the results could be more accurate. For those who are smokers, try avoiding smoking at least 24 hours before as it might affect the results.

With the advent of latest researches, now the concept of lipid profile analysis has changed and we keep adding the latest concepts based on the findings of researches. Now the latest NCEP ATP-III (Adult Treatment Panel) guidelines recommends specifically to target the levels of LDL cholesterol (LDL-C) and HDL cholesterol (HDL-C) for determining cardiovascular disease (CVD) risk and evaluating the effectiveness of lipid-lowering therapies. To be more precise there is a growing consensus that the levels of apolipoprotein (apo) B and the ratio of Apo B/ apo A-I are more accurate predictors of cardiovascular risks but it is still not sure how far the commoners would understand this consensus based on apolipoprotein guidelines. Still the general public is well aware of lipid profile and NCEP guidelines.

It would take some time for a commoner to digest this very fact and get it recognized in public. So it is wiser to continue with the already familiar and proven measurements of LDL-C/HDL-C ratio as it provides key information regarding coronary heart disease, risk and is a better predictor than LDL-C alone. The salient points one must remember is to target the levels for both LDL-C and HDL-C to understand the risk of heart disease as its substantiated with several epidemiological and clinical studies for being the excellent monitor for checking the effectiveness of lipid lowering therapies. Also if one could get the ratio of these two parameters, we could literally judge the two way traffic of cholesterol entering and leaving arterial intima.

Now the point is why we switch on to the ratio of LDL-C/HDL-C, it is because this ratio is not affected by dietary cholesterol as it increases both LDL and HDL cholesterol, with a minimal change in the LDL-C/HDL-C ratio. If to be more precise it is predicted to increase 0.01 unit per 100 milligrams/day increase in dietary cholesterol, an amount unlikely to impact cardiovascular disease risk. In a large cohort study, the use of LDL-C/HDL-C ratio did not offer any advantage over the traditional lipid ratio of TC/HDL-C in terms of measuring prediction of future coronary events.

The other important area of concern is the risk caused solely by low density lipoprotein (LDL) which is recognized as an important risk factor for coronary artery disease (CAD) and is the main target for lipid lowering therapy. The LDL particles are heterogeneous in nature respect to its size, density, chemical composition and electrical charge and certain particle of LDL being more atherogenic compared to others. Reports from several case control and prospective studies from different parts of the world have established an association between small dense LDL particles and increased risk of CHD. The association of small dense LDL is well correlated with other well-recognized risk factors such as increased plasma triglycerides and apolipoprotein B as well as decreased HDL cholesterol levels.

It is said that the atherogenecity of small dense LDL is based on a number of factors. The small dense LDL particles are highly susceptibility to oxidation and there by the affinity for their receptors decreases with more affinity to bind to the arterial wall and its permeability towards the arterial cells more readily increases. Furthermore the small dense LDL particle also has a negative effect on endothelial function.

The relative factor attributing to 30-60% of the variation in LDL particle size is mainly due to genetic factors and the rest might be due to non-genetic influences. Enlisted environmental factors like food and dietary habitat, physical activity, abdominal obesity, insulin resistance and hyperinsulinemia mainly affects the variation of LDL particle size. LDL particle size is also under the influence of a number of genes, which include: Apo E, hepatic lipase, CETP, LPL and the ApoA1/C3/A4/A5 cluster.

It is established by various research studies that Indians have a high propensity to CAD compared to other ethnic groups across the globe despite of lower prevalence of conventional risk factors among Indians.

Now let us know something about metabolic syndrome which is often talked about due to its association with cardiovascular risks. The term metabolic syndrome is now associated with cardiovascular risks. Metabolic syndrome includes a set of risk factors like abdominal obesity, decreased ability to utilize glucose or we can say insulin resistance, dyslipidemia, and hypertension. It is observed that those subjects who have these risk factors are more predisposed to developing cardiovascular disease. This syndrome can affect at any age and is more frequently observed in those individuals who are physically inactive with significant overweight, especially if the deposition of excess fat in the abdominal area.

Way back in 1998, the World Health Organization (WHO) was the first to publish this and was widely accepted along with the guidelines in the third report of NCEP ATP-III.

The following are the criteria for clinical diagnosis of Metabolic syndrome:-

Clinical measures	WHO1	ATP III2	AHA/NHLBI3
Waist Circumference	-	≥102 cm in men, ≥88 cm in women	Same as ATP III
BMI	BMI >30 kg/m2	-	-
Triglycerides	≥150 mg/dL	Same as WHO	Same as WHO
HDL-C	<35 mg/dl (♂), <39 mg/dl (♀)	<40 mg/dl (♂), <50 mg/dl (♀)	Same as ATP III
Blood Pressure	≥140/90 mm Hg	≥130/85 mm Hg	Same as ATP III
Glucose	IGT, IFG, or T2D	Fasting >110 mg/dl (IFG)	Fasting ≥100 mg/dl (IFG)
Insulin Resistance	Yes	No	No
Microalbuminuria	Yes	No	No

The primary cause of most of the metabolic syndrome is due to poor diet control and sedentary life style these days as most of them are on high profile jobs, with additional smoking and coffee drinking habits at times of stress induced in job. All these are interrelated with metabolic syndrome. Due to poor diet control, it leads to obesity and lack of exercise leads to insulin resistance. Insulin resistance has a deep impact on lipid metabolism. It increases the VLDL and LDL and TG in blood and also decreases the HDL cholesterol, which is considered to be beneficial.

This further aggravates fatty plaque deposition in the arteries which, over time, can lead to cardiovascular disease and strokes. Insulin resistance also leads to increased insulin synthesis and glucose levels in the blood. Excess insulin causes more sodium retention by the renal tubules, which further increases blood pressure and finally leading to hypertension. Chronically elevated glucose levels in turn damage blood vessels and organs, causing neuropathy, nephropathy and cataract. The products formed with additional glucose moiety are called as advanced glycosylated end products.

A physicians usually suspects a subject having metabolic syndrome by few signs and symptoms along with the supportive findings of both laboratory and non-laboratory tests. Like if the subjects have central or abdominal obesity and leads a sedentary life style without much exercise in their daily routine.

The laboratory tests which is supportive are as follows-

Blood glucose- usually fasting or sometimes post-prandial or even oral glucose tolerance test. The main objective is to analyze whether the subject is able to tolerate glucose or they have any impaired response.

Lipid Profile- Check whether it is within normal reference range or elevated.

Sometimes physicians may also call for C-peptide and Insulin assay along with microalbumin or even hsCRP, all these parameters would rule out the endogenous Insulin synthesis and the extent of renal damage and inflammation so that the risk of cardiovascular diseases can be judged.

Other tests includes-

Plasminogen activator inhibitor-1 and proinsulin

The Non- laboratory tests includes-

These include blood pressure, weight, waist circumference and hip circumference to check abdominal obesity. Apart from these, body mass index is also measured.

Apart from the lipid profile as a prognostic tool in cardiovascular diseases, the concomitant measurement of plasma hsCRP levels is highly recommended as it acts as an inflammatory marker. It is said that irrespective of different treatment strategies the basal plasma hsCRP levels are always on the higher side. So it becomes immense important to analyze both plasma hsCRP level and TC/HDL-C ratio independently to predict future cardiovascular events and confirming hsCRP for its role as a biomarkers in clinical risk stratification especially in patients undergoing medical treatment.

These two parameters are the strongest predictors of future cardiovascular events even in healthy subjects irrespective of gender. The cut-off point for hsCRP is >0.1 mg/dl and for ratio it is >4.8. If they shoot to higher levels, it is indicative of future cardiovascular events, especially in those receiving medical treatment. If this result are known well in advance in these patients than they might get benefitted by early aggressive treatment such as statin therapy to reduce vascular inflammation, as well as further normalize the lipid profile.

Research findings state an association of HDL-C and TG with the mortality in patients with heart failure. It is demonstrated that higher serum HDL and TG were associated with lower mortality in patients with symptomatic heart failure of different etiologies. The protective role of HDL-C may be explained on the basis of endotoxin- lipoprotein hypothesis, which means that serum lipoproteins modulate inflammatory immune function and HDL-c has antioxidant, anti-inflammatory and anti-thrombic properties. It has been hypothesized that serum lipids measured in the early period of stroke are predictive of stroke severity and outcome. The levels of TG and HDL-C were significantly lower in patients.

Though it is understood that dyslipidemia is associated with coronary heart diseases (CHD) but they along with inflammatory markers like hs-CRP, myeloperoxidase (MPO), lipoprotein associated phospholipase A2(Lp-PLA2), and lipid peroxides (LP) are not adequate to predict the onset, extent, and prognosis of CHD. Lipoxins (LXs), resolvins, and protectins which are derived from ω-3 fatty acids: eicosapentaenoic acid (EPA) and docosahexaenoic acid (DHA), and ω-6 arachidonic acid in the presence of aspirin; whereas nitrolipids are formed due to the interaction between polyunsaturated fatty acids and nitric oxide (NO). LXs, resolvins, protectins, and nitrolipids are endogenous anti-inflammatory lipid molecules that inhibit production of interleukin-6 (IL-6) and tumor necrosis factor- α (TNF-α), suppress free radical generation, enhance NO generation; and accelerate tissue repair. Thus, beneficial actions of EPA/DHA and aspirin in CHD could be attributed to the formation of LXs, resolvins, protectins, and nitrolipids and suggest that their plasma levels aid in the prediction and prognosis of CHD. If this proposal is true, it implies that PUFAs are not only useful in the prevention of CHD but development of stable and synthetic analogues of LXs, resolvins, and nitrolipids may form a new approach in the management of cardiovascular diseases.

Dyslipidemia is noticed in most of the patients with premature coronary disease, comprising with a familial disorder in more than half of these cases, highlighting the importance of accurate diagnosis and scope for early treatment of affected families. It is of immense importance to go for clinical assessment, incorporating review of phenotypic features, personal and family history, physical signs and laboratory tests are the fundamental modes for diagnosis.

Key tests to exclude secondary causes of dyslipidemia:

Test	Reason for test
Renal profile(sodium, potassium, creatinine, estimated GFR)	Exclude renal failure
Liver profile(total protein, albumin, ALP,ALT,GGT)	Exclude cholestasis
Thyroid profile	Exclude hypothyroidism
Fasting glucose	Exclude diabetes
Dipstick urinary protein	Exclude nephritic syndrome

* ALP = alkaline phosphatase; ALT = alanine transaminase; GFR = glomerular filtration rate; GGT = gamma-glutamyl transpeptidase.

In the first instance, it is important to exclude all the secondary causes of dyslipidemia. So diabetes mellitus, untreated hypothyroidism, nephritic syndrome and cholestasis which are associated with hyperlipidemia can be excluded by a base line tests as mentioned above to rule out the dyslipidemia due to other causes. In addition to secondary causes of dyslipidemia, there are medications which can cause dyslipidemia, some of which includes corticosteroids which increases cholesterol and triglycerides, oestrogens and retinoids which increases triglycerides, anabolic steroids which lower high-density lipoprotein cholesterol.

For most instances, the primary dyslipidemia in patients is considerably easy to manage once diagnosed. How ever it is always better to consider all the various possiblilites of a familial aetiology, especially in those patients with strong family history of coronary heart disease (CHD). With early diagnosis and usage of appropriate lipid-lowering therapy and therapeutic lifestyle changes, major cardiovascular complications can be prevented.

Familial hypercholesterolaemia (FH) is due to an autosomal genetic defect affecting the LDL-receptor pathway. The Low-density lipoprotein –derived cholesterol acts as several levels, to suppress transcription of the LDL-receptors to provide sufficient cholesterol for metabolic needs. When cholesterol levels in the cell increase, the formation and up regulation of LDL- receptors is decreased. FH is caused by mutations in genes coding for the LDL-receptor (LDLR), apolipoprotein (apo) B 100 (the LDL-receptor ligand), and a protease known as PCSK9 (proprotein convertase subtilisin/kexin type 9), which is involved in the regulation of LDL- receptor recycling.

Tendon xanthomas, characteristic of familial hypercholesterolaemia

The finding of tendon xanthomas confirms the diagnosis of FH. Although these are found in fewer than 30% of cases, greater than 80% of such cases will have a disease defining mutation in LDLR, APOB or PCSK9 genes. Research studies have confirmed the presence of this clinical sign is associated with a significant increase in cardiovascular disease risk across all age groups.

Combined hyperlipidaemia

While investigating lipid profile, when elevated LDL cholesterol, triglycerides or both when elevated are suggestive of a number of dyslipidaemias. These include familial combined hyperlipidaemia (FCH), remnant hyperlipidaemia (Type III or familial dysbetalipoproteinaemia) and dyslipidaemia associated with the metabolic syndrome, as well as milder presentations of familial hypertriglyceridaemia

Lipid profile associated with familial combined hyperlipidaemia

↑ Total Cholesterol (6.5-10.0 mmol/l)
↑ LDL Cholesterol
↑ Triglycerides (2.3-6.0 mmol/l or higher)
Apo B/ total cholesterol > 0.15
VLDL cholesterol/total triglycerides <0.69*
Small, dense, LDL
Diagnosis is commonly based on the combination of apo B >1.20 g/l+ triglycerides >1.5 mmol/l with a family history of premature cardiovascular disease

* Determined by ultracentrifugation, apo B= apolipoprotein B, LDL= low-density lipoprotein, VLDL= very low density lipoprotein

Xanthelasma represent areas of lipid-laden macrophages. The presence of these is predictive of an increased risk of coronary heart disease, atherosclerosis and mortality

Familial Combined hyperlipidemia (FCH) affects about one of hundred people. The mechanism involves overproduction of very-low-density lipoprotein (VLDL) and apoB. The genetic basis is very complex and multifactorial and is influenced by environmental factors. Since there is a vast variablility in presentation, disgnosis of FCH can often be missed in practice. It should be suspected if total cholesterol levels are in the range 6.5–8.0 mmol/l and/or triglycerides between 2.3 and 5.0 mmol/l (as shown in **Table**). Elevated levels, either alone or in combination, in patients and other family members confer a 'variable phenotype'.

Invariably ApoB is elevated and is therefore a very useful diagnostic tool, with levels >1.20 g/l, together with elevated triglycerides and family history of cardiovascular disease, strongly suggestive of diagnosis. The finding of an apoB concentration that is unexpectedly low (apoB/total cholesterol ratio <0.15 g/mmol) raises suspicion of remnant hyperlipidaemia. The presence of xanthelasma is not of diagnostic significance but represents an area of lipid-laden macrophages, which is predictive of an increased risk of CHD, atherosclerosis and mortality.

After getting to know of the various parameters of lipid profile and its efficacy in detection of cardiovascular disorders, now let's know something about the role of lipid profile as a prognostic and a diagnostic tool for diseases. There are several diseases where lipid profile could be prognostic and diagnostic. Changes in lipid profile have been associated with the structural integrity with the cellular membranes. It is observed in patients with oral premalignant lesions there is a significant decrease in plasma TC, HDLC and Apo-A1 which signifies inverse relationship between plasma lipid levels. The hypothesis is based on lowering of plasma cholesterol and other lipid constituents due to their increased utilization.

In a prospective case-control study it was found that among a panel of lipid and lipoprotein biomarkers, baseline triglycerides, very low-density lipoprotein (VLDL) size, and intermediate-density lipoprotein (IDL) particle number were significantly associated with ischemic stroke in postmenopausal women. By this information we can change lifestyle and also medications are warranted to reduce the risk of ischemic stroke in population.

Chronic hyperglycemia is also linked to subclinical myocardial injury, identified through the elevated levels of cardiac Troponin T (cTnT). The association, which existed in both diabetics and non-diabetics, suggests that hyperglycemia contributes to myocardial injury beyond its role in the development of atherosclerosis. Glycated hemoglobin (HbA1c) as a marker of chronic hyperglycemia has been associated with incident coronary heart disease (CHD) and all-cause mortality, but much less is known about any relationship between HbA1c and subclinical CHD.

Cardiac Troponin T also has been independently associated with CHD. The availability of a novel high sensitivity-cTnT assay made it possible for the authors to evaluate whether HbA1c levels would be associated with subclinical myocardial injury measured by elevated cTnT concentrations.

An expert panel formed by the National Lipid Association (NLA) currently recommends a enormous expansion in the use of new biomarkers for the diagnosis and management of cardiovascular disease. The recommendations, if widely adopted, would significantly increase not just the use of these diagnostic tests but also lead to much greater use of lipid-lowering drugs. The NLA panel recommends a greatly expanded role for 5 out of 6 new biomarkers– CRP, Lp-PLA2, Apo B, LDL particle number, and Lp(a). (HDL or LDL subfractions did not receive an expanded recommendation)

Measurement of lipid parameters, including lipoproteins, apolipoproteins, particle size, and density, beyond a standard fasting lipid profile is not recommended for cardiovascular risk assessment in asymptomatic adults.

The consensus panel recommends that the use of LDL particle number for initial clinical risk assessment of CVD is reasonable for many patients at intermediate risk, including patients with a family history of coronary heart disease (CHD) and recurrent cardiac events. In addition, LDL particle number should be considered in the risk assessment of selected patients with known CHD or CHD risk equivalent.

The panel also recommends that LDL particle number for on-treatment management of CVD risk is reasonable for many patients at intermediate risk, including patients with coronary heart disease, a CHD risk equivalent and in patients with recurrent cardiac events. LDL particle number should be considered in the management of selected patients with a family history of CHD.

Apart from cardiovascular diseases, there are many more diseases where lipid profile may serve as a prognostic factor. One such is in cancer patients. In these patients, there is drastic lowering of plasma TC, HDL-C which is considered as non-specific prognostic parameters in patients.The prognosis of women with early-stage breast cancer is affected by certain metabolic factors, namely insulin and body mass index. Higher levels of TC were observed amongst low grade tumors.

Even in leukemia and also in Hodgkin's disease, the serum level of cholesterol and HDL- cholesterol drastically decreases along with the elevated levels of TG. The inverse association between cancer and serum cholesterol may reflect a physiological response to the early stages of cancer. Thus hypocholesterolemia can be a possible prognostic factor in leukemia and Hodgkin's disease.

Hypercholesterolemia associated with enghanced atherosclerotic changes occurs in cases of systematic lupus erythematosus (SLE). The exact mechanism of atheroscelorotic pattern remains unveiled. However the immunological events in the progression of disease, the presence of anticardiolipin antibodies and hyperlipidemia contribute to development of atherosclerosis. Therefore early diagnosis, treatment and prevention of dyslipidemia are important aspects of treatment in patients with SLE.

In some malignant diseases, the serum cholesterol is altered significantly. It has been proposed that alteration in serum cholesterol in the proliferating tissues and in blood could reflect its role in carcinogenesis. The link of lipids with cancer might be affirmed as lipids have an intergral role in the maintenance of cellular integrity. Also, it is observed that antineoplastic therapies have an influence on lipid profile.

The exact mechanisms by which lipids and lipoproteins may contribute to carcinogenesis are not clearly understood. It is however suggested from research reports that the lipid peroxidation product, malondialdehyde, may cross-link DNA on the same and opposite strands via adenine and cytosine. This could link the theory of contribution of lipid peroxidation to carcinogenecity and mutagenecity in mammalian cells.

LDL-cholesterol is more susceptible to oxidation in various pathologic conditions resulting in higher LPO (lipid peroxidation) during oxidative stress. On the other hand, HDLcholesterol is able to nullify the oxidative damage of LDL-cholesterol on cell membrane and prevent LPO. It has been suggested that HDL-cholesterol prevents both enzymatic and nonenzymatic generation of O_2^-, H_2O_2 and OH· and thus acts as an anticarcinogen and a powerful antioxidant.

Apart from cancer, the low lipid levels in particular high density lipoprotein-cholesterol and total cholesterol is predictive of adverse outcomes in patients with lower respiratory tract infections. Thus reflecting the severity of disease, plasma lipid levels may be complementary tool in the diagnostic and prognostic work up of patients with lower respiratory tract infections.

The lipid profile prognostic significance can also be observed in patients with falciparum malaria. In these patients the most remarkable feature is severe elevations of serum TG and VLDL which on treatment declines.

The diagnostic importance of lipid profile changes can also be exploited in cases with acute pancreatitis. Acute pancreatitis (AP) is a common systemic inflammatory disorder of the pancreas. It is observed that the serum TG levels are severely elevated in first two days of episode. Also the level of HDL-C falls significantly in alcoholic and hypertriglyceridemic AP cases denote the severity of the disease.

Plasma lipidomics also reveals potential prognostic in cystic fibrosis patients. In these patients the variation of plasma levels of phosphotidylcholine and lysophosphotidylcholine is observed. Even in kidney transplant recipients' lipid markers could be of prognostically important in allograft survival. If elevations of TC or its subtractions and elevated TG are not associated with increased risk for patient mortality or allograft loss in these kidney transplants recipients.

Serum lipid profile could also be useful in evaluating the prognosis of decompensated cirrhosis. The usage of combined model for end-stage liver disease (MELD) and blood lipid have been useful to evaluate the prognostic implications in these patients with decompensated cirrhosis. Even though MELD score is still controversial for its ability to determine the pathogenic condition of end stage liver disease, but currently researchers are attempting to estimate the extent of pathogenesis of liver disease more accurately through MELD scores. Since liver is the main organ for synthesis, storage, transport and decomposition of lipids, including the secretion of particulate lipids. So the synthesis and secretion of any lipoprotein from the liver could be affected if the severity of the liver damage increases. It thus is indicated by reduced synthesis of HDL-C, TC, VLDL levels in death due to liver cirrhosis.

Even in cases of liver disorder the lipid parameters are affected. Since lipids are essential components of biological membranes, free molecules and metabolic regulators that control cellular function and homeostasis.Liver plays an immense role in lipid metabolism. Dyslipidemia seen in chronic liver disease differs from the other causes of secondary lyslipidemia.

Also in cases of disorders of muscle lipid metabolism, the lipid profile could be of diagnostic and therapeutic importance. All those pathways which are confined to muscle with respect to lipid metabolism would get hampered in case of muscle disorders. It involves intramyocellular triglyceride degradation, carnitine uptake, long-chain fatty acids mitochondrial transport or even fatty acid oxidation. These cause muscular weakness and are associated with severe increased muscle lipid content (lipid storage myopathies) in case of primary carnitine deficiency, neutral lipid storage disease and multiple acyl-CoA dehydrogenase deficiency.For all these lipid associated disorders the main biochemical test which gives clue for diagnosis are measurement of blood carnitine acylcarnitine and urinary organic acid profile.

Even in Duchenne muscular dystrophy, the concentration of triglycerides, phospholipids, free cholesterol, cholesterol esters and total cholesterol is elevated drastically. The ratio of free cholesterol to cholesterol esters is also significantly elevated in DMD patients.

In cases of late onset of neonatal sepsis (NLS), plasma lipid and lipoprotein is of diagnostic importance. In these case, the TC, TG, lipoprotein-a (Lp-a), HDL and apolipoprotein-A (Apo-A) and B (Apo-B) were significantly lower in the neonatal sepsis.

But amongst all parameters, Apo-A appeared to be a useful marker for detection of NLS.

Even the plasma fatty acid is also useful as diagnostic markers in autistic patients. Autism is a family of development disorders of unknown origin. The disorder is characterized by behavioral, development, neuropathological and sensory abnormalities, usually diagnosed in children aged 5-8 years. The brain is one of the most-lipid enriched tissues in the human body. Infants' brain while maturation and growth needs extensive fatty acid especially docosahexanoic acid and cholesterol which is scavenged from circulation. Thus analyzing the concentration and composition of fatty acids in circulation would be of immense diagnostic importance.

Enzyme deficiencies of fatty acid oxidation in mitochondria usually present in the neonate are accompanied with hypoketotic hypoglycaemia, metabolic acidosis, mitochondrial dysfunction, hyperammonemia, muscle weakness, cardiomyopathy, seizures, psychomotor delay, developmental regression, behavioural disorders and attention deficit disorder. Usually neonates have a poor prognosis, including cardiac arrhythmia and sudden death. The serum concentration of short chain fatty acids namely acetic, valeric, hexanoic and stearidonic acids are significantly higher in autistic patients. The acetic acid levels are indicative of gastrointestinal inflammation which is the most common clinical presentation. The most remarkable finding in autism is elevation of valeric acid which is reported to have an antioxidant property in neutralising H_2O_2 oxidative stress.

Polyunsaturated fatty acids (PUFA) are very critical for intellectual growth and development in the neonatal/ infant brain and in early childhood. PUFA could also play an important role in cognitive function in older children. In addition, PUFA have been specifically associated with dopamine activity in the frontal lobes of the brain. Diets rich in saturated fats may increase brain uptake of intact free fatty acids from the plasma through the blood brain barrier (BBB).

Thus, it could be realized that just by simple measurement of lipid profile, we can arrive with so many diagnostic features of it and its clinical usefulness too. In a nutshell only little have been discovered about the lipids and many more are awaited from the future researches with respect to its diagnostic and prognostic implications in management of diseases.

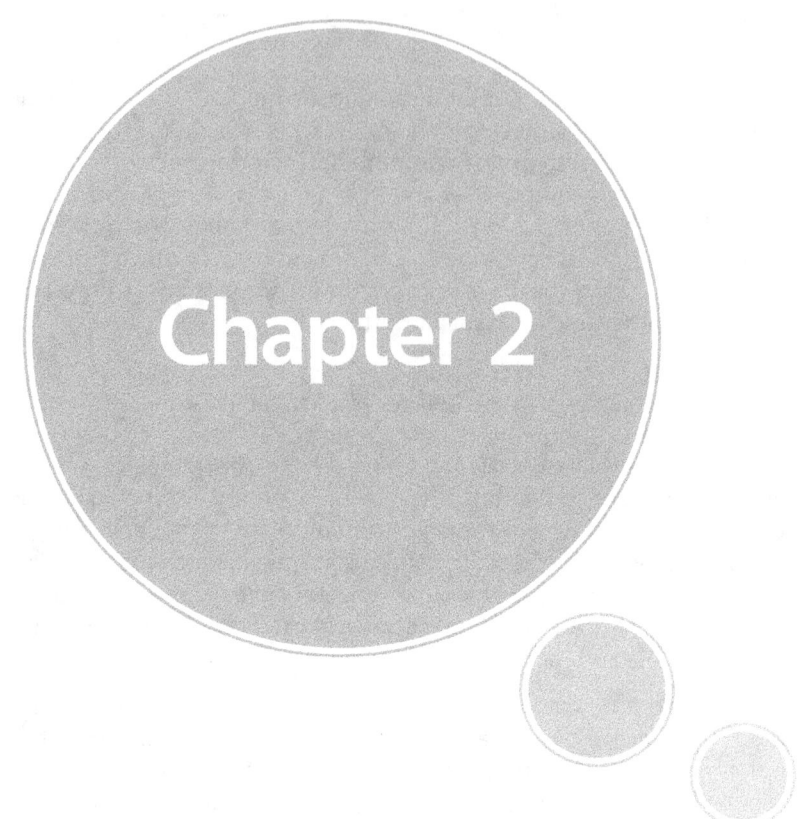

Chapter 2

Anthropometric measurement in myocardial infract patients with normal lipid profile

Abstract

Objectives: To observe if there any changes noticed in anthropometric variables in patients of myocardial infarction with normal lipid profiles compared to normal healthy control.

Materials and Methods: The study was conducted at University of Peradeniya, Department of Biochemistry, Faculty of Medicine, Peradeniya, Sri Lanka. The study subjects were categorized into two groups – one being control and the other being normolipaedemic AMI patients. The control group and study group consist of 165 healthy age and sex matched subjects where as 165 age sex matched normolipaedemic AMI patients. The physical examination emphasized measurement of height, weight, waist circumference, hip circumference, waist-hip ratio, mid arm circumference, biceps skin fold thickness and triceps skin fold thickness. Height was measured in centimeters and weight in kilograms using calibrated spring balance. Supine waist girth was measured at the level of umbilicus with a person breathing silently and standing hip girth was measured at inter-trochanteric level. Mid arm circumference was measured half way between the acromion process of the scapula and the tip of the elbow. Triceps skin fold thickness (TSFT) measurements were made at a point over the triceps muscle mid way the acromion and olecranon process on the posterior aspect of the arm.

Results: The present study observed highly significant changes (p<0.001) in weight, waist circumference, hip circumference, biceps and triceps skin fold thickness in cases compared to healthy age-sex matched control.

Conclusion: Waist-to-hip ratio is a marker for determining the patients of myocardial infarction. The importance of anthropometric measurement should be implemented in ruling out the patients of high risk groups apart from considering the conventional risk factors.

Key words: Anthropometric measurement, normal lipid profile, myocardial infarction.

Introduction: Coronary artery disease is a major cause of mortality and morbidity in the industrialized world. Recent research in this area focused primarily on the management of patients with overt disease, but there has been an increasing emphasis on the identification and early detection of factors that predispose to the development and progression of coronary artery disease. As a result research efforts are no longer directed solely towards management but toward early detection and prevention as well. Coronary artery disease (CAD) develops through the chain of events. The presence certain risk factors elicit changes in the heart and vascular, some of which may initially be beneficial but may be maladaptive or become pathogenic when they progress. Cardiac biochemistry- hyperlipidemia a subject of rapidly growing importance in Indian and Sri Lankan population. In fact, on account of neglect and ignorance, this extremely important subject has not received any attention at all [1]. Due to economical variations there is a major demographic shift of the population from rural to urban areas. The urban population has rapidly acquired many of the adverse factors for CAD. There is change from traditional vegetarian food habits to a mixed food pattern consisting of intake of excess saturated fats also in the form of "fast foods" [2]. In addition there is a considerable exposure to stress of day to day living, especially in metropolitan cities, living little or no time for physical exercise and causing excess smoking, alcohol consumption with acquisition of these additives habits a complex interaction of inherited and acquired risk factors are likely to operate, leading to insulin resistance and accelerated atherosclerosis. Recent research focused on the anthropometric variables in assessing the risk of heart attack as these could be an additive factor apart from the conventional risk factors involved in the etiology of myocardial infarction. Recent studies on anthropometric measurement focused on waist-to-hip ratio, irrespective of other heart disease risk factors. Until now, researchers and doctors have used body mass index (BMI) to judge someone is overweight but a global study found waist girth divided by hip circumference would more accurately predicted the people who would suffer heart attacks. According to the researchers, the danger point was more than 0.85 for women and more than 0.9 for men. This is because fat stored around the waist is more likely to affect lipids in the blood and clog up arteries than fat stored around the thighs and hips. It is more likely that apple shape physic is more risky than pear shape. The researchers found that BMI was only slightly higher in heart attack patients than in the others, with no difference for people from the Middle East and southern Asia. But heart attack patients had "strikingly higher" waist-to-hip ratios, irrespective of other heart disease risk-factors. This observation was also found to be consistent in men and women across all ages, and in all regions of the world. A larger waist size was found to be harmful, whereas larger hip size - possibly indicating lower-body muscle mass - was protective. With a view of the above studies, the present study was undertaken to assess the effect of anthropometric variables of patients with myocardial infarction with normal lipid profile irrespective of the effects of dyslipidemia.

Materials and Methods: The study was conducted at University of Peradeniya, Department of Biochemistry, Faculty of Medicine, Peradeniya, Sri Lanka. The study subjects were categorized into two groups – one being control and the other being Normolipidemic AMI patients. The control group and study group consist of 165 healthy age and sex matched subjects where as 165 age sex matched normolipaedemic AMI patients. The subjects chosen as control for the study underwent the given criterion for being classified as normal individuals:

i. One hundred sixty-five healthy males and 165 healthy females between the age of 48 and 69 years.
ii. Normal and healthy persons not suffering from any physiological and pathological illness.
iii. Their lipid profiles were normal.
iv. A proforma was prepared that incorporated information regarding demographic, anthropometric and clinical variation.

The physical examination emphasized measurement of height, weight, waist circumference, hip circumference, waist-hip ratio, mid arm circumference, biceps skin fold thickness and triceps skin fold thickness. Height was measured in centimeters and weight in kilograms using calibrated spring balance. Supine waist girth was measured at the level of umbilicus with a person breathing silently and standing hip girth was measured at inter-trochanteric level.

Mid arm circumference was measured half way between the acromion process of the scapula and the tip of the elbow. Triceps skin fold thickness (TSFT) measurements were made at a point over the triceps muscle mid way the acromion and olecranon process on the posterior aspect of the arm.

Diagnostic criteria: Body Mass Index (Weight in kg/height in meters)[2] was calculated and obesity defined as BMI≥25kg/m2. Truncal obesity was diagnosed when waist-hip ratio was >0.9 in male and >0.8 in female.

Normal lipid profile was defined if LDL-C was less than 160 mg/dl, HDL-C ≥ 35mg/dl and TG < 200 mg/dl [3]. Isolated low HDL-C (IL- HDL-C) was defined if levels of HDL-C were less than 35 mg/dl, LDLC less than 160 mg/dl and TG less than 200 mg/dl [4]. Isolated high LDL (IL-LDL-C) was defined if the LDL-C was ≥ 160, TG <200 mg/dl, HDL-C ≥ 35 mg/dl. Isolated high TG (IH-TG) was defined if the TG was ≥200 mg/dl, LDL-C less than 160 mg/dl, HDL-C ≥ 35 mg/dl.

The study was further preceded by collecting blood samples, after an overnight fast. Five ml of blood sample was collected from each patient in a sterilized vial from the anticubital vein avoiding venostasis. The blood sample was stored in heparinized vial for antioxidant studies. The parameters mainly observed were Lipid Profiles.

Plasma total cholesterol, HDL-cholesterol and triglycerides were assayed using an enzymatic estimation kit (Randox Laboratories Limited, Crumlin, UK). Plasma LDL-cholesterol was determined from the values of total cholesterol and HDL-cholesterol using the following formulae:

$$\text{LDL-cholesterol} = \text{Total cholesterol} - \frac{\text{Triglycerides}}{5} - \text{HDL-cholesterol (mg/dl)}$$

For statistical analysis two-sample t-test was performed and the results were expressed as mean ± SD, P≤0.05 was considered significant.

Results: The findings of the present study are shown in **Table 1, 2, 3** and **4 Table 1** and **2** depicts the lipid profile measurement in controls and cases and gender-wise analysis. **Table 3** and **4** shows the findings of the anthropometric variables in cases of myocardial infracted subjects with normal lipid profiles. The present study observed highly significant changes in weight, waist circumference, hip circumference, Biceps and Triceps skin fold thickness when controls and cases were compared.

Table 1. Lipid Profile in Control and Case of Myocardial Infarct subjects.

Variables	Control (n = 165)	Case (n = 165)	P value
Age (Mean ± SD)	60.55 ± 3.98	61.84 ± 3.80	p>0.1
Total Cholesterol (mg/dl)	168.58 ± 12.16	186.44 ± 13.95	p<0.001
HDL-Cholesterol (mg/dl)	50.51 ± 6.78	41.27 ± 4.62	P<0.001
TC: HDL-C ratio	3.39 ± 0.36	4.57 ± 0.58	P<0.001
Triglycerides (mg/dl)	107.84 ± 11.51	128.96 ± 12.19	P<0.001
LDL-Cholesterol (mg/dl)	83.59 ± 11.95	119.37 ± 14.05	P<0.001
LDL:HDL-C ratio	1.90 ± 0.31	2.93 ± 0.51	P<0.001
TG: HDL-C ratio	2.17 ± 0.35	3.16 ± 0.49	p>0.1

Table 2. Lipid Profile in Males and Females of Control and Case of Myocardial Infarct subjects.

Variables	Control		Case	
	Male(n=123)	Female(n=42)	Male(n=123)	Female(n=42)
Age (Mean ± SD)	60.68 ± 4.14	60.52 ± 2.93	61.53 ± 3.28	62.73 ± 4.97
P value			p>0.1	p>0.1
Total Cholesterol (mg/dl)	168.09 ± 12.10	170.00 ± 12.35	183.84 ± 13.65	194.03 ± 13.03
P value			p<0.001	p<0.001
HDL-Cholesterol (mg/dl)	49.90 ± 7.30	52.31 ± 4.58	41.78 ± 4.88	39.77 ± 3.37
P value			p<0.5	p<0.001
TC: HDL-C ratio	3.42 ± 0.30	3.28 ± 0.47	4.45 ± 0.58	4.96 ± 0.44
P value			p<0.001	p<0.001
Triglycerides (mg/dl)	105.02 ± 10.31	116.11 ± 10.96	126.22 ± 11.74	136.99 ± 9.81
P value			p<0.001	p<0.001
LDL-Cholesterol (mg/dl)	79.88 ± 7.98	94.47 ± 14.81	116.82 ± 13.76	126.86 ± 12.22
P value			p<0.001	p>0.1
LDL:HDL-C ratio	1.92 ± 0.25	1.83 ± 0.44	2.84 ± 0.52	3.21 ± 0.40
P value			p<0.001	p>0.1
TG:HDL-C ratio	2.15 ± 0.37	2.23 ± 0.28	3.06 ± 0.47	3.47 ± 0.41
P value			p<0.01	p<0.001

Table 3. Anthropometric variables in Control and Cases of Myocardial Infarct
subjects.

Variables	Control (n=165)	Case (n=165)	P value
Age (Mean ± SD)	60.55 ± 3.98	61.84 ± 3.80	p>0.1
Height (cm)	1.63 ± 0.04	1.64 ± 0.05	p>0.1
Weight (kg)	68.34 ± 3.97	72.01 ± 5.37	p<0.001
BMI (kg/m^2)	25.40 ± 1.20	26.16 ± 1.45	p<0.01
Waist Circumference(cm)	93.70 ± 3.63	100.77 ± 6.06	p<0.001
Hip Circumference (cm)	100.01 ± 3.16	105.72 ± 5.23	p<0.001
Waist: Hip ratio	0.93 ± 0.01	0.95 ± 0.01	p<0.02
Mid Arm Circumference(cm)	29.70 ± 1.47	30.63 ± 1.87	p<0.05
Biceps skin fold thickness (mm)	6.95 ± 1.05	7.5 ± 1.38	p<0.001
Triceps skin fold thickness (mm)	11.97 ± 1.27	12.89 ± 1.69	p<0.001

Table 4. Anthropometric variables in males and females in Control and Cases of
Myocardial Infarct subjects.

| Variables | Control | | Case | |
	Male(n=123)	Female(n=42)	Male(n=123)	Female(n=42)
Age (Mean ± SD)	60.68 ± 4.14	60.52 ± 2.93	61.53 ± 3.28	62.73 ± 4.97
P value			p>0.1	p>0.1
Height (cm)	1.64 ± 0.04	1.61 ± 0.03	1.66 ± 0.05	1.59 ± 0.04
P value			p>0.1	p>0.1
Weight (kg)	68.64 ± 3.78	67.47 ± 4.41	71.68 ± 5.28	72.45 ± 5.69
P value			p<0.001	p<0.001
BMI (kg/m^2)	25.33 ± 1.06	25.63 ± 1.54	26.02 ± 1.34	26.57 ± 1.69
P value			p>0.1	p>0.1
Waist Circumference (cm)	93.38 ± 3.37	94.64 ± 4.21	100.18 ± 5.69	102.50 ± 6.82
P value			p<0.001	p<0.001
Hip Circumference (cm)	99.73 ± 2.89	100.80 ± 3.75	105.28 ± 4.98	107.00 ± 5.78
P value			p>0.1	p<0.001
Waist: Hip ratio	0.93 ± 0.01	0.93 ± 0.01	0.95 ± 0.01	0.95 ± 0.01
P value			p>0.1	p<0.001
Mid Arm Circumference (cm)	29.62 ± 1.30	29.95 ± 1.88	30.44 ± 1.80	31.17 ± 2.00
P value			p<0.001	p<0.001
Biceps skin fold thickness (mm)	6.88 ± 1.01	7.17 ± 1.15	7.43 ± 1.30	7.69 ± 1.59
P value			p>0.1	p>0.1
Triceps skin fold thickness (mm)	11.86 ± 1.18	12.30 ± 1.50	12.82 ± 1.61	13.08 ± 1.93
P value			p<0.001	p>0.1

Discussions: Coronary artery disease remains the major cause of morbidity and mortality in all developed and developing countries in the world like India and Sri Lanka. It has already climbed the charts from 14th to 4th place only behind tuberculosis, communicable disease and malnutrition. Lipid and lipoproteins are the major risk factors for CAD; however they do not account for the disease in 30%- 40% of the population with CAD [5]. Other risk factors include smoking, hypertension, diabetes mellitus etc.

Major CAD risk factors do not predict subsequently myocardial infarction accurately and do not fully explain social class differences in South Asians as these have high incidence of CAD which is not fully explained by conventional risk factors. Present study focus on those group of patients who had MI even being their lipid profiles were normal. As mentioned earlier subjects selected for the study were divided two groups. Control group comprising of 165 subjects (48-69 years of age) and Patients (48-71 years of age). Anthropometric measurements were taken for both the control and MI. The anthropometric measurement in control and myocardial infarct patients are shown in **Table 1**. The observations reveals very minimal changes in anthropometric measurements except the observations on Body weight, Waist circumference(WC), Biceps skin fold thickness (BSFT) and Triceps skin fold thickness (TSFT) where the changes were highly significant ($p < 0.0001$). The observations made therefore conclude that as far as anthropometric measurements are concerned, the major changes were observed in Body weight, WC, BSFT and TSFT and are statistically significant.

Earlier study [6] reported that waist to hip ratio is a dominant independent, predictive variable for CVD and CHD deaths in Australian men and women. They stressed on the assessment of obesity by waist-hip ratio which is a better predictor of CVD and CHD mortality than waist circumference, which in turn, is a better predictor than BMI. The recognition of central obesity is clinically important, as life style intervention is likely to provide significant health benefits. In another study [7] it was reported that high hip circumference, relative to body size and waist circumference predicts low incidence of CVD and CHD and total deaths in women but not in case of men; BMI and WC were the strongest independent predictors. In present study we found both larger hip circumference (HC) and WC the data were highly significant in both genders of patients for waist circumference but only females had significant differences in hip circumference.

In another study conducted[8] on the clinical usefulness of waist-to-hip ratio (WHR) for predicting the risk of cardiovascular events, estimated with models based on the data from Framingham and Prospective Cardiovascular Munster (PROCAM) studies was evaluated. A total of 552 men and 160 women, asymptomatic and at risk for CVD, aged 30-74 years were recruited from an ongoing risk factor screening program conducted at worksites. They found abdominal fat was a strong predictor of cardiovascular complications in subjects whose WHR was in the top quintile (>0.98 for men and >0.091 for women). The estimated percentage rate of coronary heart disease (CHD, $p < 0.01$) and death ($p < 0.01$), myocardial infarction ($p < 0.01$), stroke ($p < 0.01$), total CVD ($p < 0.01$) increased with increasing quintile of WHR in men and women. In the highest WHR, the number of subjects exceeding a 15% risk of developing a coronary event over the next 10 years was more than two-fold greater than in the lowest WHR quintiles. They concluded abdominal deposition of fat assessed by WHR may be strong clinical value for predicting high risk of cardiovascular events.

In another study reported [9] that even though the prevalence of obesity is not high in Asians Indians, the cardiovascular risk factors have been reported. It was a cross-sectional study that involved 639 subjects (170 men and 469 women) from low socioeconomic stratum residing in urban slums of New Delhi, reported approximately 68% of men and 88% of women had at least one risk factor for CVD. They concluded that Asian Indians have excess cardiovascular risk at BMI and WC values considered "normal". They suggested that the definitions of "normal" ranges of BMI and WC need to be revised for Asian Indians. The findings of the present study is not agreeable to the earlier study [10] where the prevalence of 13.6% of overweight and 2.2% of obesity in myocardial infarct subjects. 45.5% of them had normal weight and 38.4% were underweight. 11.4% had waist-hip ratio $\geq$ 92. They found positive correlation between BMI and Waist –Hip ratio (WHR). In present study we found the mean value of all the subjects was above 25.0 tending towards overweight, but the differences were insignificant in control and study. Present study reports that the waist-hip ratios were above 0.93 in all the subjects and the values were significant only in females. The evaluation of central obesity by way of the WHR has been recognized as a substantial component in the assessment of CVD risk factor due to a positive association between high WHR and hypertension. In a study [11] worked on survivors of acute myocardial infarction (MI) with respect to their weight changes reported significant weight changes occur in patients not given nutritional or weight management advice after MI.

After reviewing above studies and reports it is concluded that WHR is considered these days, a better predictor of CVD than BMI and same is observed in our study. We found that BMI were almost insignificant in both the test and control subjects but the variations were observed only in WHR. Various studies conducted in different countries with different races of population resulting with the mixed results were observed. We could not find any literature comprising of triceps skin fold thickness in relation to myocardial infarction.

Conclusion: Apart from considering the various conventional risk factors for myocardial infarction, it is important for clinicians and researchers to go for non-invasive anthropometric measurement to rule out cases going for myocardial infarction. The importance of anthropometric measurement needs to be stressed as these variables could predict the majority of the cases. A large-scale work needs to be done on community based studies as this study was a hospital based study on that group of patients who had myocardial infarction with normal lipid profile.

References

1. Mendis, S. and Wissler, R. A Nutritional experiment to study short term effects of coconut in diet on serum cholesterol and platelet factor 4 in man. International Congress on Coronary Heart Disease 18th to 21st February 1988, Bombay, India.
2. Reddy, K.S., Pandit, K., Nagtilak, S., Pajnu, A., Karmarkar, M.G.,Srivastava, U. and Wasir, H.S. Biochemical coronary risk profile of urban and rural population samples: Interim results of a cross sectional survey. Indian Heart Journal. 1992; 44::336.
3. National Cholesterol Education Programme. Second report of the expert panel on detection, evaluation and treatment of high blood cholesterol in adults (Adult Panel II).(1994).
4. Harper, ER. and Jacobson, T.A. New Perspectives on the management of low levels of high-density lipoprotein cholesterol. Arch Intern Med. 1999; 159:1049-57.
5. Stringer,M.D., Gorog,P.G., Freeman,A. and Kakkar,V.V. Lipid peroxides and atherosclerosis. Br. Med.J. 1989; 98:281-284.

6. Welborn,T.A., Dhaliwal, S.S. and Bennett, S.A.Waist-hip ratio is the dominant risk factor predicting cardiovascular death in Australia. Med J Aust; 2003;179:580–5.

7. Heitman, B.L., Frederickson, P. and Lissner, L. Hip Circumference and Cardiovascular Morbidity and Mortality in Men and Women. Obesity Research 2004; 12: 482-487.

8. Megnien J.L., Denarie, N., and Cocaul, M. Predicitve value of Waist-to-hip ratio on Cardiovascular Risk Events. Int J Obes Relat Metab Disord. 1999;23:90-97.

9. Vikram N.K., Pandey R.M., Misra A., Sharma R., Devi J.R and Khanna N. Non-Obese (body mass index<25kg/m2) Asians Indians with normal waist circumference have high cardiovascular risk. Nutrition.2003; 19(6):503-9.

10. Shahbazpour, N. Prevalence of Overweight and Obesity and Their Relation to Hypertension in Adult Male University Students in Kerman, Iran. Int J Endocrinol Metab. 2003; 2:55-60.

11. Hankey, C.R., Leslie, W.S., Currall, J.E., Matthews, D. and Lean, M.E. Weight change after myocardial infarction: statistical perspectives for future study. J Hum Nutr Diet. 2002; 15(6):439-44.

Chapter 3

Analysis of cardiovascular risk factors in normolipidemic acute myocardial infarct patients on admission based on aging -A case controlled study from South Asia

Abstract

The goal of the present study was to address the various risk factors associated in normolipidemic acute myocardial infarction (AMI) patients admitted to the intensive coronary care unit (ICCU). The study compared serum lipid profiles, lipid peroxidation markers, antioxidants and inflammatory markers in acute myocardial infarction (AMI) patients and age/sex-matched controls. The risk variables were analysed age wise with patients <60 years and >60 years of age.

A lipid profile, lipid peroxidation, enzyme antioxidants, endogenous antioxidants, ischemia modified-albumin (IscMA), ceruloplasmin, C-reactive protein (CRP), fibrinogen, lipoprotein (a) and paraoxonase-1 activities were analyzed in 165 acute myocardial infarction (AMI) patients of which 45 patients were <60 years of age.

Lower superoxide dismutase (p=0.002), catalase (p=0.002) and arylesterase activity (p= 0.005) were observed and was statistically significant in >60 years age of acute myocardial infarction patients. Higher levels of C-reactive protein (p=0.003) were observed among the >60 years age patients compared to <60 years. Other biochemical findings were not statistically significant.

During the process of aging the risk factors vary as lowering of antioxidants is due to decreased free radical scavenging properties.

Introduction

Coronary heart disease (CHD) is increasing progressively in developing countries and it is presumed to be the largest killer in India by 2020 [1, 2]. Traditional risk factors like smoking, hypertension, diabetes, hypertriglyceridaemia, truncal obesity, low levels of HDL-C, high levels of LDL-C, low levels of antioxidants, sedentary lifestyle in totality accounts only for 50% of the prevalence and severity of the disease [3, 4]. During the last twenty years the fight against CHD to reduce its incidence, prevalence and outcomes has led to the discovery of the newly emerging risk factors. Now it is well established that CHD is multifactorial disease. Though there are evidences that even the subjects who are completely free from the traditional risk factors are also susceptible to coronary heart disease. Despite of our study reported earlier [5, 6, 7, 8] currently we did risk factor analysis based on age group on the cardiovascular risk factors in >60 years and <60 years of age irrespective of gender on acute myocardial infarct patients and tried to rule out whether all the emerging risk factors are similar in both young and elderly acute myocardial infarct patients.

Earlier studies conducted on young acute myocardial infarct patients of acute myocardial infarction (AMI) established some risk factors but do these similar risk factors exists in elderly AMI patients was the main objective of the current study. Literature search reveals no such study based on normolipidemia is reported so far, so the current study will highlight the risk factors associated with acute myocardial infarction in elderly patients.

Setting Design and Patients

The study consisted of 165 patients (123 men and 42 women) with AMI. The diagnosis of AMI was established according to diagnostic criteria: chest pain lasting for ≤3 hours, electrocardiographic (ECG) changes (ST elevation ≥ 2 mm in at least two leads) and elevation in enzymatic activities of serum creatine phosphokinase and aspartate aminotransferase. The design of this study was pre-approved by the institutional ethical committee. Informed consent was taken from the subjects or from their relatives who participated in the study.

Inclusion criteria were patients with a diagnosis of AMI with normal lipid profile. Patients with diabetes mellitus, renal insufficiency, current and past smokers, hepatic disease or taking lipid lowering drugs or antioxidant vitamin supplements were excluded from the study.

Normolipidemic status was judged by the following criteria: LDL≤160 mg/dl; HDL, ≥35 mg/dl; total cholesterol (TC), <200 mg/dl; and triglycerides (TG), <150 mg/dl [9]. For biochemical studies, 10 ml of blood was collected from the patients soon after admission to intensive care unit and the time period of collection of blood sample from the patient after experiencing the symptoms of chest pain was around three hours.

Lipid Profile TC, TG and HDL-cholesterol were analyzed enzymatically using kit obtained from Randox Laboratories Limited, Crumlin, UK. Plasma LDL-cholesterol was determined from the values of total cholesterol and HDL-cholesterol using friedwalds formula [10]:

$$LDL\text{-}cholesterol = TC - \frac{TG}{5} - HDL\text{-}cholesterol \ (mg/dl)$$

Serum albumin Serum albumin was measured by Bromocresol green binding method [11].

Other assays- All chemicals of analytical grade were obtained from Sigma-Aldrich Company, New Delhi. Serum uric acid was estimated by the method of Brown based on the development of a blue color due to tungsten blue as phosphotungstic acid is reduced by uric acid in alkaline medium.[12] Serum ascorbic acid was estimated by method of Roe and Kuether.[13] Serum total bilirubin was estimated by the method of Jendrassik and Grof [14]. Serum aryl esterase activity was determined by cleavage of phenyl acetate resulting in phenol formation. Aryl esterase activity is measured by the rate of enzymatic hydrolysis of 4 mM phenyl acetate to phenol in 1 mM $CaCl_2$ in 20 mM Tris/HCl (pH 8.0). The amount of phenol generated is monitored with a continuously recording spectrophotometer by the increase in absorbance at 270 nm and 25°C. The amount of phenol generated was calculated from molar absorbitivity at pH 8.0. One unit of aryl esterase activity caused the formation of 1 µmol of phenol/min at ph 8.0 at 25°C.

Serum caeruloplasmin concentration was determined by Ravin [15] erythrocyte superoxide dismutase activity was determined by INT dye binding method and erythrocyte glutathione peroxidase was determined by Paglia and Valentine method [16]

Erythrocyte catalase activity was determined by Beers and Sizer method. [17] Plasma fibrinogen was estimated by TE Clot Fib Kit 10 (TECO GmbH, Dieselstr, 1, 84088 Neufahrn NB Germany). Serum C-reactive protein was determined by ELISA. Lipoprotein (a) was determined by Latex enhanced turbidimetric method.

Malondialdehyde (MDA) derived from lipid peroxides was determined as a thiobarbituric acid (TBA)-reactive substance.[18] Conjugated dienes (CD) were measured according to the method of Recknagel and Glende. [19]

Statistical analysis: The data from patients and controls were compared by Student's *t*-test. Values are expressed as mean ± standard deviation (SD). Microsoft Excel for Windows 2003 was used for statistical analysis. *P*-value <0.05 was considered to indicate statistical significance.

Results: Lipid profile of acute myocardial infarction (AMI) patients below and above sixty years is statistically not significant (**Table 1**). The other biochemical variables are shown in **Table 2**. Significant difference in superoxide dismutase (p=0.002), catalase (p=0.002), arylesterase activity (p= 0.005) and C-reactive protein (p=0.003) were observed among the two groups of patients.

Table 1. Lipid variables in AMI patients below and above sixty years of age.

Lipid variables	Age <60 years (n= 45)	Age >60 years (n=120)	P values
Total cholesterol (mg/dl)	186.77 ± 13.51	186.31 ± 14.16	0.425
HDL-cholesterol (mg/dl)	41.57 ± 4.91	41.15 ± 4.52	0.306
Triacylgycerol (mg/dl)	129.97 ± 12.68	128.58 ± 12.04	0.258
LDL-cholesterol (mg/dl)	119.20 ± 14.05	119.44 ± 14.11	0.462
LDL-C/ HDL-C ratio	2.91 ± 0.53	2.94 ± 0.51	0.373
TG/HDL-C ratio	3.17 ± 0.52	3.16 ± 0.48	0.441

All the parameters are statistically not significant.

Table 2. Biochemical parameters in AMI patients below and above sixty years of age.

Biochemical variables	Age <60 years (n=45)	Age >60 years (n=120)	P values
Albumin (g/dl)	4.25 ± 0.40	4.23 ± 0.32	0.338
Uric acid (mg/dl)	4.38 ± 0.90	4.30 ± 0.90	0.298
Ascorbic Acid (mg/dl)	2.90 ± 0.78	2.78 ± 0.69	0.178
Bilirubin –total (mg/dl)	0.68 ± 0.22	0.66 ± 0.19	0.273
Superoxide dismutase (U/gHb)	889.46 ± 185.81	785.64 ± 210.85	0.002
Glutathione Peroxidase (U/gHb)	41.31 ± 6.57	43.03 ± 6.25	0.060
Catalase (k/gHb)	205.77 ± 38.56	188.30 ± 33.75	0.002
Arylesterase activity (kU/L)	72.86 ± 10.18	68.45 ± 9.89	0.005
Caeruloplasmin (mg/dl)	52.18 ± 2.61	51.29 ± 2.22	0.016
Plasma fibrinogen (mg/dl)	358.91 ± 24.50	357.38 ± 22.76	0.353
Ischemia modified albumin (U/ml)	94.93 ± 10.95	98.46 ± 11.89	0.042
C-reactive protein (mg/l)	2.59 ± 1.02	3.12 ± 1.11	0.003
Lp (a) (mg/l)	11.11 ± 2.17	10.78 ± 2.24	0.200
Malondialdehyde (nmol/l)	14.76 ± 1.33	14.82 ± 1.78	0.414
Conjugated diene (µmol/l)	48.52 ± 5.74	48.20 ± 5.41	0.370

Discussion: The current study analyzed the risk variables in normolipidemic acute myocardial infarct patients. The study observed several emerging risk factors (as shown in **Table 1** and **2**) in the patients at the time of admission ($\approx$ 3 hours after chest pain) in hospital.

We analyzed the risk variables in two groups of patients depending on their age and evaluated major risk factors in elderly patients (>60 years) compared to other patients (<60 years).

Of the risk variables observed in both group of patients, serum lipid profile, serum ascorbic acid, serum uric acid, serum total bilirubin, erythrocyte glutathione peroxidase, plasma fibrinogen, serum ischemia modified albumin, lipoprotein (a), malondialdehyde and conjugated diene were not significantly altered. The risk variables which were significantly altered among the two groups were superoxide dismutase (p=0.002), catalase (p=0.002), aryl esterase (p=0.005) and C-reactive protein (p=0.003).

Involvement of free radicals in the pathophysiology of inflammation, ischemia and in reperfusion damage in a number of organs and tissues have been reported earlier [20,21] Indirect evidence of free radical generation in AMI patients is validated by the presence of lipid peroxidation products, such as malondialdehyde (MDA) and conjugated diene (CD). The serum concentration of MDA and CD are reported to be higher in AMI patients but not significantly differed among the two groups.

It is believed that free radicals are generated particularly in early stage of AMI and antioxidants are involved in the reduction of free radicals, resulting in a decrease in their activities during that period [22, 23]. In the present study, low activities of superoxide dismutase, glutathione peroxidase and catalase were observed in elderly (>60 years) AMI patients as compared to those with younger age group (<60 years).

Thus, the present study is suggestive of imbalance between oxidant and antioxidants in AMI patients which is mainly due to increased oxidative stress, but it is prominent in elderly patients.

The serum antioxidants, mainly superoxide dismutase and catalase are significantly decreased in elderly patients compared to the younger ones (**Table 2**).

The current study also observed reduction in albumin, uric acid, total bilirubin, ascorbic acid in AMI patients but the observations were prominent in elderly patients compared to younger ones with not statistically significant differences among the two groups.

The present study is in good agreement with those conducted by Verma et al [24] and Kharb [25] where they demonstrated a significant drop in serum antioxidants as observed in the current study, more over the difference was significant in antioxidants status among the two groups of patients.

In the present study, we observed a significant association between high baseline levels of serum caeruloplasmin and the subsequent risk of myocardial infarction in both groups and was statistically significant but the younger patients (<60 years) has more risk compared to those of elderly patients.

This indicates that the antioxidant system combating oxidative stress and inflammation is severely impaired in AMI patients. The findings of the present study indicate that the existence of an abnormal balance between the oxidative and protective mechanisms in patients can be a causative factor for the occurrence of AMI.

The elevated levels of C-reactive protein in AMI patients suggests inflammation leading to an acute clinical event by the induction of plaque rupture. Atherosclerosis seems to be a chronic inflammatory condition that can be converted to an acute clinical event by the induction of plaque rupture, which in turn leads to thrombosis. Hence inflammation occurs during all phases of atherosclerosis, although it must smolder for decades before resulting in a clinical event such as AMI.[26] The elevated C-reactive protein in AMI patients justifies the above facts as observed in our study.

The levels of IscMA in AMI patients was significantly higher than in controls as observed in the present study is similar to previous reports [27, 28, 29] Even though determination of IscMA is promising for the prediction of AMI, its use should be limited until further studies reveal its validity as a biomarker for AMI and usefulness in constructing treatment plans in acute coronary syndrome patients. An extensive study with increased number of patients would be required to compare IscMA with other markers such as troponins and myoglobin. Whether IscMA can be an additional parameter along with troponins to boost the confidence of clinicians in ruling out cardiac ischemia would be of particular interest.

Limitations of the current study

The samples for lipid profile and other variables were collected within 3 hours at the time of admission of patients admitted in intensive coronary care unit, which does not obey the normal criteria of standardized sampling pattern of 12 hours fasting for sample analysed for lipid profile studies. As the patients were very vulnerable and were at high risk at the time of admission so we didn't follow the standard criteria of sample collection.

Conclusion: AMI is a multi factorial disease that can arise even in normolipidemic subjects. Hence, earlier concepts of maintaining lipid profile within normal limits to prevent MI may be overruled. The present study suggests that measuring serum antioxidants and IscMA in normolipidemic patients will aid better prognosis and management of patients with acute coronary syndromes. Oxidative stress appears an etiological factor for MI as a consequence of free radical scavengers namely antioxidants which tends to be lower in AMI patients.

Future research including measurement of parameters of oxidative stress and inflammatory markers should be carried out as the role of inflammatory markers like C-reactive proteins, Caeruloplasmin are emerging which could be possibly be a causative factor for atherosclerosis.

References

1. Gupte,M.D., Ramachandran Vidya., Mutatkar, R.K. Epidemiological profile of India: Historical and contemporary perspectives. Journal of Bioscience, 2001; 26(4) Suppl: 437-464.
2. Singh, S.P., Sen, P. Coronary Heart Disease: The Changing Scenario. Indian Journal of Preventive and Social Medicine, 2003; 34: 74-80.
3. Reddy KS. Rising burden of cardiovascular disease in India. In: Sethi KK (ed). Coronary artery disease in Indians: a global perspective. Mumbai, Cardiological-Society-of-India 1998; Dec 10–13: 63-72.
4. Rissam, H.S., Kishore, S. & Trehan, N. Coronary Artery Disease in Young Indians-The Missing Link. Journal of Indian Academy of Clinical Medicine, 2001; 2 (3): 128-132.
5. Kumar, A., Sivakanesan, R. Singh, S. Oxidative stress, Endogenous Antioxidant and Ischemia modified albumin in Normolipidemic Acute Myocardial Infarction Patients. Journal of Health Science, 2008; 54(4):482-487.
6. Kumar, A., Sivakanesan, R. Serum Caeruloplasmin as a Coronary Risk Factor in patients with Acute Myocardial Infarction with normal lipid profile. Journal of Health Science, 2008; 54(5):567-570.
7. Kumar, A., Nagtilak, S., Sivakanesan, R., Gunasekera,S. Cardiovascular risk factors in elderly normolipidemic acute myocardial infarct patients: A Case Controlled study from India. The South East Asian Journal of Tropical Medicine and Public Health, 2009; 40(3); 581.
8. Kumar, A., Sivakanesan, R. Does plasma fibrinogens and C - reactive protein predicts the incidence of myocardial infarction in patients with normal lipids profile? Pakistan Journal of Medical Sciences, 2008; 24(2): 336-339.
9. Executive Summary of the Third Report of The National Cholesterol Education Program (NCEP) Expert Panel on Detection, Evaluation, and Treatment of High Blood Cholesterol in Adults (Adult Treatment Panel III). Expert Panel of Detection, Evaluation, and Treatment of High Blood Cholesterol in Adults. JAMA 2001; 285(19):2486-97.
10. Friedewalds, W.T., Levy, R.I. and Fredrickson, D.S. Estimation of the concentration of low density lipoprotein cholesterol in plasma without the use of preparative ultracentrifuge. Clinical Chemistry; 1972; 18: 499-502.
11. Perry, B.W & Doumas, B.T. Effect of heparin on albumin determination by use of bromocresol green and bromocresol purple. Clinical Chemistry, 1979; 25:1520-1522.
12. Brown H. The determination of uric acid in human blood. Journal of Biological Chemistry, 1945; 158:601-608.
13. Roe, J.H. & Kuether, C.A. The determination of ascorbic acid in whole blood and urine through the 2,4-dinitrophenylhydrazine derivative of dehydroascorbic acid. Journal of Biological Chemistry, 1943; 147:399-407.
14. Jendrassik, J. & Grof P.Vereinfachte photometrische Methoden Zur Beetimmung des Blutbilirubin. Biochem. Z., 1938;297; 81-89.
15. Ravin, H.A. An improved colorimetric enzymatic assay of caeruloplasmin. Journal of Laboratory Medicine,1961;58:161-168.
16. Paglia, D.E., & Valentine, W.N. Studies on the quantitative and qualitative characterization of erythrocyte glutathione peroxidase. Journal of Laboratory and Clinical Medicine, 1967; 70:158-169.
17. Beers, R. F., & Sizer, I. W. A spectrophotometric method for measuring the breakdown of H_2O_2 by catalase. Journal of Biological Chemistry, 1952; 195:133-140.

30

18. Bernheim, S., Bernheim, M.L.C. & Wilbur, K.M. The reaction between thiobarbituric acid and the oxidant product of certain lipids. Journal of Biological Chemistry, 1948; 174: 257-264.

19. Recknagel, R.O & Glende, E.A. Spectrophotometric detection of lipid conjugated dienes. Methods of Enzymology, 1984; 105:331-337.

20. Frei B, Stocker R, Ames BN. Antioxidant defenses and lipid peroxidation in human blood plasma. Proc Natl Acad Sci USA 1988; 85: 9748-9752.

21. Beutler E, Duron O, Kelly B. An improved method for the determination of blood glutathione. J Lab Clin Med 1963; 61: 822-826.

22. Recknagel RO, Glende EA. Spectrophotometric detection of lipid conjugated dienes. Methods Enzymol 1984; 105:331-337.

23. Uhling S, Wendel A. The physiological consequences of glutathione variations. Life Sci 1992; 51: 1083-94.

24. Verma V.K., Ramesh, V., Tewari,S., Gupta, R.K., Sinha,N.& Pandey,C.M. Role of Bilirubin, Vitamin C and Ceruloplasmin as antioxidants I Coronary Artery Disease (CAD). Indian J Clin Biochem 2005 20(2): 68-74.

25. Kharb S. Low blood glutathione levels in acute myocardial infarction. Indian J Med Sci 2003; 57 (8): 335-7.

26. Libby P. Vascular biology of atherosclerosis: Overview and state of art. Am J Cardiol 2003;91(Suppl):3A-6A.

27. Sinha, M.K., Roy, D., Gaze, D.C. Collinson, P.O., Kaski, J.C. Role of Ischemia Modified Albumin", a new biochemical marker of myocardial Ischaemia, in the early diagnosis of acute coronary syndromes. Emerg Med J 2004; 21:29-34.

28. Collinson,P.O., Gaze,D.C., Bainbridge, K., Morris, F., Morris,B., Price,A. and Goodacre, S. Utility of admission cardiac troponin and "Ischemia Modified Albumin" measurements for rapid evaluation and rule out of suspected acute myocardial infarction in the emergency department. Emerg Med J 2006; 23: 256-261.

29. Bar-Or, D., Lau, E., Rao, N., Bampos, N., Winkler, J.V. and Curtis, C.G. Reduction in the cobalt binding capacity of human albumin with myocardial ischemia. Ann Emerg Med 1999; 34:556.

Chapter 4

Serum Caeruloplasmin as a Coronary Risk Factor in Patients with Acute Myocardial Infarction with Normal Lipid Profile

Abstract

There have been studies demonstrating that serum caeruloplasmin acts as an antioxidant in cardiovascular disease. However, several studies have demonstrated that it acts as an independent risk factor in patients with cardiovascular disease. To ascertain the role of caeruloplasmin in normolipidemic acute myocardial infarction patients, we investigated the correlation between the serum caeruloplasmin level and incidence of cardiovascular disease in individuals with normal lipid profiles. The levels of caeruloplasmin were significantly higher in patient sera than in those of controls ($p < 0.001$) and the difference in the lipid profiles was also significant ($p < 0.001$). These results suggest that caeruloplasmin may act as a prooxidant and appears to be a risk factor in this disease.

Key words: acute myocardial infarction, normal lipid profile, caeruloplasmin.

Introduction

Coronary artery disease is a major cause of mortality and morbidity in the industrialized world [1]. Elevated serum caeruloplasmin levels have been found in patients with cardiovascular disorders including arteriosclerosis, abdominal aneurysms, unstable angina, and vasculitis and peripheral artery disease [2]. Several prospective studies have indicated that the serum copper or caeruloplasmin level may be an independent risk factor for cardiovascular disease [3-5].The increased risk has been attributed to the prooxidant function of caeruloplasmin, and recent experimental studies demonstrating the ability of caeruloplasmin to oxidatively modify low-density lipoprotein (LDL) [6] seem to underline this concept. However, the question has been raised whether elevated caeruloplasmin is not merely an indicator of inflammation, given its acute-phase protein property. Studies have demonstrated the antioxidant property of caeruloplasmin through its oxidase activity, which is directed toward ferrous ions (ferroxidase activity) [7]. Studies have also demonstrated the inhibition of lipid peroxidation by ferrous ion which is also known to be involved in the decomposition of lipid peroxides [8]. Due to mixed results of the studies conducted earlier, the present study was undertaken. Moreover, earlier studies investigated the association between caeruloplasmin or copper and cardiovascular disorders in patients with hyperlipidemia, but in the present study, the serum caeruloplasmin levels in normolipidemic acute myocardial infarction (AMI) patients were studied due to the dearth of reports related to caeruloplasmin concentration in Normolipidemic individuals.

Patients and controls

Setting design and patients: The study was conducted among 165 patients (123 men and 42 women) with AMI. The diagnosis of AMI was established according to the following diagnostic criteria: chest pain lasting for up to 3 hr; electrocardiogram changes (ST elevation of 2 mm or more in at least two leads); and elevation of serum creatine phosphokinase (CPK-MB) and aspartate aminotransferase levels. The control group consisted of 165 age sex and matched healthy volunteers (123 men and 42 women). Informed consent was given from all before enrollment in the study, and the protocol was approved, by the Ethical committee of the institute.

Inclusion criteria: Patients with a diagnosis of AMI with normal lipid profiles were enrolled.

Exclusion criteria: Patients with diabetes mellitus, renal insufficiency, or hepatic disease, or who were taking lipid lowering drugs or antioxidant vitamin supplement and current or past smokers were excluded from the study.

Criteria for Normolipidemics: A normal lipid profile was defined as LDL < 160 mg/dl, high-density lipoprotein (HDL) ≥ 35 mg/dl, total cholesterol (TC) < 200 mg/dl and triglycerides (TG) < 150 mg/dl. [9]

For biochemical assays 5 ml of blood was collected after an overnight fast. The serum was separated and used for the determination of lipid profiles and caeruloplasmin levels.

Lipid profile TC, TG, and HDL were analyzed enzymatically using kits obtained from Randox Laboratories Limited (Crumlin, UK). Plasma LDL was determined from the values of TC and HDL using the following formula:

$$LDL = TC - \frac{TG}{5} - HDL \ (mg/dl)$$

Serum caeruloplasmin assay: The caeruloplasmin assay was performed using the p-phenylene diamine method [10]. The serum caeruloplasmin assay was performed using the p- phenylenediamine method. The principle of the assay is based on the oxidation of p-phenylenediamine to produce a purple-colored complex with an absorption peak at 530 nm. All chemicals of analytical grade were obtained from Sigma Chemicals, India.

Results and discussion

Demographic data on controls and AMI patients are shown in **Tables 1** and **2**). The differences in age, height, and body mass index (BMI) in control and AMI patient were not significant. The weight and waist circumference were greater in AMI patients than those in the control group ($p < 0.001$) (**Tables 1** and **2**). Systolic and diastolic blood pressure was significantly higher in AMI patients than in controls ($p < 0.05$) (**Tables 1** and **2**).

The lipid profiles and serum caeruloplasmin concentrations are shown in **Tables 3** and **4**).The TC and TC:HDL ratio, TG, LDL and LDL:HDL ratio, and serum caeruloplasmin were significantly higher ($p < 0.001$) in AMI patients compared with controls (**Table 3**). A significant difference ($p < 0.001$) was also observed in HDL levels between AMI patients and controls. TC, TC:HDL ratio, TG, and serum caeruloplasmin were significantly higher ($p < 0.001$) in both genders of AMI patients compared with controls (**Table 4**). A significant difference ($p < 0.001$) in HDL levels between AMI patients and controls was seen only among women (**Table 4**). LDL and LDL:HDL ratio were significantly higher ($p < 0.001$) in AMI male patients compared with controls (**Table 4**).

In the present study, we observed a significant association between high baseline levels of serum caeruloplasmin and the subsequent risk of myocardial infarction. Comparable findings of an elevated risk of myocardial infarction[5] and incidence of coronary heart disease (CHD) [11] among individuals with high levels of serum caeruloplasmin have been reported. Several other studies reported associations of high levels of serum Cu with an elevated risk of increased carotid intima-media thickness[12], myocardial infarction[13], mortality from CHD or cardiovascular disease[3,4]. The present studies along with the findings of previous ones indicate that caeruloplasmin could be a prooxidant in normolipidemic AMI patients.

The Pro-oxidant property of caeruloplasmin involves lipid peroxidation. Studies indicate that caeruloplasmin by itself can oxidize LDL *in vitro* and possibly *in vivo* [6, 14]. However, accessory factors derived from vascular cells may be modulatory or requisite during lipoprotein oxidation within the vessel wall[2]. Studies have reported about the cardioprotective nature of caeruloplasmin[15] which could protect the myocardial tissue against the deleterious effects of oxygen free radicals. Studies observing the role of transition metal ion-mediated oxidation of LDL molecules centered on the role of human caeruloplasmin in this oxidative process as it is the principal coppercontaining protein in serum. Biochemical studies showed that caeruloplasmin is a potent catalyst of LDL oxidation in vitro. The prooxidant activity of caeruloplasmin requires an intact structure, and a single copper atom at the surface of the protein, near His (426), is required for LDL oxidation. Under conditions where an inhibitory protein (such as albumin) is present, LDL oxidation by caeruloplasmin is optimal in the presence of superoxide, which reduces the surface copper atom of caeruloplasmin. Cultured vascular endothelial and smooth muscle cells also oxidize LDL in the presence of caeruloplasmin. Superoxide released by these cells is a critical factor regulating the rate of oxidation. The role of caeruloplasmin in lipoprotein oxidation and atherosclerotic lesion progression in vivo has not been directly assessed and is an important area for future studies[16]

Studies have demonstrated significantly higher levels of caeruloplasmin copper and antioxLDL in AMI patients. High concentrations of anti-oxLDL suggest an increase in oxidative stress that would contribute to disease severity. The observed correlation of caeruloplasmin with anti-oxLDL suggests the possible prooxidative activity of caeruloplasmin in patients with cardiovascular disease[17]

Table 1. Baseline Variables in Controls and AMI Patients (mean ±SD).

Variable	Control (n = 165)	Patients (n = 165)
Age	60.6 ± 4.0	61.8 ± 3.8†
Height (cm)	1.6 ± 0.1	1.6 ± 0.1 ‡
Weight (kg)	68.3 ± 4.0	72.0 ± 5.4 §
BMI (kg/m^2)	25.4 ± 1.2	26.2 ± 1.5‖
Waist circumference (cm)	93.7 ± 3.6	100.8 ± 6.1 §
Hip circumference (cm)	100.0 ± 3.2	105.7 ± 5.2 §
Waist : Hip*	0.9	1.0 ¶
Systolic blood pressure (mm Hg)	113 ± 8	136 ± 2 **
Diastolic blood pressure (mm Hg)	85 ± 7	95 ± 10 **

* Ratio †(p = 0.0037) ; ‡(p = 0.2919); § (p < 0.001); ‖(p < 0.01); ¶(p < 0.02); **(p < 0.05)

Table 2. Baseline Variables in Men and Women in the Control and AMI Patient Groups (mean ± SD).

Variable	Control		Patients	
	Men(n=123)	Women(n=42)	Men(n=123)	Women(n=42)
Age	60.7 ± 4.1	60.5 ± 2.9	61.5 ± 3.3 †	62.7 ± 4.97 **
Height (cm)	1.6 ± 0.1	1.6 ± 0.1	1.6 ± 0.1‡	1.6 ± 0.1 ††
Weight (kg)	68.6 ± 3.8	67.5 ± 4.4	71.7 ± 5.3 §	72.5 ± 5.7 §
BMI (kg/m^2)	25.3 ± 1.1	25.6 ± 1.5	26.0 ± 1.3 ‖	26.6 ± 1.7 ‡‡
WC(cm)	93.4 ± 3.4	94.6 ± 4.2	100.2 ± 5.7 §	102.5 ± 6.8 §
HC (cm)	99.7 ± 2.9	100.8 ± 3.8	105.3 ± 5.0 ¶	107.0 ± 5.8 §
Waist : Hip*	0.9 ± 0.0	0.9 ± 0.0	1.0 ± 0.0¶	1.0 ± 0.0 §
SBP (mm Hg)	114 ± 7	118 ± 8	136 ± 13 ¶	132 ± 17 ¶
DBP(mm Hg)	86 ± 8	87 ± 9	95 ± 15 ¶	94 ± 13 ¶

* Ratio †p=0.0366; ‡p = 0.0081; §p<0.001; ‖p=1.5085; ¶p<0.05; **p = 0.0356; ††p=0.0170; ‡‡p=0.0001.

Table 3. Lipid Profile and Serum Caeruloplasmin in the Control and AMI Patient Groups (mean ± SD).

Variable	Controls (n=165)	Patients (n=165)
Total cholesterol §	168.6 ± 12.2	186.4 ± 14.0 †
HDL-cholesterol §	50.5 ± 6.8	41.3 ± 4.6 †
TC : HDL-C*	3.4 ± 0.4	4.6 ± 0.6 †
Triglycerides §	107.8 ± 11.5	129.0 ± 12.2 †
LDL-cholesterol §	83.6 ± 11.9	119.4 ± 14.1 †
LDL:HDL-C*	1.9 ± 0.3	2.9 ± 0.5 †
TG:HDL-C*	2.2 ± 0.4	3.2 ± 0.5 ‡
Caeruloplasmin §	20.5 ± 2.3	51.5 ± 2.3 †

* Ratio †p<0.001; ‡p = 1.0008; §mg/dl.

Table 4. Lipid Profile and Serum Caeruloplasmin in the Control Group and Male and Female AMI Patients (mean ± SD).

Variable	Control (n =165)		Patients (n =165)	
	Men(n=123)	Women(n=42)	Men(n=123)	Women(n=42)
Total cholesterol **	168.1 ± 12.1	170.0 ± 12.4	183.8 ± 13.6 †	194.0 ± 13.0 †
HDL-cholesterol **	49.9 ± 7.3	52.3 ± 4.6	41.8 ± 4.8 ‡	39.8 ± 3.4 †
TC : HDL-C*	3.4 ± 0.3	3.3 ± 0.5	4.5 ± 0.6 †	5.0 ± 0.4 †
Triglycerides **	105.0 ± 10.3	116.1 ± 11.0	126.2 ± 11.7 †	137.0 ± 9.8 †
LDL-cholesterol **	79.9 ± 8.0	94.5 ± 14.8	116.8 ± 13.8 †	126.9 ± 12.2 ||
LDL:HDL-C*	1.9 ± 0.3	1.8 ± 0.4	2.8 ± 0.5 †	3.2 ± 0.4 ¶
TG:HDL-C*	2.2 ± 0.4	2.2 ± 0.3	3.1 ± 0.5 §	3.5 ± 0.4 †
Caeruloplasmin **	20.5 ± 2.4	20.5 ± 2.2	51.7 ± 2.5 †	51.1 ± 1.9 †

* Ratio † $p<0.001$; ‡ $p=1.7609$; § $p=2.53035$; || $p=1.2743$; ¶ $p=1.0255$; ** mg/dl.

References

1. Mendis, S. and Wissler, R. (1988) A nutritional experiment to study short term effects of coconut in diet on serum cholesterol and platelet factor 4 in man. *Proceedings of the International Congress on Coronary Heart Disease Conference,* Feb 18-21, Bombay, India.
2. Fox, P. L., Mukhopadhyay, C. and Ehrenwald, E. (1995) Structure, oxidant activity, and cardiovascular mechanisms of human caeruloplasmin. *Life Sci.,* 56, 1749-1758.
3. Kok, F. J., van Duijin, C. M., Hofman, A., van der Voet, G. B., de Wolff, F. A., Paays, C. H., et al. (1988) Serum copper and zinc and the risk of death from cancer and cardiovascular disease. *Am. J. Epidemiol.,* 128, 352-359.
4. Salonen, J. T., Salonen, R., Korpela, H., Suntioiun, S. and Tuomilehto, J. (1991) Serum copper and the risk of acute myocardial infarction: a prospective study in men in Eastern Finland. *Am.J. Epidemiol.,* 134, 268-276.
5. Reunanen, A., Knekt, P. and Aaran, R. K. (1992) Serum caeruloplasmin level and the risk of myocardial and stroke. *Am. J. Epidemiol.,* 136, 1082-1090.
6. Ehrenwald, E., Chisolm, G. M. and Fox, P. L. (1994) Intact human caeruloplasmin oxidatively modifies low density lipoprotein. *J. Clin. Invest.,* 93, 1493-1501.
7. Holmberg,C. and Laurell, C. (1951) Investigations in serum copper III. Caeruloplasmin as an enzyme. *Acta Chem. Scand.,* 5, 476-481.
8. Osaki, S., Johnson, D. and Frieden, E. (1966) The possible significance of the ferrous oxidase activity of caeruloplasmin in normal human serum. *J. Biol. Chem.,* 241, 2746-2751.
9. National Cholesterol Education Programme. (1994) Second report of the expert panel on detection,evaluation and treatment of high blood cholesterol in adults (Adult Panel II).
10. Ravin, H.A. (1961) An improved colorimetric enzymatic assay of caeruloplasmin. *J. Lab. Med.,* 58, 161-168.
11. Manttari, M., Manninen, V., Huttunen, J. K., Palosno, T., Ehnholm, C., Heinonen, O. P., et al. (1994) Serum ferritin and caeruloplasmin as coronary risk factors. *Eur Heart J.,* 15, 1599-1603.
12. Salonen, J. T., Salonen, R., Seppanen, K., Kantola, M., Suntioinen, S. and Korpela, H. (1991) Interactions of serum copper, selenium, and low density lipoprotein cholesterol in atherogenesis. *BMJ,* 302, 756-760.

13. Reunanen, A., Knekt, P., Marneimi, J., Maki, J., Maatela, J.and Aromaa, A.(1996) Serum calcium, magnesium, copper and zinc and risk of cardiovascular death. *Eur. J. Clin. Nutr.*, 50, 431-437.

14. Craig, W. Y., Poulin, S. E., Palomaki, G. E., Neveux, L. M., Ritchie, R. F.and Ledue, T. B. (1995) Oxidation-related analytes and lipid and lipoprotein concentrations in healthy subjects. *Arterioscler Thromb Vasc. Biol.,* 15, 733-739.

15. Mateeseu, M., Chahine, R., Roger, S.and Atanasiu, R. (1995) Protection of myocardial tissue against deleterious effects of oxygen free radicals by caeruloplasmin. *Arzneim. Forsch. Drug. Res.*, 45, 476-580.

16. Fox, P. L., Mazumder, B., Ehrenwald, E. and Mukhopadhyay, C. K. (2000) Ceruloplasmin and cardiovascular disease. *Free Radic. Biol. Med.,* 28, 1735-1744.

17. Awadallah, S. M., Hamad, M., Jbarah, I., Salem, N. M., and Mubarak, M. S. (2006) Autoantibodies against oxidized LDL correlate with serum concentrations of caeruloplasmin in patients with cardiovascular disease. *Clin. Chim. Acta.,* 365, 330-336.

Chapter 5

Cardiovascular Risk Factors in Normolipidemic Acute Myocardial Infarct Patients on Admission – Do Dietary Fruits and Vegetables Offer Any Benefits?

Abstract

Background: Myocardial Infarction (MI) is a leading cause of death in India. Whether dietary vitamins could reduce risk of cardiovascular disease among Indians is still not clear and very few studies have addressed the association between dietary vitamin acting as an antioxidant or pro-oxidant and its effect on risk reduction or aggravation in normolipidemic AMI patients.

Objective: The goal of the current study was to address the association between dietary vitamin and cardiovascular risk in normolipidemic acute myocardial infarct patient compared with healthy control.

Design: Dietary intake of vitamins was assessed by 131 food frequency questionnaire items in both AMI patients and age/sex-matched control. The associated changes in risk factors due to antioxidant vitamins intake was also assessed in normolipidemic acute myocardial patients and was compared with controls.

Results: Dietary intake of vitamin A, B1, B2, B3 was significantly higher in AMI patients compared to healthy control but the intake of vitamin C was significantly higher in control compared to AMI patients. Even though the vitamins intake was higher in patients, the associated cardiovascular risk factors were not reduced compared to control. The total cholesterol, LDL-c, TAG were significantly higher ($p<0.001$) in AMI patients except HDL-c which was significantly higher ($p<0.001$) in controls.

The endogenous antioxidants were found to be significantly lowered in patients compared to controls in spite of higher vitamin intake. Similarly the enzymatic antioxidants were also significantly lowered in patients. The mean serum Lipoprotein (a) malondialdehyde (MDA) and conjugated diene (CD) levels in patients were significantly elevated compared with controls. The levels of caeruloplasmin, C-reactive protein, fibrinogen, ischemia-modified albumin were significantly higher but arylesterase activities were lowered in patients.

Conclusion: Diets rich in vegetables and fruits does not reduce the cardiovascular risk in normolipidemic AMI patients among Indians and Sri Lankans.

Key Words: Dietary vitamins, acute myocardial infarction, cardiovascular risk factors, Normolipidemia, India and Sri Lanka.

Introduction

Cardiovascular disease (CVD) is a major cause of morbidity and mortality in Western World. In the recent years its steep rise have alarmed common man and raised its importance internationally among scientists and researchers, and it is going to be the major cause of mortality in the globe by 2020 [1]. It is a multifactorial disease associated with factors like hereditary, hyperlipidemia, obesity, hypertension, environmental and life style variables like stress, smoking, alcohol consumption, etc [2].

The World Health Organization predicts that deaths due to CVD are projected to double between 1985 and 2015 [3, 4]. Asian Indians living abroad indicates a 40% higher risk of ischemic heart disease (IHD) mortality than that for Europeans [5]. Researchers across the world are emphasizing their researches to prevent or minimize this increase in the death rate due to CVD. When it comes to line of prevention and regression of this disease, dietary management comes as the first line of prognosis and emphasis are placed on rich antioxidant dietary regimen [6]. It is believed that oxidative stress is involved in the pathogenesis of atherosclerosis, while a variety of antioxidants has been used in clinical trials and studies during the past few years but very clear cut message is still awaited from the studies [7]. American Heart Association has taken long standing commitment to provide information related to nutritional role in risk reduction of future episode of CVD [8]. No clear cut dietary regimen in antioxidant vitamins and guidelines have still been provided for prevention of this disease as vitamins even though act as antioxidants but at times it can also acts as pro-oxidants and nullify the antioxidants effect of other antioxidants if consumed in the form of cock tail [9]. In the present study, the dietary antioxidants vitamins were assessed in AMI patients and were compared with healthy controls. The study also aimed to observe the variation is risk factors in patients and controls due to variation in dietary vitamins intake which was estimated using three 24-hour dietary records from the food stuffs which are generally consumed among Indians and Sri Lankans. The study also measured anthropometric details among the two groups along with risk factors which could be associated in causation of myocardial infarction. The data presented in this paper is an outcome of the study.

Materials and Methods

Cases

Eligible cases were all patients aged 48-69 y hospitalized with a diagnosis of first incident acute myocardial infarction (MI) in Peradeniya Hospital, Faculty of Medicine, Peradeniya, Sri Lanka. The definitive diagnosis of AMI was established according to diagnostic criteria: chest pain lasting for ≤3 hours, electrocardiographic (ECG) changes

(ST elevation ≥ 2 mm in at least two leads) and elevation in enzymatic activities of serum creatine phosphokinase and aspartate aminotransferase. The control group consisted of 165 age/sex-matched healthy volunteers (123 men and 42 women).

Inclusion criteria were patients diagnosed of AMI with normal lipid profile. Patients were excluded if they had any previous history of MI or IHD (including bypass surgery, angina, or stroke) because such prior diagnoses may alter behaviors, including diet. Patients with diabetes mellitus, renal insufficiency, hepatic disease or taking lipid lowering drugs or antioxidant vitamin supplements were also excluded from the study. We also excluded patients if they were pregnant, had a history of cancer, gastrointestinal tract infection, or thyroid, because these conditions may have affected dietary intake. The patients were interviewed on average 2–5 d after admission. The eligibility criteria were met by 245 cases, and 165 were included in the study. The reasons for exclusion were death (n = 19) or discharge (n = 27) before the interviews could be completed, being too sick to be interviewed (n = 16), and not giving consent to participate (n = 18).

Controls For each case subject, 2 control subjects matched by age (within 5 y), sex, and hospital were obtained from noncardiac outpatient clinics or inpatient wards. The same exclusion criteria used for cases were applied for control selection. We identified ≈ 165 eligible control subjects. Controls were selected by using predominantly any of these two methods depending on the hospital. In the first method, we accompanied a particular physician during an outpatient clinic, according to a weekly schedule of clinics and wards. At the end of each consultation, the physician or the physician's assistant invited the patient to speak with us about his or her lifestyle and diet. Patients matching the required age and sex profile were eligible according to study criteria and were then informed of the study and asked to participate. In these situations, participation was 100%. In the second method, we independently identified control patients from clinics and wards. We attempted to approach all individuals present during a particular outpatient clinic or in a specified ward. In large clinics, patients were screened for eligibility and invited to participate according to their queue number (highest number first). This method was used to prevent bias in the selection of controls. Overall participation was high, ≈ 98%. Basic demographic information was collected from all persons who were approached. If an individual fit the required age and sex profile and was eligible, we briefly explained the study and asked whether the patient was willing to participate.

Criteria for Normolipidemics: Normal lipid profile was defined if LDL was <130mg/dl, HDL ≥ 35 mg/dl, Total cholesterol (TC) <200 mg/dl and Triglycerides (TG) <150 mg/dl [10].

Data Collection

Interviews were conducted in hospital wards or clinics by us and lasted ≈ 30 min. Informed consent was obtained from all study subjects. This included various life style factors such as education, socio-economic status, income and type of job. Details of major cardiovascular risk factors such as smoking, alcohol intake, diabetes, obesity and hypertension were also obtained. We also collected data on socioeconomic status; smoking history; history of hypertension, diabetes, and hypercholesterolemia; family history of cardiovascular disease (including IHD, angina, MI, hypertension, diabetes, stroke, sudden death, and bypass surgery); dietary intake; types of fat or oils used in cooking; nutritional supplement use; and physical activity.

Dietary Intake by 24-hour dietary record[11]**:** The patients and controls were given the food items which they were supposed to mark including the quantity consumed. This was carried for three times in the same subjects to avoid biasness and to get more accuracy in intake. The dietary intake was tabulated and the amount of vitamins was calculated from the food consumed.

Anthropometric measurements: Anthropometric measures (height, weight, and hip and waist circumferences) were obtained and body mass index (weight in kg divided by height in meters squared) and waist-to-hip ratio were calculated. Their height, weight, waist-hip ratio and blood pressure were recorded. Height was measured in centimeters and weight in kilograms using calibrated spring balance. Supine waist girth was measured at the level of umbilicus with a person breathing silently and standing hip girth was measured at inter-trochanteric level. Waist and hip measures were assessed by using a standardized tape measure, with waist measures taken at the midpoint between the costal margin and ileac crest and hip measures taken at the widest circumference.

Blood Pressure: The blood pressure was measured using standard mercury manometer. At least two readings at 5 minutes intervals as per World Health Organization guidelines were recorded [12]. If high blood pressure ($\geq$140/90 mmHg) was noted a third reading was taken after 30 minutes. The lowest of the three readings was taken as blood pressure.

Electrocardiogram: Electrocardiogram (12 lead) was performed on all persons using proper standardization.

Collection of Samples

Blood (10 ml) was collected after overnight fasting in different containers.

EDTA vial: 5.0 ml of blood was taken. Red cells were washed 3-4 times with ice-cold normal saline and used for estimation of glutathione peroxidase, superoxide dismutase and catalase.

Plain vial: Remaining blood was allowed to clot and serum separated by centrifugation for 5 min at 5000 rpm and was used for determination of lipid profile, malondialdehye and conjugated dienes, and other assays as described.

For IscMA analysis, 2 ml of blood was collected from the patients immediately after admission to intensive care unit.

Lipid profile -Total cholesterol, triglycerides, and HDL-cholesterol were estimated by enzymatic methods using the kits obtained from Randox Laboratories Limited, Crumlin, UK. Plasma LDL-cholesterol was determined from the values of total cholesterol and HDL-cholesterol using the following formulae:

$$LDL\text{-}C = T\,C - \frac{TG}{5} - HDL\text{-}C \text{ (mg/dl)}$$

All chemicals of analytical grade were obtained from Sigma chemicals, India.

Serum Albumin: Serum Albumin was measured by Bromocresol green dye binding method [13].

Serum Uric acid: Serum uric acid was estimated by the method of Brown based on the development of a blue color due to tungsten blue as phosphotungstic acid is reduced by uric acid in alkaline medium [14].

Serum total bilirubin: Serum total bilirubin was estimated by Jendrassik and Grof method [15].

Glutathione peroxidase: The glutathione peroxidase activity was determined by the procedure of Paglia and Valentine [16].

Superoxide dismutase (SOD): Superoxide dismuatse enzyme activity was measured by SOD assay kit using rate of inhibition of 2-(4-indophenyl)-(4-Nitrophenol)-5-phenyltetrazolium chloride (I.N.T) reduction method modified by Sun et al [17].

Catalase: Catalase activity was measured spectrophotometrically as described by Beutler [18,19].

MDA - MDA levels were estimated by thiobarbituric acid (TBA) reaction [20].

Conjugated dienes (CD): CD levels were measured by Recknagel and Glende method [21] with little modification.

Serum Ceruoplasmin: The caeruloplasmin assay was done by *p*-phenylene diamine method [22].

All chemicals of analytical grade were obtained from Sigma Chemicals, India.

Ischemia Modified Albumin (IscMA): IscMA concentration was determined by addition of a known amount of cobalt (II) to a serum sample and measurement of the unbound cobalt (II) by the intensity of colored complex formed after reacting with dithiothreitol (DTT) by colorimeter [23,24].

Lipoprotein (a), Lp(a): The Lp(a) levels were determined by Latex- Enhanced Turbidimetric method.

Aryesterase /Paraoxonase assay: Serum Arylesterase/Paraoxonase was estimated using Zeptometrix Assay Kit obtained from Zeptometrix Corp, New York, 14202 based on the cleavage of phenyl acetate resulting in phenol formation. The rate of formation of phenol is measured by monitoring the increase in absorbance at 270 nm at 25°C.

Ascorbic acid: Estimation of Vitamin C was carried out by Roe and Kuether method [25].

Measurement of High sensitive C- Reactive protein (hs-CRP): The hsCRP ELISA is based on the principle of a solid phase enzyme-linked immunosorbent assay.

Plasma fibrinogen: TEClot Fib Kit 10 (TECO GmbH, Dieselstr. 1, 84088 Neufahrn NB Germany) was used for the estimation of fibrinogen.

Results

Dietary vitamins intake was higher in AMI patients excepting for ascorbic acid which was higher in controls as shown in **Table 1**. Anthropometric variables in acute myocardial infarction (AMI) patients showed highly significant differences in weight, BMI, waist circumference, hip circumference, waist-hip ratio, mid-arm circumference, biceps and triceps skin fold thickness as shown in **Table 2**. The total cholesterol, LDL-c, TG were significantly higher (p<0.001) in AMI patients except HDL-c which was significantly higher (p<0.001) in controls as shown in **Table 3**. The cardiac markers enzymes are shown in **Table 4**. The serum endogenous antioxidants were significantly decreased in patients compared to controls. Similarly the enzyme antioxidants were also significantly lowered in patients. The mean serum Lipoprotein (a) malondialdehyde (MDA) and conjugated diene (CD) levels in MI patients were higher compared with controls as shown in **Tables 5** and **6**. Serum fibrinogen, caeruloplasmin, ischemia- modified albumin and C-reactive protein were significantly elevated whereas arylesterase activities were significantly lowered in cases compared with controls as shown in **Table 7**.

Table 1. Mean dietary intakes of vitamins in Control and AMI Patients.

	Control (n=165)	AMI Patients (n=165)	P value (95%CI)
Vitamin A (µg)	2102.3 ± 425.2	2638.6 ± 154.3	<0.01(2611.33-2665.87)
Vitamin B1 (mg)	1.8 ± 0.3	2.2 ± 0.3	<0.05 (2.15-2.24)
Vitamin B2 (mg)	1.7 ± 0.2	1.9 ± 0.3	<0.001(1.85-1.94)
Vitamin B3 (mg)	19.0 ± 3.6	25.3 ± 3.6	<0.001 (24.79-24.80)
Vitamin C (mg)	460.8 ± 85.3	304.0 ± 101.5	<0.001(289.67-318.32)

Values are in Mean ± SD.

Table 2. Anthropometric data of control and AMI patients (mean ± SD).

	Control (n=165)	AMI patients (n=165)	P- value (95%CI)
Age (years) Range (years)	60.5 ± 3.4 *(48-69)*	61.8 ± 3.8 *(48-69)*	0.0037 (61.26-62.33)
Height (m)	1.63 ± 0.04	1.64 ± 0.59	0.2919 (1.55-1.72)
Weight (kg)	68.34 ± 3.97	72.01 ± 5.37	<0.01 (71.25-72.76)
BMI (kg/m²)	25.40 ± 1.20	26.16 ± 1.45	<0.01 (25.95-26.36)
Waist Circumference (cm)	93.70 ± 3.63	100.77 ± 6.06	<0.01 (99.91-101.62)
Hip Circumference (cm)	100.01 ± 3.16	105.72 ± 5.23	<0.01 (104.82-106.45)
Waist-Hip ratio	0.93 ± 0.01	0.95 ± 0.01	<0.001 (0.94-0.95)
Mid Arm Circumference (cm)	29.70 ± 1.47	30.63 ± 1.87	<0.01 (30.36-30.89)
Biceps skin fold thickness (mm)	6.95 ± 1.05	7.5 ± 1.38	<0.001 (7.30-7.69)
Triceps skin fold thickness (mm)	11.97 ± 1.27	12.89 ± 1.69	<0.001 (12.65-13.12)

Systolic blood pressure (mmHg)	121.06 ± 4.19	134.32 ± 11.65	<0.05 (132.67-135.96)
Diastolic blood pressure (mmHg)	79.90 ± 3.64	86.04 ± 4.25	<0.05 (85.44-86.63)

Table 3. Lipid profile in AMI patients and healthy controls (mean ± SD).

Variables	Controls (n=165)	AMI patients (n=165)	P-value (95%CI)
Age	60.55 ± 3.98	61.84 ± 3.80	0.0037(61.26-62.42)
Total Cholesterol †	168.58 ± 12.16	186.44 ± 13.95	<0.001(184.31-188.56)
HDL-Cholesterol †	50.51 ± 6.78	41.27 ± 4.62	<0.001(40.56-41.97)
Triglycerides †	107.84 ± 11.51	128.96 ± 12.19	<0.001(127.10-130.82)
LDL-Cholesterol †	83.59 ± 11.95	119.37 ± 14.05	<0.001(17.22-21.51)

* ratio † (mg %).

Table 4. Cardiac Enzyme Markers in Control subjects and AMI patients.

	Control (n=68)	AMI patients (n=97)	P value (95%CI)
Troponin I (ng/ml)	0.23 ± 0.11	1.56 ± 1.03	<0.0001(1.41-1.70)
Troponin T (ng/ml)	0.04 ± 0.03	0.64 ± 0.42	<0.0001(0.58-0.69)
Myoglobin (ng/ml)	20.64 ± 6.37	180.87 ± 120.31	<0.0001(163.89-197.87)
CK-Total (IU/L)	0.97 ± 0.53	314.78 ± 221.13	<0.0001(283.57-345.98)
CK-MB (IU/L)	0.13 ± 0.07	67.11 ± 54.64	<0.0001(59.39-74.82)

Values are in Mean ± SD.

Table 5. Antioxidant status in Control subjects and AMI patients.

	Control (n=165)	AMI patients (n=165)	P value (95%CI)
Serum albumin (g/dl)	4.4 ± 0.3	4.2 ± 0.3	<0.0001(4.15-4.24)
Serum uric acid (mg/dl)	5.8 ± 1.2	4.3 ± 0.9	<0.0001(4.17-4.42)
Serum ascorbic acid (mg/dl)	5.3 ± 1.2	2.8 ± 0.7	<0.0001(2.70-2.89)
Serum Total bilirubin (mg/dl)	0.8 ± 0.2	0.7 ± 0.2	<0.0001(0.67-0.72)
Serum superoxide dismutase (U/gHb)	1826.5 ± 31.9	813.9 ± 208.9	<0.0001 (784.42-843.37)
Serum glutathione peroxidase (U/gHb)	61.3 ± 3.9	42.6 ± 6.3	<0.0001 (41.71- 43.48)
Serum catalase (k/gHb)	256.2 ± 26.7	193.1 ± 35.9	<0.0001 (188.03-198.16)

Values are in Mean ± SD.

Table 6. Lp (a) and Lipid Peroxidation levels in Control subjects and AMI patients.

	Control (n=165)	AMI patients (n=165)	P value (95%CI)
Serum Lipoprotein (a) (mg/dl)	3.0 ± 1.1	10.9 ± 2.2	<0.0001 (10.58-11.21)
Serum malondialdehyde (nmol/L)	5.7 ± 1.0	14.8 ± 1.7	<0.0001 (14.56-15.03)
Serum conjugated dienes (µmol/L)	31.0 ± 2.7	48.3 ± 5.5	<0.0001 (47.52-49.07)

Values are in Mean ± SD.

Table 7. Other Biochemical parameters in Control subjects and AMI patients.

	Control (n=165)	MI patients (n=165)	P value (95% CI)
Plasma fibrinogen (mg/dl)	237.5 ± 17.4	357.8 ± 23.2	<0.0001 (354.52 -361.07
Serum caeruloplasmin (mg/dl)	20.4 ± 2.3	51.5 ± 2.4	<0.0001 (51.16-51.83)
Serum Arylesterase activity (kU/L)	98.4 ± 6.2	69.7 ± 10.0	<0.0001(68.28-71.11)
Serum Ischemia modified albumin (U/ml)	81.9 ± 3.9	97.5 ± 11.7	<0.001(95.84-99.15)
Serum C-reactive protein (mg/dl)	1.1 ± 0.3	3.0 ± 1.1	<0.0001(2.84-3.15)

Values are in Mean ± SD.

Discussion

Coronary artery disease (CAD) remains the major cause of morbidity and mortality in all developed and developing countries in the world including India [26]. Various risk factors have been identified among which dyslipidemia is one of the major modifiable risk factors [27, 28, 29].

The coronary artery disease (CAD) risk factors do not predict the occurrence of acute myocardial infarction (AMI) as variation in risk factors is observed in South Asian population due to varied dietary habits and life style [30]. The search for various conventional risk factors among Asians could be helpful in recognizing the future events of stroke as always there are some missing links between cardiovascular disease (CVD) and risk factors associated with them. These curiosities prompted us to identify the newer risk factors and to observe the variations in risk factors due to variation in antioxidant vitamins intake with respect to Indian and Sri Lankan population.

Even though antioxidants and vitamins are efficient in cardio-protection and delays the progression of CVD which is highlighted by the outcome of researches but the search for the newer risk factors continues and now investigations are on the line to exploit the role of inflammatory markers and other potential risks factors which could link with acute myocardial infarction (AMI).

In this prospective case-control study, only Normolipidemic acute myocardial infarction (AMI) patients were selected. The study was designed to identify and evaluate potential risk factors in Normolipidemic acute myocardial infarction (AMI) patients with respect to their antioxidants intake. The subjects selected for the study comprised of 165 controls, 48-69 y and 165 acute MI patients, 48-69 y.

Antioxidants intake

The current study observed higher antioxidant vitamins consumption in patients compared to controls, excepting for vitamin C which was higher in controls. The matter of debate arises why the antioxidant status was comparatively lower in patients and risk factors observed were higher in them compared to controls even though they had higher exogenous intake of antioxidants through the food stuffs. The basis could be partially explained with the nullifying effect of these vitamins by various inter-plays of oxidants and pro-oxidants which could have been higher in patients, that failed to provide adequate protection from oxidants [31]. Earlier studies have emphasized to increase the antioxidants in diet and clinical trials have shown effective results. Though a beneficial role for vitamins in CVD has long been explored but the data are still inconsistent and it is not affirmative with several findings. Studies shows that intake of fruits and vegetables does not prevent but can cause metabolic syndrome and type II diabetes which are considered as a major risk factor in cardiovascular diseases. The beneficial effects though supported by observational studies and randomized controlled clinical trials have not yet supported in the prevention of CVD rather indicated higher mortality in those with late-stage atherosclerosis.

Studies have suggested that a combination therapy is superior over single supplementation but ongoing trials are yet to confirm. Further studies have indicated that beta-carotene neutralizes the beneficial effects mediated by other vitamins as it acts as pro-oxidants when given in supplementation cocktail. The trials that used a combination of vitamins that include beta-carotene have been disappointing. However, ascorbic acid along with vitamin E in combination have shown some good results as long term anti-atherogenic effects but their combined effect on clinical endpoints has been inconsistent. Research data suggest that vitamins would be beneficial to individuals who are deficient of antioxidants or exposed to increased levels of oxidative stress such as in smokers, diabetics and elderly patients. Through defining the right population group and the optimal vitamin combination we could potentially find a future role for vitamins in CVD.

Anthropometric variables

Anthropometric variables in acute myocardial infarction (AMI) patients showed highly significant differences in waist/hip ratio and biceps skin fold thickness. Study reported [32] that waist /hip ratio is a dominant, independent and predictive variable of cardiovascular disease and coronary heart disease deaths in Australian men and women. Megnien et al [33] also reported high hip circumference relative to weight and waist circumference is a better predictor of low incidence of cardiovascular disease and coronary heart disease. The present study is in good agreement with the observations of the above studies. Among Indians the cardiovascular risk is high even the prevalence of obesity is minimal [33]. In the present study the mean body mass index and waist / hip ratio in all subjects was 26.56 and 0.96 respectively, showing a significantly higher body mass index and weight /hip ratio in patients compared with control.

Based on the observations of the aforementioned studies and further supported by the present study it could be concluded that weight/hip ratio is a better predictor of cardiovascular disease (CVD) than body mass index. So it is better tool for identifying the future risk of acute myocardial infarction (AMI) in subjects by non-invasive procedures.

Observations of lipid profile

The mean total cholesterol level of the controls compared with acute myocardial infarction patients (186.44 ± 13.95 mg/dl) was significantly (p<0.001) higher compared with controls (168.58 ± 12.16 mg/dl). The mean high density lipoprotein-cholesterol level in the patients was significantly lower (p<0.001) compared with controls. Triglyceride (TG) values observed in acute myocardial infarction (AMI) patients was (129mg/dl) significantly higher than controls (107.8mg/dl). The mean low density lipoprotein-cholesterol (LDL-c) levels in patients was (119.4mg/dl) significantly higher than controls (83.6 mg/dl). The total cholesterol / high density lipoprotein – cholesterol ratio in acute myocardial infarct patients (4.6) was significantly (p<0.001) higher compared with controls (3.4). The present study observed significantly higher ratio (2.9) in acute myocardial infarction patients compared with control (1.9).

Earlier studies in lipid profile analysis conducted on acute myocardial infarction patients [34,35,36,37,38,39,40,41,42,43,44,45] observed higher total cholesterol, triglyceride, low-density lipoprotein –cholesterol and lower levels of high-density lipoprotein-cholesterol in patients compared to controls.

Also higher ratio of total cholesterol to high density lipoprotein-cholesterol, low-density lipoprotein-cholesterol to high-density cholesterol-lipoprotein and higher triglyceride to high-density cholesterol-lipoprotein was observed in the present study. The present study concludes the importance of assessing the lipid ratios even in normolipidemic subjects as it is one of the atherogenic factors for development of myocardial infarction and other coronary complications. The practice of computing the ratio should be implemented even in a normal health check up packages. In the final analysis it appears that myocardial infarction and coronary artery disease are not always associated with an elevated serum total cholesterol concentration. The major concern of this observation is that subjects who maintain desirable total cholesterol concentration also are targets for myocardial infarction (MI) and coronary artery disease (CAD) and therefore analysis of other risk factors that are non-conventional and newly emerging will be of immense important in the eventual assessment of the risk status. The existing literature and the results of the present study all point out that acute myocardial infarction and coronary artery disease patients have significantly higher total cholesterol concentration whether the values are in the desirable range or elevated.

Antioxidant status

The serum endogenous antioxidants were decreased in acute myocardial infarction compared to controls. Similarly the enzyme antioxidants were also significantly lowered in patients.

Study conducted [46, 47] in acute myocardial infarction patients, reported significantly lower (p<0.0001) albumin and bilirubin (p<0.0001), where as lower levels of uric acid [48, 49, 50] and ascorbic acid [35, 51, 52, 53, 54] in acute myocardial infarct patients were reported.

The aforementioned studies suggested the expected risk of acute myocardial infarction is increased where these endogenous antioxidants are lowered due to enhanced utilization during oxidative stress in patients. Though, uric acid is well established antioxidant, but at times it can also act as a pro-oxidant, which might increase the risk of myocardial infarction. Aulinskas et al, [55] established the role of ascorbic acid as up regulator of low density –lipoprotein (LDL) receptors, facilitating the clearance of low density –lipoprotein (LDL). The low levels of ascorbic acid in acute myocardial infarction (AMI) patients in the present study might be due to enhanced utilization of ascorbic acid during oxidative stress in patients.

The enzymatic antioxidants namely superoxide dismutase, catalase and glutathione peroxidase are also lowered in patients compared with controls. The findings of the present study concurs to earlier studies [35, 43, 52, 56, 57, 58, 59] where lower activities of superoxide dismutase, catalase and glutathione peroxidase. Studies conducted [37, 44, 56, 58, 59, 60] also reported reduced activities of glutathione peroxidase in patients compared with controls. These studies are based on the hypothesis of decreased antioxidants due to oxidative insult in myocardial infarct patients. Thus it is indicative that low levels of both endogenous and enzyme antioxidants in circulation may be due to its in creased utilization to scavenge toxic lipid peroxides.

Lipoprotein (a) and lipid peroxidation

The mean serum Lipoprotein (a) malondialdehyde (MDA) and conjugated diene (CD) levels in MI patients were higher compared with controls. Earlier studies conducted [39, 58, 61, 62] also observed higher Lipoprotein (a) in AMI patients where as Nascetti et al, [63] did not observed any change in Lipoprotein (a) levels in cardiovascular disease (CVD) patients and concluded lipoprotein (a) not to be considered as an independent risk factor in cardiovascular disease (CVD) patients.

Studies conducted [35, 37, 44, 52, 53, 56, 59] reported higher levels of malondialdehyde (MDA) in myocardial infarct patients.

Other biochemical parameters

The levels of caeruloplasmin, C-reactive protein, fibrinogen, ischemia-modified albumin were higher and arylesterase activities were lowered in patients. Studies conducted [60, 64, 65, 66] observed significantly higher (p<0.001) levels of caeruloplasmin where as [42, 67, 68, 69 70] observed higher levels of C-reactive protein in patients. Shukla et al, [71] stated elevated levels of caeruloplasmin as a risk factor for acute myocardial infarct patients.

The reactive oxygen species disrupts copper binding to caeruloplasmin thus impairing its antioxidant property and further promoting oxidative pathology. Studies conducted on plasma fibrinogen levels in acute myocardial infarct patients [42, 72, 73, 74] reported rise in plasma fibrinogen as the present study. Earlier study conducted [23, 24] in acute myocardial infarct patients also reported higher levels in patients as observed by the present study. Studies on arylesterase activities in acute myocardial infarct patients [75, 76, 77, 78, 79, 80, 81] also observed lower activities as concurrent to the current study. Increased C-reactive protein (CRP) concentrations in patients with unstable angina and acute myocardial infarct might induce the production by the monocytes of the tissue factor which initiates the coagulation process. C-reactive protein together with fibrinogen acts as a chemotactic factor. Fibrinogen is responsible for the adhesion of macrophages to the endothelial surface for their migration into the intima. The elevated c-reactive protein levels have been found to be related to the occurrence of cardiovascular complications such as sudden cardiac death or AMI [82].

Conclusions

Our study concluded dietary vitamin could not decrease the risk of acute myocardial infarction. There might be number of additional risk factors interplaying in Acute Myocardial Infarction patients which have not given adequate protection against AMI, in spite of higher vitamin intake by them.

Limitatations of the study

The sample size is not adequate to draw definitive conclusion. Future studies should be carried out with large scale patients sample size.

Conflicts interest: The author does not have any conflict interest from the study.

References

1. Avezum A, Braga J, Santos I, Guimaraes HP, Marin-Neto JA, Piegas LS. Cardiovascular disease in South America: current status and opportunities for prevention. Heart 2009; 95:1475-1482 doi:10.1136/hrt.2008.156331.
2. Reddy KS. Cardiovascular disease in India. World Health Stat Q 1993; 46:101-7.
3. Chopra V, Wasir H. Implications of lipoprotein abnormalities in Indian patients. Journal Assoc Physicians of India 1998; 46:814-8.
4. Reddy KS, Yusuf S. Emerging epidemic of cardiovascular disease in developing countries. Circulation1998; 97:596–601.
5. Bulatao RAO, Stephens PW. Demographic estimates and projections, by region, 1970-2015. In: Jamison DT, Mosley WH, eds. Disease control priorities in developing countries. Washington, DC: World Bank, 1990. (Health sector priorities review no. 13.)
6. Mack T. Ruffin IV and Cheryl L. Rock. Do antioxidants still have a role in the prevention of human cancer? Current Oncology Reports 2001; 3:306-313 doi:10.1007/s11912-001-0082-8.
7. Ludwig S, Shen GX. Statins for diabetic cardiovascular complications. Curr Vasc Pharmacol 2006; 4:245-251.
8. Penny M. Kris-Etherton, Alice H. Lichtenstein, Barbara V. Howard, Daniel Steinberg, Joseph L. Witztum. Antioxidant Vitamins Supplements and Cardiovascular Disease. Circulation 2004; 110:637-641.

9. Harold E. Seifried, Darrell E. Anderson, Barbara C. Sorkin, Rebecca B. Costello. Free Radicals: The Pros and Cons of Antioxidants J. Nutr 2004; 134:3143S-3163S.

10. National Cholesterol Education Program. Detection, evaluation and treatment of high blood cholesterol in adults (Adult Treatment Panel III). Circulation 2002; 106:3143-3421.

11. International Epidemiological Association. Relative validity and reproducibility of a diet history questionnaire in Spain. III. Biochemical markers. EPIC Group of Spain. European Prospective Investigation into Cancer and Nutrition. International Journal of Epidemiology 1997; 26: S110-S117.

12. Rose GA, Blackburn H, Gillum RF, Prineas RJ. Cardiovascular Survey Methods. 2nd Ed. WHO Monograph Series No. 56. Geneva. World Health Organisation; 1982.

13. Perry BW, Doumas BT. Effect of heparin on albumin determination by use of bromocresol green and bromocresol purple. Clin Chem 1979; 25:1520-1522.

14. Brown H. The determination of uric acid in human blood. Journal of Biological Chemistry, 1945; 158:601-608.

15. Jendrassik, J. & Grof P.Vereinfachte photometrische Methoden Zur Beetimmung des Blutbilirubin. Biochem. Z., 1938;297; 81-89.

16. Paglia DE, Valentine WN. Studies on quantitative and qualitative characterization of erythrocyte glutathione peroxidase. J Lab Clin Med 1967;70: 158-69.

17. Sun Y, Oberly LW, Li Y. A simple method for clinical assay of superoxide dismutase. Clin Chem 1988; 34: 497-500.

18. Beutler E. Red Cell Metabolism: A Manual of Biochemical Methods, 3rd edition. New York, Grune and Stratton, 1984; 105.

19. Beutler E, Duron O, Kelly B. An improved method for the determination of blood glutathione. J Lab Clin Med 1963;61: 822-826.

20. Bernheim S, Bernheim MLC, Wilbur KM. The reaction between thiobarbituric acid and the oxidant product of certain lipids. J Biol Chem 1948; 174: 257-264.

21. Recknagel RO, Glende EA. Spectrophotometric detection of lipid conjugated dienes. Methods Enzymol 1984; 105:331-337.

22. Ravin HA. An improved colorimetric enzymatic assay of caeruloplasmin. J. Lab. Med 1961; 58, 161-168.

23. Chawla R, Goyal N, Calton R, Goyal S. Ischemia modified albumin: A novel marker for acute coronary syndrome. Indian Journal of Clinical Biochemistry 2006; 21(1):77-82.

24. Auxter S. Cardiac Ischemia testing: a new era in chest pain evaluation. *Clin Lab News* 2003; 29, 1-3.

25. Roe, J.H. & Kuether, C.A. The determination of ascorbic acid in whole blood and urine through the 2,4-dinitrophenylhydrazine derivative of dehydroascorbic acid. Journal of Biological Chemistry, 1943; 147:399-407.

26. Reddy KS, Yusuf S. Emerging epidemic of cardiovascular disease in developing countries. Circulation 1998; 97:596–601.

27. Chopra V, Wasir H. Implications of lipoprotein abnormalities in Indian patients. The Journal Assoc Physicians of India 1998; 46:814-8.

28. Malhotra P, Kumari S, Singh S, Verma S. Isolated Lipid Abnormalities in Rural and Urban Normotensive and Hypertensive North-West Indians. The Journal of Assoc Physicians of India 2003; 51:459-463.

29. Vasisht S, Narula J, Awtade A, Tandon R, Srivastava LM. Lipids and lipoproteins in normal controls and clinically documented coronary heart disease patients. Ann Natl Acad Med Sci (India) 1990; 26:57-66.

30. Mishra, A., Luthra, K. and Vikram, N.K. Dyspipidemia in Asian Indians: Determminants and Significance. The Journal of Assoc Physicians of India 2005; 52:137-142.

31. Nanda N, Zachariah B, Hamide A. Oxidative Stress and protein glycation in primary hypothyroidism. Male/Female difference. Clinical and Experimental Medicine 2009; 8:101-108. doi:10.1007/s10238-008-0164-0.

32. Heitman BL, Frederickson P, Lissner L. Hip Circumference and Cardiovascular Morbidity and Mortality in Men and Women. Obesity Research 2004; 12:482-487.

33. Megnien JL, Denarie N, Cocaul M. Predicitve value of Waist-to-hip ratio on Cardiovascular Risk Events. Int J Obes Relat Metab Disord 1999; 23:90-97.

34. Mishra TK, Routray SN, Patnaik UK, Padhi PK, Satapathy C, Behera M. Lipoprotein (a) and Lipid Profile in Young Patients with Angiographically Proven Coronary Artery Disease. Indian Heart Journal 2001; 53 :(5) Article No. 60.

35. Das S, Yadav D, Narang R, Das N. Interrelationship between lipid peroxidation, ascorbic acid and superoxide dismutase in coronary artery disease. Current Science 2002; 83:488-491.

36. Goswami K Bandyopadhyay. Lipid profile in middle class Bengali population of Kolkata. Indian Journal of Clinical Biochemistry 2003; 18:127-130.

37. Kharb S. Low Glutathione levels in acute myocardial infarction. Ind J Med Sci 2003; 57; Issue8: 335-7.

38. Malhotra, P., Kumari, S., Singh, S. and Varma, S. Isolated Lipid Abnormalities in Rural and Urban Normotensive and Hypertensive North-West Indians. The Journal of Association of Physicians of India 2003; 51:459-463.

39. Burman A, Jain K, Gulati R, Chopra V, Agrawal DP, Vaisisht S. Lipoprotein (a) as a marker of Coronary Artery Disease and its Association with Dietary Fat. The Journal of Assoc Physicians of India 2004; 52:99-102.

40. Rajasekhar D., Srinivasa Rao P.V., Latheef S.A., Saibaba K.S., and Subramanyam G. Association of serum antioxidants and risk of coronary heart disease in South Indian population. Indian J Med Sci 2004; 58(11):465-71.

41. Rani, S.H., Madhavi, G., Ramachandra Rao, V., Sahay, B.K. and Jyothy, A. Risk factors for coronary heart disease in type II diabetes. Indian J Clin Biochem 2005; 20(2):75-80.

42. Sivaraman S K, Zachariah G, Annamalai PT. Evaluation of C - reactive protein and other Inflammatory Markers in Acute Coronary Syndromes. Kuwait Medical Journal 2004; 36(1):35-37.

43. Patil N, Chavan V, Karnik N.D. Antioxidant Status in patients with Acute Myocardial Infarction. Indian Journal of Clinical Biochemistry 2007;22:45-51.

44. Shinde S, Kumar P, Patil N. Decreased Levels Of Erythrocyte Glutathione In Patients With Myocardial Infarction. The Internet Journal of Alternative Medicine 2005; 2:1.

45. Yadhav AS, Bhagwat VR, Rathod IM. Relationship of Plasma homocysteine with lipid profile parameters in Ischemic Heart disease. Indian Journal of Clinical Biochemistry 2006; 21(1):106-110.

46. Olusi SO, Prabha K, Sugathan TN. Biochemical Risk factors for Myocardial Infarction Among South Asian Immigrants and Arabs. Annals of Saudi Medicine 1999; 19: 147-149.

47. Djousse L, Rothman KJ, Cupples LA, Levy D, Ellison RC. Effect of serum albumin and bilirubin as a risk factor for Myocardial infarction. Am J Cardiol 2003; 91: 485- 488.

48. Jing F, Alderman M H. Serum uric acid and cardiovascular mortality. JAMA 2000; 283: 2404-2410.

49. Brand FN, Mcgee DL, Kannel WB, Stokes J, Castelli W P. Hyperuricemia as a risk factor of coronary heart disease: The Framingham Study. American Journal of Epidemiology 1985; 121: 11-18.

50. Niskanen LK, Laaksonen DE, Nyyssonen K, Alfthan G, Lakka H M, Lakka TA, Salonene JT. Uric acid level as a risk factor for cardiovascular and all- cause moratlity in middle-aged men: a prospective study. Arch Intern Med 2004; 164:1546-51.

51. Nyyssonen K, Markku TP, Salonen R, Tuomilehto J, Salonen JT. Vitamin C deficiency and risk of myocardial infarction: prospective population study of men from eastern Finland. BMJ 1997; 314:634.

52. Bhakuni P, Chandra M, Misra MK. Levels of free radical scavengers and antioxidants in post perfused patients of myocardial infarction. Current Science 2005; 89: 168-170.

53. Bhakuni P, Chandra M, Misra MK. Oxidative stress parameters in erythrocytes of post-reperfused patients with myocardial infarction. J Enzyme Inhib Med Chem 2005; 20(4):337-81.

54. Kurl S, Tuomainen TP, Laukkanen JA, Nyyssonen K, Lakka T, Sivenius J, Salonen JT. Plasma Vitamin C Modifies the Association Between Hypertension and Risk of Stroke. Stroke 2002; 33:1568.

55. Aulinskas TH, Vander Westhuyzen DR, Coetzee G A. Ascorbate increases the number of low density lipoprotein receptors in cultured arterial smooth muscle cells. Atherosclerosis 1983; 47(2):159-171.

56. Senthil S, Veerappan RM, Ramakrishna RM, Pugalendi KV. Oxidative stress and antioxidants in patients with cardiogenic shock complicating acute myocardial infarction. Clin Chim Acta 2004; 348 (1-2):131-7.

57. Jain A, Gupta HL. Hyperfibrinogenemia in patients of diabetes mellitus in relation to glycemic control and urinary albumin excretion rate. The Journal of Association of Physicians of India 2001; 49:227-230.

58. Rajasekhar D, Srinivasa Rao PV, Latheef SA, Saibaba KS, Subramanyam G. Association of serum antioxidants and risk of coronary heart disease in South Indian population. Indian Journal of Medical Sciences 2004; 58(11):465-471.

59. Gupta M, Chari S. Proxidant and Antioxidant status in patients of type II Diabetes Mellitus with IHD. Indian Journal of Clinical Biochemistry 2006; 21(2):118-122.

60. El- Badry I, Abon El N, Yehia T K, Zakhari MM. Free radicals activity in Acute Myocardial Infarction. The Egyptian Heart Journal 1995; 47: 71-78.

61. Guha S, Chatterjee S, Mazumder R, Sadek Ali SK, Guha S, Chatterjee N, Biswas S, Bhattacharya GC. Lipoprotein (a), Lipid Tetrad Index and Coronary Artery Disease: A Correlative Study.Indian Heart Journal 2001; 53 (5) Article No. 28.

62. Bal BS, Bhangu MS, Chhabra N, Sandhu PS, Mahajan M, Batra K S. Incidence of Raised Lipoprotein (a) Level in Cases of Angina with Hyperhomocysteinemia and Normal Lipid Profile. Indian Heart Journal 2001; 53: (5) Article No. 47.

63. Nascetti S, D' Addato S, Pascarelli N, Sangiorgi Z, Grippo MC, Gaddi A. Cardiovascular disease and Lp(a) in the adult population and in the elderly: the Brisighella study. Riv Eur Sci Med Farmacol 1996; 18(5-6):205-12.

64. Grobusch KK, Grobbee DE, Koster JF, Lindemans J, Boeing H, Hofman A, Witteman Jacqueline C.M. Serum caeruloplasmin as a coronary risk factor in the elderly: the Rotterdam Study. British Journal of Nutrition 1999; 81:139-144.

65. Awadallah SM, Hamad M, Jbarah I, Salem NM, Mubarak MS. Autoantibodies against oxidized LDL correlate with serum concentrations of caeruloplasmin in patients with cardiovascular disease. Clin Chim Acta 2006; 365: 330-336.

66. Giurgea N, Constantinescu MI, Stanciu R, Suciu S, Muresan A. Caeruloplasmin- acute –phase reactant or endogenous antioxidant? The case of cardiovascular disease. Med Sci Monit 2005; 11: RA 48-51.

67. Berton G, Cordiano R, Palmieri R, Pianca S, Pagliara V, Palatini P.C-Reactive Protein in Acute Myocardial Infarction: Association With Heart Failure. American Heart Journal 2003; 145(6):1094-1101.

68. Bhagat S, Gaiha M, Sharma VK, Anuradha S. A Comparative Evaluation of C - reactive protein as a Short-Term Prognostic Marker in Severe Unstable Angina- A Preliminary Study. The Journal of the Association of Physicians of India 2003; 51:349-354.

69. Kulsoom B, Nazrul SH. Association of serum C - reactive protein and LDL: HDL with myocardial infarction. Journal of Pakistan Medical Association 2006; 56(7):318-322.

70. Boncler M, Luzak B, Watala C. Role of C-reactive protein in atherogenesis. Postepy Hig Med Dosw 2006; 60:538-46.

71. Shukla N, Maher J, Masters J, Angelini G D, Jeremy JY. Does oxidative stress change ceruloplasmin from a protective to a vasculopathic factor? Atherosclerosis 2006; 187: 238-250.

72. Harkut PV, Sahashrabhojney VS, Salkar RG. Plasma fibrinogen as a marker of major adverse cardiac events in patients of type 2 Diabetes with unstable angina. Int J Diab Dev Countries 2004; 24: 69-74.

73. Coppola G, Rizzo M, Maurizio GA, Corrado E, Alberto DG, Braschi A, Braschi G, Novo S. Fibrinogen as a predictor of mortality after acute myocardial infarction: a forty-two-month follow up study. Ital Heart J 2005; 6:315-322.

74. Beg M, Nizami A, Singhal KC, Mohammed J, Gupta A, Azfar SF. Role of serum fibrinogen in patients of ischemic cerebrovascular disease. Nepal Med Coll J 2007; 9: 88-92.

75. Aviram M, Rosenblat M, Billecke S, Eroul J, Sovenson R, Bisaier CL. Human serum paraoxonase (PON1) is in activated by oxidized low density lipoprotein and preserved by antioxidants. Free Radic Biol Med 1999; 26:892-904.

76. Ayub A, Mackness MI, Sharon A, Mackness B, Patel J, Durrington PN. Serum Paraoxonase After Myocardial Infarction. Arteriosclerosis, Thrombosis, and Vascular Biology 1999; 19:330-335.

77. Azizi F, Rahmani M, Raiszadeh F, Solati M, Navab M. Associations of lipids, lipoproteins, apolipoproteins and paraoxonase enzyme activity with premature coronary artery disease. Coronary Artery Dis 2002; 13(1): 9-16.

78. Jarvik GP, Tsai NT, Mckinstry LA, Wani R, Victoria HB, Richter RJ, Schellenberg GD, Heagerty PJ, Hatsukami TS, Furlong CE. Vitamin C and E Intake Is Associated With Increased Paraoxonase Activity. Arteriosclerosis, Thrombosis, and Vascular Biology 2002; 22:1329.

79. Sarkar PD, TMS Madhusudhan B. Association between paraoxonase activity and lipid levels in patients with premature coronary artery disease. Clin Chim Acta 2006; 373:77-81.

80. Richard JW, Leview I, Righetti A. Smoking Is Associated With Reduced Serum Paraoxonase Activity and Concentration in Patients With Coronary Artery Disease Circulation 2000; 101:2252-2257.

81. Singh S, Venketesh S, Verma JS, Verma M, Lellamma CO, Goel RC. Paraoxonase (PON11) activity in northwest Indian Punjabis with coronary artery disease & type II diabetes mellitus. Indian J Med Res 2007; 125:783-7.

82. Pepys MB and Hirschfield G M. C-reactive protein: a critical update. J Clin Invest 2003; 111(12): 1805-1812. doi: 10.1172/JCI200318921.

Chapter 6

Cardiovascular Risk factors in elderly Normolipidemic Acute Myocardial Infarct patients- A Case Controlled Study from India

Abstract

Background: Myocardial Infarction (MI) is a leading cause of death in India. Cardiovascular risk factor varies with persons and location. Early detection and identification could reduce the cost effectiveness of high coronary care unit costs. Only few studies have addressed the cardiovascular risk factors among Indians.

Objective: The goal of the present study was to address the various risk factors associated in Normolipidemic AMI patients admitted in Intensive Coronary care unit after heart attack. The study also evaluated the serum lipid peroxidation markers and antioxidants enzyme status among the two groups consisting of AMI patients and age/sex- matched controls.

Design: Lipid profile (TC, TG, HDL-C, LDL-C), MDA, CD, SOD, GPx, Cat activities were analyzed in 330 subjects, which included 165 AMI patients and 165 age-sex matched control. Apart from that IMA, caeruloplasmin, fibrinogen, HDL-PON activities were also analyzed.

Results: We observed a significant and dose-dependent inverse association between vegetable intake and IHD risk. The inverse association was stronger for green leafy vegetables; in multivariate analysis, persons consuming a median of 3.5 servings/wk had a 67% lower relative risk (RR: 0.33; 95% CI: 0.17, 0.64; P for trend = 0.0001) than did those consuming 0.5 servings/wk. Controlling for other dietary covariates did not alter the association. Cereal intake was also associated with a lower risk. Use of mustard oil, which is rich in α-linolenic acid, was associated with a lower risk than was use of sunflower oil [for use in cooking: RR: 0.49 (95% CI: 0.24, 0.99); for use in frying, RR: 0.29 (95% CI: 0.13, 0.64)].

Conclusion: Diets rich in vegetables, fruits and use of mustard oil could contribute to the lower risk of AMI among Indians.

Key Words: Dietary vitamin, nutrition, acute myocardial infarction, India, foods, vegetables, green leafy vegetables, oils, malondialdehyde, conjugated diene, superoxide dismutase, catalase, glutathione peroxidase, normolipidemia.

Introduction

With the explosive rise in the incidence of Coronary Artery disease (CAD) it is projected to be the leading cause of morbidity and mortality among Indians by the year 2015 (1). The World Health Organization predicts that deaths due to circulatory system diseases are projected to double between 1985 and 2015 (2, 3). Asian Indians living abroad indicates a 40% higher risk of ischemic heart disease (IHD) mortality than that for Europeans (4).

It is a multifactorial disease associated with factors like hereditary, hyperlipidemia, obesity, hypertension, environmental and life style variables like stress, smoking, alcohol consumption, etc (5). Lipoprotein profile has been investigated extensively in recent years, which is deranged in large proportion of CAD patients; especially Asians showing a mixed picture of dyslipidemia (6). Literature survey reveals the chances of myocardial infarction in dyslipidemic persons are more due to increased free radical generation and ischemia and is a conventional risk factor as reported (7-14). Lowering of High density lipoprotein- cholesterol (HDL-C) is a common phenomenon observed in MI patients supported by previous studies (7-13). HDL is the most important independent protective factor for arteriosclerosis which underlies coronary heart disease (CHD). HDL associated Paraoxonase (PON1) enzyme is protective against lipid peroxidation (15). Numerous cohort studies and clinical trials have confirmed the association between a low HDL-C and increased risk of CHD. Low density lipoprotein-cholesterol (LDL-C) is considered as the most important risk factor of CAD and its oxidized form promotes foam cells formation which initiates the process of atherosclerosis by its accumulation in sub-endothelium leading to fatty streaks and complex fibro fatty or atheromatous plaques (16). The oxidation of LDL can be limited by antioxidant enzyme system, including superoxide dismutase, catalase, glutathione peroxidase and antioxidant vitamins C, A, E and other carotenoids. Among the endogenous antioxidant system, includes albumin, uric acid, and total bilirubin. Imbalance of this reaction either due to excess free radical formation or insufficient removal by antioxidants leads to oxidative stress (17, 18, 19).

Various other risk factors have been identified apart from dyslipidemia are caeruloplasmin, C-reactive proteins, Lp (a), plasma fibrinogen, etc. Since we have encountered myocardial infarct patients with normal serum lipid concentration, we conducted a case-control study to evaluate the levels of antioxidant enzymes, extent of lipid peroxidation as a marker of oxidative stress and other risk factors associated with acute MI.

Materials and methods

Cases

Eligible cases were all patients aged 48-69 y hospitalized with a diagnosis of first incident acute myocardial infarction (MI). The definitive diagnosis of AMI was established according to diagnostic criteria: chest pain lasting for ≤3 hours, electrocardiographic (ECG) changes (ST elevation ≥ 2 mm in at least two leads) and elevation in enzymatic activities of serum creatine phosphokinase and aspartate aminotransferase. The control group consisted of 165 age/sex-matched healthy volunteers (123 men and 42 women).

Inclusion criteria were patients with a diagnosis of AMI with normal lipid profile. Patients were excluded if they had any previous history of MI or IHD (including bypass surgery, angina, or stroke) because such prior diagnoses may alter behaviors, including diet. Patients with diabetes mellitus, renal insufficiency, hepatic disease or taking lipid lowering drugs or antioxidant vitamin supplements were also excluded from the study. We also excluded patients if they were pregnant, had a history of cancer, gastrointestinal tract infection, or thyroid, because these conditions may have affected dietary intake. The patients were interviewed on average 2–5 d after admission. The eligibility criteria were met by 245 cases, and 165 were included in the study. The reasons for exclusion were death (n = 19) or discharge (n = 27) before the interviews could be completed, being too sick to be interviewed (n = 16), and not giving consent to participate (n = 18).

Controls

For each cases, control subjects matched by age (within 1 y), sex, and hospital were obtained from noncardiac outpatient clinics or inpatient wards. The same exclusion criteria used for cases were applied for control selection. We identified ≈ 165 eligible control subjects.

Criteria for normolipidemics: Normal lipid profile was defined if LDL was <130mg/dl, HDL ≥ 35 mg/dl, Total cholesterol (TC) <200 mg/dl and Triglycerides (TG) <150 mg/dl (20).

Data collection

Interviews were conducted in hospital wards or clinics by us and lasted ≈ 30 min. Informed consent was obtained from all study subjects. This included various life style factors such as education, socio-economic status, income and type of job. Details of major cardiovascular risk factors such as smoking, alcohol intake, diabetes, obesity and hypertension were also obtained. We also collected data on socioeconomic status; smoking history; history of hypertension, diabetes, and hypercholesterolemia; family history of cardiovascular disease (including IHD, angina, MI, hypertension, diabetes, stroke, sudden death, and bypass surgery) and physical activity.

Anthropometric measurements

Anthropometric measures (height, weight, and hip and waist circumferences) were obtained and body mass index (weight in kg divided by height in meters squared) and waist-to-hip ratio were calculated. Their height, weight, waist-hip ratio and blood pressure were recorded. Height was measured in centimeters and weight in kilograms using calibrated spring balance. Supine waist girth was measured at the level of umbilicus with a person breathing silently and standing hip girth was measured at inter-trochanteric level. Waist and hip measures were assessed by using a standardized tape measure, with waist measures taken at the midpoint between the costal margin and ileac crest and hip measures taken at the widest circumference.

Blood pressure

The blood pressure was measured using standard mercury manometer. At least two readings at 5 minutes intervals as per World Health Organization guidelines were recorded (21). If high blood pressure (≥140/90 mmHg) was noted a third reading was taken after 30 minutes. The lowest of the three readings was taken as blood pressure.

Electrocardiogram

Electrocardiogram (12 lead) was performed on all persons using proper standardization.

Collection of samples

Blood (10 ml) was collected after overnight fasting in different containers.

EDTA vial: 5.0 ml of blood was taken. Red cells were washed 3-4 times with ice-cold normal saline and used for estimation of glutathione peroxidase, superoxide dismutase and catalase.

Plain vial: Remaining blood was allowed to clot and serum separated by centrifugation for 5 min at 5000 rpm and was used for determination of lipid profile, malondialdehye and conjugated dienes, and other assays as described.

For IscMA analysis, 2 ml of blood was collected from the patients immediately after admission to intensive care unit.

Lipid profile

Total cholesterol, triglycerides, and HDL-cholesterol were estimated by enzymatic methods using the kits obtained from Randox Laboratories Limited, Crumlin, UK. Plasma LDL-cholesterol was determined from the values of total cholesterol and HDL-cholesterol using the following formulae (22):

$$LDL\text{-}C = T\,C - \frac{TG}{5} - HDL\text{-}C \ (mg/dl)$$

All chemicals of analytical grade were obtained from Sigma chemicals, India.

Serum albumin: Serum Albumin was measured by Bromocresol green dye binding method (23).

Serum uric acid: Serum uric acid was estimated by the method of Brown based on the development of a blue color due to tungsten blue as phosphotungstic acid is reduced by uric acid in alkaline medium (24).

Serum total bilirubin: - Serum total bilirubin was estimated by Jendrassik and Grof method (25).

Glutathione peroxidase: The glutathione peroxidase activity was determined by the procedure of Paglia and Valentine (26).

Superoxide dismutase (sod): Superoxide dismuatse enzyme activity was measured by SOD assay kit using rate of inhibition of 2-(4-indophenyl)-(4-Nitrophenol)-5-phenyltetrazolium chloride (I.N.T) reduction method modified by Sun et al (27). CATALASE- Catalase activity was measured spectrophotometrically as described by Beutler (28).

MDA - MDA: levels were estimated by thiobarbituric acid (TBA) reaction (29).

Conjugated dienes (CD): CD levels were measured by Recknagel and Glende method (30) with little modification.

Serum ceruloplasmin: The caeruloplasmin assay was done by *p*-phenylene diamine method (31).

All chemicals of analytical grade were obtained from Sigma Chemicals, India.

Ischemia modified albumin (IscMA): IscMA concentration was determined by addition of a known amount of cobalt (II) to a serum sample and measurement of the unbound cobalt (II) by the intensity of colored complex formed after reacting with dithiothreitol (DTT) by colorimeter (32).

Lipoprotein (a), Lp(a): The Lp(a) levels were determined by Latex- Enhanced Turbidimetric method.

Arylesterase / paraoxonase assay

Serum Arylesterase/Paraoxonase was estimated using Zeptometrix Assay Kit obtained from Zeptometrix Corp, New York, 14202 based on the cleavage of phenyl acetate resulting in phenol formation. The rate of formation of phenol is measured by monitoring the increase in absorbance at 270 nm at 25°C.

Ascorbic acid: Estimation of Vitamin C was carried out by Roe and Kuether method (33).

Measurement of high sensitivity c- reactive (hs-CRP): The C-reactive protein were determined using high sensitivity enzyme Immunoassay kit11 manufactured by Life Diagnostics,inc., Catalog Number: 2210. The principle of the assay was based on a solid phase enzyme-linked immunosorbent assay (34).

Plasma fibrinogen: The plasma fibrinogen was determined using kit12 which was obtained from TEClot Fib Kit 10 Catalog No: 050-500, manufactured by TECO GmbH, Dieselstr. 1, 84088 Neufahrn NB Germany (34).

Results

The study involved 165 myocardial infarct patients and 165 age/sex-matched controls. The mean (± SD) age of the controls were 60.5 ± 3.4 y and in AMI cases and 61.26 ± 3.80 y in controls (**Table 1**).

Anthropometric variables

Anthropometric examination revealed no significant differences of height in cases compared with controls (**Table 1**).

Most (80%) of the cases were overweight compared to controls (69.7%) and had significant difference between them (p<0.001). The Body Mass Index (BMI) in all study subjects were ≥ 25. However the cases were significantly heavier than controls.

Table 1. Anthropometric data of control and patients.

	Control (n=165)	MI patients (n=165)
Age (years)	60.5 ± 3.4	61.8 ± 3.8
Range (years)	(48-69)	(48-69)
Height (m)	1.63 ± 0.04	1.64 ± 0.59
Weight (kg)	68.34 ± 3.97[a]	72.01 ± 5.37[b]
BMI (kg/m^2)	25.40 ± 1.20[c]	26.16 ± 1.45[d]
Waist Circumference (cm)	93.70 ± 3.63[e]	100.77 ± 6.06[f]
Hip Circumference (cm)	100.01 ± 3.16[g]	105.72 ± 5.23[h]
Waist-Hip ratio	0.93 ± 0.01[i]	0.95 ± 0.01[j]
Mid Arm Circumference (cm)	29.70 ± 1.47[k]	30.63 ± 1.87[l]
Biceps skin fold thickness (mm)	6.95 ± 1.05[m]	7.5 ± 1.38[n]
Triceps skin fold thickness (mm)	11.97 ± 1.27[o]	12.89 ± 1.69[p]
Systolic blood pressure (mmHg)	121.06 ± 4.19[q]	134.32 ± 11.65[r]
Diastolic blood pressure (mmHg)	79.90 ± 3.64[s]	86.04 ± 4.25[t]

Values are in Mean ± SD
Values with different superscripts in a row, [a,b,c,d,e,f,g,h] (<0.01) [i,j](<0.001), indicate significantly different,

The mean values of waist-hip circumference were higher in cases compared with controls and were highly significant ($p<0.001$) (**Table1**).

Only 16.3% of controls had their waist-hip ratio >0.95 compared with cases (69.9%) showed values >0.95. The mean values of waist-hip ratio was higher in cases compared with controls and the differences was found to be highly significant ($p<0.001$).

The mean values of mid-arm circumference was significantly higher ($p<0.001$) among cases compared with controls (**Table 1**). A comparison of the mean values of triceps skin fold thickness in cases and controls showed a higher mean values in cases and was statistically significant ($p<0.001$).

Altogether, the body weight, waist circumference, hip circumference, waist-hip ratio and mid arm circumference were significantly higher ($p<0.0001$) in cases compared with controls Therefore it can be concluded from the present study that body weight, waist circumference, hip circumference, waist-hip ratio and mid arm circumference, which reflect the body fat content could be possibly a risk for developing myocardial infarction. Further more the waist-hip ratio is a reliable index than BMI for assessing the risk of subjects who is prone to develop MI since the study revealed that the statistically significant difference was observed only in waist-hip not in body mass index. The relative risk of MI was increased by 2.6 folds in subjects whose waist-hip ratio was ≥0.95 compared to those with normal waist-hip ratio.

Table 2. Lipid profile in patients and healthy controls (mean ± SD).

Variables	Controls (n=165)	Patients (n=165)	P-value (95%CI)
Age	60.55 ± 3.98	61.84 ± 3.80	0.0037(61.26-62.42)
Total Cholesterol †	168.58 ± 12.16	186.44 ± 13.95	<0.001(184.31-188.56)
HDL-Cholesterol †	50.51 ± 6.78	41.27 ± 4.62	<0.001(40.56-41.97)
Triglycerides †	107.84 ± 11.51	128.96 ± 12.19	<0.001(127.10-130.82)
LDL-Cholesterol †	83.59 ± 11.95	119.37 ± 14.05	<0.001(17.22-21.51)

* ratio † (mg %)

Lipid profile analysis

Serum parameters in cases and control are shown in **Table 2**. Total cholesterol, its ratio to HDL-cholesterol (TC/HDL-C), LDL-cholesterol, triglycerides was significantly higher in cases compared with control (**Table 2**). Significant difference for HDL-cholesterol between AMI and control was observed (Table 2). On the other hand, LDL-cholesterol and its ratio to HDL-cholesterol (LDL-C/HDL-C) were higher in cases compared with controls (**Table 3**). No statistically significant difference was observed in TG/HDL-C ratio among cases with controls. Also, significantly lower HDL-C concentration was observed in cases than in the controls (p<0.001).

The analysis based on the ratio of TC/HDL-cholesterol, TG/HDL-cholesterol and LDL-cholesterol/HDL-cholesterol is shown in **Table 4**. Higher ratio of TC/HDL-C, TG/HDL-C and LDL-C/HDL-C was observed in cases compared to controls (**Table 4**).

Cardiac Markers

The serum cardiac marker enzymes were significantly (p<0.0001) different in cases compared with the controls as presented in **Table 5**.

Table 3. TC/HDL-C, LDL-C/HDL-C and TG/HDL-C ratio in patients and healthy controls (mean ± SD).

Variables	Controls (n=165)	Patients (n=165)	P-value (95%CI)
TC: HDL-C*	3.39 ± 0.36	4.57 ± 0.58	<0.001(4.48-4.65)
LDL:HDL-C*	1.90 ± 0.31	2.93 ± 0.51	<0.001(2.85-3.00)
TG: HDL-C*	2.17 ± 0.35	3.16 ± 0.49	0.3149(3.086-3.234)

* ratio † (mg %)

Table 4. Distribution pattern of TC/HDL-C, TG/HDL-C and LDL-C/HDL-C ratio in patients and healthy controls (mean ± SD).

Ratio	Controls (n=165)	Patients (n=165)
TC/HDL-C		
2-3	2.90 ± 0.09 (n=28)	-
3-4	3.44 ± 0.25 (n=129)	3.70 ± 0.20 (n=31)
4-5	4.19 ± 0.22 (n=8)	4.53 ± 0.27 (n=90)
5-6	-	5.26 ± 0.23 (n=44)
TG/HDL-C		
1-2	1.77 ± 0.13 (n=56)	-
2-3	2.38 ± 0.23 (n=109)	2.65 ± 0.27 (n=59)
3-4	-	3.42 ± 0.26 (n=99)
4-5	-	4.22 ± 0.19 (n=7)
LDL-C/HDL-C		
1-2	1.71 ± 0.17 (n=106)	1.86 ± 0.15 (n=5)
2-3	2.23 ± 0.21 (n=59)	2.57 ± 0.27 (n=81)
3-4	-	3.32 ± 0.21 (n=74)
4-5	-	4.11 ± 0.12 (n=5)

Table 5. Cardiac Enzyme Markers in Control subjects and AMI patients

	Control (n=68)	MI patients (n=97)	P value (95%CI)
Troponin I (ng/ml)	0.23 ± 0.11	1.56 ± 1.03	<0.0001(1.41-1.70)
Troponin T (ng/ml)	0.04 ± 0.03	0.64 ± 0.42	<0.0001(0.58-0.69)
Myoglobin (ng/ml)	20.64 ± 6.37	180.87 ± 120.31	<0.0001(163.89-197.87)
CK-Total (IU/L)	0.97 ± 0.53	314.78 ± 221.13	<0.0001(283.57-345.98)
CK-MB (IU/L)	0.13 ± 0.07	67.11 ± 54.64	<0.0001(59.39-74.82)

Values are in Mean ± SD

Table 6. Behavioral Pattern in cases and control subjects.

		Control Group	Study Group
Hyperactive	yes	39 (23.63)	68 (41.21)
	no	126 (76.36)	97 (58.78)
Triffle thinker	yes	30 (18.18)	99 (60.00)
	no	135 (81.81)	66 (40.00)
Irrelevant thinker	yes	50 (30.30)	106 (64.24)
	No	115 (69.69)	59 (35.75)

yes	14 (8.48)	62 (37.57)	63
Familial history of CVD			
No	151 (91.51)	103 (62.42)	

Numbers in parentheses are percent unless mentioned otherwise

Table 7. Distribution of Acute Myocardial Infarction (AMI) risk factors among case and control subjects.

	AMI Cases (n=165)	Controls (n= 165)
Age (y)	61.84 ± 3.80	60.55 ± 3.98
BMI (kg/m^2)	26.16 ± 1.45	25.40 ± 1.20
Waist-to-hip ratio	0.95 ± 0.11	0.93 ± 0.08[1]
Alcohol intake (servings/d)	0.36 ± 0.68	0.15 ± 0.34[1]
Physical activity (MET-min/d)	56.23 ± 123.8	97.83 ± 174.8[1]
Current cigarette smokers (%)	14.45	3.6[2]
Current bidi smokers (%)	23.67	12.31[3]
Family history of MI (%)	37.57	8.48[4]
Hypertension (%)	49.09	1.8[5]
Alcoholics (%)	47.87	20.60[6]

Values are in Mean ± SD [1, 2, 3, 4, 5, 6] Significantly different from cases (*t* test for matched data): [1, 2, 3] $P \leq 0.001$, [4, 5] $P \leq 0.0001$, [6] $P \leq 0.003$ [7] $P \leq 0.05$.

Analysis of Behavioral Patterns

The behavioral pattern and familial history of cardiovascular disease is presented in **Table 6**. Sixty-eight (41.2%) were hyperactive, ninety-nine (60%) were trifle thinkers, one hundred six (64.2%) were irrelevant thinkers among cases. Sixty-two (37.6%) of cases had the family history of CVD compared with controls (8.5%) (**Table 6**).

Distribution of Risk factors among cases

The mean and percentage values of various cofactors among the cases and controls are presented in **Table 7**. In our study population, case subjects had higher body mass indexes, waist-to-hip ratios, and alcohol intakes and a significantly higher prevalence of history of hypertension, and family history of myocardial infarction. However, cases participated in less exercise than did control subjects. They also had slightly higher body mass indexes and were less likely to smoke bidis. The relative risk (RR) of AMI according to potential risk factors is presented in **Table 8**. In age- and sex-adjusted analyses and in multivariate-adjusted analyses, cigarette and bidi smoking, body mass index, waist-to-hip ratio, leisure-time physical exercise, family history of IHD, history of hypertension, and education were significant predictors of AMI in this population. The subjects were classified into lower, middle and upper class depending on monthly income of the family. Subjects whose monthly income was Rs.≤ 5000/month, Rs. 5000-15000 /month and Rs. ≥15000/month respectively were categorized as lower, middle and higher

Table 8. Relative risk (RR) of Acute Myocardial Infarction (AMI) according to potential risk factors[1].

	No. of cases N	No. of controls N	Age- and sex-adjusted RR (95% CI)[2]	Multivariate RR (95% CI)[3]
Cigarette smoking				
Never smoker	120	136	1.0	1.0
>10 cigarettes/d	36	6	7.8 (4.9, 13.5)	7.4 (4.3, 15.2)
Bidi smoking				
Never smoker	120	136	1.0	1.0
> 10 bidis/d	49	8	8.2 (5.2, 14.2)	6.5 (3.9, 12.9)
BMI (kg/m2)				
20-24.9	30	51	1.0	1.0
≥ 25	135	114	2.7 (1.8,4.1)	2.9 (1.6, 5.1)
Waist –to-hip ratio				
≤ 0.95	52	137	1.0	1.0
> 1.0	113	28	3.9 (2.1, 6.3)	2.8 (1.6, 5.7)
Family history of MI				
No	97	151	1.0	1.0
Yes	62	14	2.1(1.6, 2.7)	2.7 (1.8, 3.8)
History of Hypertension				
No	136	142	1.0	1.0
Yes	29	23	2.1 (1.7, 3.2)	1.9 (1.4, 2.9)
Education level				
Highest level of education	25	27	1.0	1.0
None	101	132	3.1 (1.3, 5.1)	3.6 (1.0, 6.2)
Type of Family				
Split	20	64	1.0	1.0
Joint	145	101	4.5 (1.5- 2.9)	3.9 (1.2-2.6)
Civil Status				
Lower Class	10	19	1.0	1.0
Middle Class	119	131	3.4 (4.3, 6.7)	2.8 (3.7, 5.9)
Higher Class	36	15	4.7 (4.9, 7.2)	3.8 (3.1, 4.7)
Leisure –time exercise				
Non-exerciser	82	58	1.0	1.0
≥ 145 MET-min/d	83	107	0.76 (0.4, 0.8)	0.68 (0.4, 0.7)
Household income				
>10 000 rupees/month	155	146	1.0	1.0
<5000 rupees/month	10	19	1.8 (1.2, 2.7)	1.7 (1.0, 3.1)

Hindu religion				
No	33	12	1.0	1.0
Yes	132	153	0.8 (0.6, 1.1)	0.9 (0.7, 1.3)

1 MET, metabolic equivalent. RR estimates were obtained by using conditional logistic regression analysis controlled for the matching factors (age, sex, and hospital) and then additional potential risk factors.
2 Also adjusted for hospital.
3 Covariates controlled for in the multivariate model were as follows: age; sex; hospital; cigarette smoking [never, current (≤10 cigarettes/d, >10 cigarettes/d)]; bidi smoking [never, current (≤10 bidis/d, >10 bidis/d)]; BMI, in kg/m² (20-24.9, ≥25); waist-to-hip ratio (≤0.95, >1.0); leisure time physical exercise (none, < 145 MET-min/d, ≤145 MET-min/d); history of hypertension (no, yes); history of diabetes (no, yes); history of high cholesterol (no, yes); family history of IHD (no, yes); education (none, primary school, middle, secondary, higher secondary, college, graduate or professional); household income (<5000, 5000-10000, 10000-15000,>10000 rupees/mo); and Hindu religion (no, yes).

class. The study observed that most of the MI cases belonged to the middle class. Among the cases, 85 males (69.1%) and 32 females (76.2%) belonged to middle class. Further 113 (91.9%) males and 32 (76.2%) females belonged to joint family, where all the member of the family remained together even after marriage. The subjects were classified according to the educational status depending on the highest degree they possessed (**Table 3** and **4**). It was observed that 75 (61%) males and 26 (62%) females were graduates. The educational qualification reflected the type of job profile of the subjects. The percentages of male MI patients with mild and moderated physical activity were 48% and 52% respectively. Among the female MI patients 54.8% were mildly and 45.2% were moderately active. Most of the female patients (67.4%) were involved in household jobs. During questioning and filling up the questionnaire, it was found that most of the subjects switched from moderate to mild type of work after they had the myocardial infarction.

Among the MI patients, only the males were smokers. The incidence of smoking habit was not found in female patients. The study classified the smokers into two categories, depending on the number of cigarettes they smoked/day. Thirty six male MI patients (29.3%) were chronic smokers and smoked ≥ 10 cigarettes /day, and 45(36.6%) MI patients were smokers compared to 29 smokers (23.6%) in control group. When chi-square test was applied, smokers were higher in MI patients compared to controls and were statistically significant. The incidence of alcohol consumption was observed only in males of both groups. Seventy nine MI patients (64.2%) and 45 (27.6%) controls were alcoholics. The study observed more alcoholics (64.2%) than smokers (36.6%), among the MI patient. Of the seventy nine alcoholics, most (87.6%) consumed alcohol occasionally and were not in the regular habit of drinking. Chi square methods of statistical evaluation revealed a higher number of MI patients were alcoholics compared to the controls and differences was significant.

Antioxidant status in cases and control

The antioxidant status among the cases and control are presented in **Table 9**.The mean serum albumin concentration in cases (4.2 mg/dl) was significantly lower (p<0.0001) compared to controls (4.4 mg/dl). The mean serum uric acid concentration in cases

Table 9. Antioxidant status in Control subjects and AMI patients.

	Control (n=165)	AMI patients (n=165)	P value (95% CI)
Serum albumin (g/dl)	4.4 ± 0.3	4.2 ± 0.3	<0.0001 (4.15-4.24)
Serum uric acid (mg/dl)	5.8 ± 1.2	4.3 ± 0.9	<0.0001 (4.17-4.42)
Serum ascorbic acid (mg/dl)	5.3 ± 1.2	2.8 ± 0.7	<0.0001 (2.70-2.89)
Serum Total bilirubin (mg/dl)	0.8 ± 0.2	0.7 ± 0.2	<0.0001 (0.67-0.72)
Serum superoxide dismutase (U/gHb)	1826.5 ± 31.9	813.9 ± 208.9	<0.0001 (784.42-843.37)
Serum glutathione peroxidase (U/gHb)	61.3 ± 3.9	42.6 ± 6.3	<0.0001 (41.71- 43.48)
Serum catalase (k/gHb)	256.2 ± 26.7	193.1 ± 35.9	<0.0001 (188.03-198.16)

Values are in Mean ± SD.

(4.3 mg/dl) was significantly lower ($p<0.0001$) compared with controls (5.8 mg/dl). The mean serum ascorbic acid concentration in cases were significantly lower ($p<0.0001$) than controls. The mean serum total bilirubin concentration in cases were significantly lower ($p<0.0001$) compared with controls. Serum activity of superoxide dismutase, glutathione peroxidase and catalase were significantly lower ($p<0.0001$) in cases compared with control.

Lp(a) and Lipid Peroxidation

The lipoprotein (a) concentration in cases was 3 fold higher than control and was highly significant ($p<0.0001$). Serum malondialdehyde and conjugated dienes were significantly ($p<0.0001$) increased in cases compared with controls (**Table 10**).

Other biochemical parameters

The other biochemical parameters observed in cases and controls are presented in **Table 12**. The mean plasma fibrinogen and caeruloplasmin levels was significantly higher ($p<0.0001$) in cases compared with controls. There was almost two fold increase in fibrinogen levels in cases. The mean arylesterase activity in cases were significantly lower ($p<0.0001$) than controls. The levels of ischemia modified albumin and C-reactive protein were also significantly higher ($p<0.001$) in cases compared with controls.

Table 10. Lp(a) and Lipid Peroxidation levels in Control subjects and AMI patients

	Control (n=165)	AMI patients (n=165)	P value (95%CI)
Serum Lipoprotein (a) (mg/dl)	3.0 ± 1.1	10.9 ± 2.2	<0.0001 (10.58-11.21)
Serum malondialdehyde (nmol/L)	5.7 ± 1.0	14.8 ± 1.7	<0.0001 (14.56-15.03)
Serum conjugated dienes (μmol/L)	31.0 ± 2.7	48.3 ± 5.5	<0.0001 (47.52-49.07)

Values are in Mean ± SD.

Table 11 Other Biochemical parameters in Control subjects and AMI patients.

	Control (n=165)	MI patients (n=165)	P value (95% CI)
Plasma fibrinogen (mg/dl)	237.5 ± 17.4	357.8 ± 23.2	<0.0001 (354.52 -361.07
Serum caeruloplasmin (mg/dl)	20.4 ± 2.3	51.5 ± 2.4	<0.0001 (51.16-51.83)
Serum Arylesterase activity (kU/L)	98.4 ± 6.2	69.7 ± 10.0	<0.0001 (68.28-71.11)
Serum Ischemia modified albumin (U/ml)	81.9 ± 3.9	97.5 ± 11.7	<0.001 (95.84-99.15)
Serum C-reactive protein (mg/dl)	1.1 ± 0.3	3.0 ± 1.1	<0.0001 (2.84-3.15)

Values are in Mean ± SD.

Dicussion

Coronary artery disease (CAD) remains the major cause of morbidity and mortality in all developed and developing countries in the world including India (2). Dyslipidemia is one of the major modifiable risk factors for CAD (5, 6, 7).

The CAD risk factors do not predict the occurrence of MI as varying risk factors is observed in South Asian population (8). The search for variations in conventional risk factors among Asians could be helpful in recognizing the future events of stroke, irrespective of conventional risk factors. These facts prompted us to identify the newer risk factors, with respect to Indian population.

The search for the newer risk factors continues and researchers are investigating the role of inflammatory markers and other potential risks factors which could link with MI.

In this case-control study in India, only Normolipidemic acute MI patients were selected. The study was designed to indentify and evaluate potential risk factors in Normolipidemic acute MI patients. The subjects selected for the study comprised of 165 controls, 48-69 y and 165 acute MI patients, 48-69 y.

The anthropometric data of control and myocardial infarct patients are shown in **Table 1**. The body weight (W), waist circumference (WC), mid upper-arm circumference (MUAC), hip circumference (Hp), waist-hip ratio (W/H) ratio were significantly (p<0.0001) higher in patients compared with controls. Study reported (36) that (W/H) ratio is a dominant, independent and predictive variable of CVD and CHD deaths in Australian men and women. They stressed that the assessment of obesity by W/H ratio rather than BMI would be better in predicting CVD and CHD risks (36). Another study reported high hip circumference relative to W and WC is a better predictor of low incidence of CVD and CHD (37). The present study is in good agreement with the observations of the above studies.

The clinical usefulness of W/H ratio for predicting the risk of cardiovascular events was assessed with data from Framingham and Prospective Cardiovascular Munster (PROCAM) studies. Cardiovascular risk factors have been reported in Asian Indians even the prevalence of obesity is minimal (37). In the present study the mean BMI and W/H ratio of all the subjects was 26.56 and 0.96 respectively, tending to be overweight and higher W/H ratio, with a significantly higher BMI and W/H ratio in patients compared with controls.

Based on the observations of the aforementioned studies and further supported by the present study it could be concluded that W/H ratio is a better predictor of CVD than BMI. So it is better tool for indentifying the future risk of MI in subjects by non-invasive procedures.

Observations of Total Cholesterol

The lipid profile pattern in Normolipidemic AMI patients and control were studied and the variation in patterns was compared. The mean TC level of the controls compared with AMI patients (186.44 ± 13.95 mg/dl) was significantly (p<0.001) higher compared with controls (168.58 ± 12.16 mg/dl).

Earlier study also observed higher (189.70 mg/dl) TC in normal subjects compared with controls of the present study (Goswami, et al., 2003) (38). In a study on MI patients, a mean TC level of (196.60 mg/dl) was reported and it was 5.3% higher than the TC of MI patients of the present study.

Higher values for TC (196.60 mg/dl) (39) and (215.70 mg/dl) (40) have been reported by previous studies in MI patients compared with controls. These values were 5.3% and 15% greater than the values observed for TC in AMI patients in the present study.

The TC levels observed (199.80 mg/dl) were slightly higher than the present study have been reported by Sivaraman et al., 2004 (41) in patients with acute coronary syndrome. They also reported a significant higher values (p<0.001) when compared to the controls in their study.

Similarly, significant differences (p<0.001) were observed in young CAD patients compared with control (9). The result of the present study was in agreement with their observation.

Lower levels of TC (181mg/dl) in MI patients was observed by Shindhe, et al., 2005 (42), Rajashekhar, et al., 2004 (12) and Kharb, et al., 2003 (43) in studies on Indian population compared with the present study.

Though the TC levels of the subjects selected in the present study were within the normal lipid profile, the mean levels of TC in MI patients was greater and was in concurrence with the observations of earlier studies though they have reported greater or lower levels of TC in MI patients than the TC levels in the present study.

Observations of High Density Lipoprotein-Cholesterol

The mean serum HDL-C level observed in patients (41.3 mg/dl) was significantly lower (p<0.001) compared with controls (50.5mg/dl). In a study on Normolipidemic subjects in the age group 21-70 years, mean HDL-C levels of 52.9 mg/dl was reported, which is 28.1% higher than the present study (38).

HDL-C levels similar to the present study have been reported (39.5mg/dl) (38) (42.11mg/dl) (8) in patients with heart disease. Similar levels of HDL-C were reported in many studies (7, 11, 40, 42). Therefore, most of the research evidences supported drastic lowering of HDL-C levels in AMI patients.

Observations of Triglycerides

Triglyceride (TG) values observed in MI patients was (129mg/dl) significantly higher when compared with controls (107.8mg/dl). A similar level of TG has been reported (38, 42) in Normolipidemic AMI patients as observed in the present study. However 22.3% and 18% higher levels of HDL-C in MI patients was observed and reported (39, 40).

Furthermore, significantly higher levels of TG (149 mg/dl) (15.5%) (43) and (140.5 mg/dl) (8.5%) (13) have been observed compared with the observations of the present study.

The findings of the above data confirms that elevated TG levels are associated with the incidence of heart diseases and that is even so when they are within the normal levels.

Observations of Low Density Lipoprotein-Cholesterol

The mean serum level of LDL-C in the patients was (119.4mg/dl) significantly higher than control (83.6 mg/dl). In a study of healthy subjects with age group of 21-70 years, significantly higher value was reported and it was very much similar to the LDL-C level of the MI patients of the present study (38).

In earlier studies on MI patients, higher values of LDL-C were reported by several researchers (8, 42), some reported lower values (11) than observed in the present study. However similar levels of LDL-C in MI patients were also reported in several studies (14, 39, 40).

Observations of TC/HDL-C ratio

The TC/HDL-C ratio in MI patients (4.6) was significantly (p<0.001) higher compared with controls (3.4). Similar TC/HDL-C ratio (3.6) has been observed in normal subjects of the age group 21-70 years by Goswami, et al., 2003 (38). Lower ratio of TC/HDL-C were observed in AMI patients were reported elsewhere (39).

Similar ratio (4.6) was reported in MI patients by study conducted elsewhere (11, 40, 42, 43). Higher ratio of TC/HDL-C is reported in MI patients (13, 40, 42) compared with the present study. A cut of level of 3.3 has been suggested (20).

These data indicate though the TC levels were within the normal level; the TC/HDL-C ratio was elevated significantly in MI patients indicating the importance of assessing TC/HDL-C ratio even in Normolipidemic subjects.

Observations of LDL-C/HDL-C ratio

Increased LDL-C and reduced HDL-C are considered to be highly atherogenic. Thus the increased level of LDL-C/HDL-C would indicate an increased risk of developing atherosclerosis. A cut of level of 1.6 has been suggested (20).

The present study observed significantly higher ratio (2.9) in AMI patients compared with control (1.9).

Reports of the earlier studies were inconsistent, as some studies reported higher ratios (8), similar ratio (39) and lower ratios (44) of LDL-C/HDL-C compared to the present study.

Observations of TG/HDL-C ratio

Increased TG and decreased HDL-C are also thought to be atherogenic and thus increased ratio of TG/HDL-C would indicate an increased atherogenic risk. The present study observed significantly ($p < 0.001$) higher ratio (3.2) in patients compared with control (2.2). A slightly higher ratio (2.5) has been reported in healthy subjects earlier (38). The data reported in previous studies in MI patients were inconsistent to the present study. Some studies have reported higher ratios (13, 39, 40, 41, 43) and some reported similar ratios (42) as the present study. As per NCEP ATP-111 a cut of level of 2.5 has been suggested.

The present study concludes the importance of assessing the lipid ratios even in a normal individual as it is one of the atherogenic factors for development of myocardial infarction and other coronary complications. The practice of computing the ratio should be practiced even in a normal health check up packages.

Antioxidant status

The mean serum albumin levels in MI patients was 4.2 mg/dl compared to controls (4.4 mg/dl), 4.8% lower in patients and the difference was significant ($p < 0.0001$). The mean serum total bilirubin concentration in MI patients was 0.8 mg/dl compared to controls (0.7 mg/dl) and were significantly lower ($p < 0.0001$) to controls.

Study conducted by Olusi, et al., (1999) (45) in MI patients, reported significantly lower ($p < 0.0001$) albumin and higher ($p < 0.0001$) bilirubin. Djousse, et al., (2003) (46) suggested lower albumin and bilirubin levels are associated with greater than expected risk of MI. In another study (Hopkins, et al., 1996) (47) suggested slight increase in bilirubin could be protective and reduces the risk of MI by acting as an antioxidant. The decrease albumin and bilirubin in MI patients in the present study tends to concur in some respect to previous studies. Albumin and bilirubin are known to possess antioxidant potential (Djousse, et al., 2003) (46) and their lowering could have contributed to MI.

The mean serum uric acid concentration in MI patients (4.3 mg/dl) was significantly lower (p<0.0001) compared with controls (5.8 mg/dl). Study conducted by Jing, et al., (2000) (48), (Brand, et al., 1985)(49) and Niskanen, et al., (2004) (50) showed the positive correlation of serum uric acid with the incidence of MI. Bruce, et al., (1999) (51) did not show any correlation with the serum uric acid levels and the incidence of MI. Though, uric acid is well established antioxidant, but it can also be a pro-oxidant, which might increase the risk of MI. The findings of the present study do not concur with the findings of those studies reported earlier. In the present study, the decreased levels of uric acid levels in MI patients might be due to increased free radical toxicity at time of ischemia.

The mean serum ascorbic acid in MI patients was 2.8 mg/dl compared with controls (5.3 mg/dl) which was 89.3% lower with significant (p<0.0001) difference. In a prospective study carried out by (Nyossen et al, 1997) (52) in Finland comprising of 1605 subjects without any CVD problems at the time of enrollment. In eight years of follow up, 70 men had a fatal or non-fatal MI due to decreased ascorbic acid. The study concluded low serum ascorbic acid as a risk factor for Coronary Heart Disease.

Lower ascorbic acid levels have been reported (Bhakuni, et al 2006) (53) (Das, et al., 2002) (44) in AMI patients which concurs to the present study. The observation of present study is also in good agreement with the findings of Nyyosonen, et al (1997) (52) and (Kurl, et al., 2002) (54) where they reported the higher risk in MI patients due to decreased ascorbic acid. Aulinskas, et al., (1983) (55) reported the beneficial role of ascorbic acid against the toxic peroxides and up regulation of LDL receptors on arterial smooth cells, thus facilitating lipoprotein cholesterol clearance.

The findings of the present study are similar to the findings of earlier studies. The low levels of ascorbic acid in AMI patients in the present study might be due to enhanced utilization of ascorbic acid during oxidative stress in patients.

The mean serum superoxide dismutase (SOD) activity in MI patients was 55.4% lower compared with controls and was highly significant (p<0.0001). Earlier studies reported Senthil, et al., (2004) (56), Bhakuni, et al., (2006) (57), Jain, et al., (2000) (58), Rajashekhar, et al., (2004) (12), Das, et al., (2002) (44) and Patil, et al., (2007) (11) significantly reduced activities of SOD in MI patients compared with controls. In another study (Gupta, et al., 2006) (59) conducted also reported reduced SOD activities in Type II diabetes patients with IHD. The findings of the present study are in good agreement with the earlier studies. Observations made from all the above studies related to SOD activities and lipid peroxides levels in AMI patients, reveals reduced activities might be due to increased utilization of SOD to combat the increased oxidative stress due to enhance formation of lipid peroxidation products in AMI patients.

The mean serum Glutathione Peroxidase (GPx) activity in MI patients was 42.6 (U/gHb) compared with controls (61.3 U/gHb) showing reduced activities in MI patients with highly significant (p<0.001) difference with controls. Senthil, et al., (2004) (56), Shindhe, et al., (2005) (42), (Rajasekhar, et al., 2004) (12), (El-Badry, et al., 1995) (60), (Gupta, et al., 2006) (59) and Kharb (2003)(43) reported reduced activities of erythrocyte

GPx and reduced glutathione in MI patients compared with controls. Shindhe (2005) (42) observed two folds, Kharb (2003) (43) observed four folds lower activities of GPx in acute MI patients compared with controls.

The results of the present study also observed lower activities of GPx in acute MI patients, could be due to increased utilization of GPx to scavenge lipid peroxidation products produced in MI patients.

The means serum Catalase activity in MI patients was 193.1 (k/gHb) compared to the controls (256.2k/gHb) which was 24.6% lower compared to control and was highly significant (p<0.001). Earlier studies conducted (Senthil, et al., 2004) (56), (Chandra, et al., 1994) (61) reported reduced activities of erythrocyte catalase in AMI patients compared with controls. They concluded from their observations that decreased catalase activity is a cause of elevated lipid peroxides in AMI patients. Further studies conducted by Dusinovic, et al., (1998) (62) and Pandey, et al., (2000) (63) reported lower activity of catalase in AMI patients. In another study conducted by Bhakuni, et al., (2005) (57), the effect of reperfusion therapy in MI patients was analyzed for antioxidant enzymes, thiols, malondialdehyde, and ascorbate levels. They reported significant lower catalase activity in post-perfused MI patients which is indicative of oxidative stress wherein anti-oxidant mechanisms become less effective in coping with the oxidative insult. This was further substantiated by significant rise in MDA levels in AMI patients. Observations made from all the above studies related to antioxidants and lipid peroxidation in AMI patients reveals lowering of antioxidants could be due to increased utilization of antioxidants due to increased oxidative stress as evidenced from the higher MDA levels.

Lipoprotein (a) and Lipid Peroxidation

The mean serum Lp (a) levels in MI patients was 10.9 mg/dl which was 2.6 folds higher levels compared with controls (3.0 mg/dl). Earlier studies conducted (Burman, et al., 2004) (39) on CHD patients reported 6 folds higher Lp(a) in AMI patients. Guha, et al (2001) (64) observed 2 folds rise in Lp(a) levels in IHD patients. Studies conducted by Bal, et al., (2001) (65) and Rajashekhar, et al., (2004) (12)reported 2.6 folds higher Lp(a) in angina patients.

In all the above studies, higher Lp(a) levels in AMI patients compared with controls. The studies concluded Lp(a) as an independent risk factor multiplying the magnitude of CAD.

On the contrary, a 14 –year follow up study conducted by Nascetti, et al., (1996) (66) observed no increase in Lp(a) levels in CVD patients and concluded, Lp(a) cannot be considered as independent risk factor for CVD patients.

The concentration of malondialdehyde (MDA) and conjugated diene (CD) was significantly higher (p<0.001) in MI patients compared with controls. Studies conducted by Senthil, et al., (2004)(56), Das, et al., (2002) (44), Kharb (2003) (43), Bhakuni, et al., (2006) (57) and Shindhe, et al., (2005) (42) reported 3 fold higher levels of MDA in AMI patients.

Study conducted by Gupta, et al., (2006)(59) and El-Badry, et al., (1995) (60) on AMI patients reported 2 fold increase in MDA, where as Patil, et al., (2006) (11) reported 1.9 fold and Jain, et al., (2000) (58) reported 1.5 folds rise in patients.

Other Biochemical parameters

The mean serum caeruloplasmin concentration was significantly higher (p<0.0001) in MI patients (155%) compared to controls. Studies conducted by Grobusch et al., (1999) (67), El-Badry, et al., (1995)(60) and Awadallah, et al., (2006) (68) observed significantly higher (p<0.001) levels of caeruloplasmin in AMI patients as observed in the present study.

Giurgie, (2005) (69) reviewed the role of caeruloplasmin in involvement in CVD, though it is widely accepted for counteracting oxidative stress in CVD. The review reported a dual effect of caeruloplasmin, both as an oxidant and as antioxidant.

In another study (Shukla, et al., 2006) (70) suggested even caeruloplasmin posses antioxidant properties, but its elevated levels in CVD is a risk factor. They suggested due to its copper content, it promotes vasculopathic effects causing lipid oxidation which further enhances formation of reactive oxygen species (ROS). The ROS in turns disrupts copper binding to caeruloplasmin, thereby impairing its antioxidant property and further promote oxidative pathology. The role of caeruloplasmin in lipoprotein oxidation and atherosclerotic lesion progression in vivo has not been directly assessed and is an important area for future studies.

The serum C-reactive proteins (CRP) levels in the present study was 3 folds higher in MI patients compared with controls and was significant (p<0.0001).

Studies conducted by Berton, et al., (2003) (71), Bhagat, et al., (2003)(72) and Sivaraman, et al., (2004) (41) reported 4 fold rise, where as Beg, et al., (2006) (73) and Kulsoom, et al., (2006) (74) reported 3 fold and 2.4 fold rise in CRP levels in AMI patients respectively.

Boncler, et al., (2006) (75) stated CRP as a direct contributor in atherosclerosis, which was formerly considered as inflammatory marker. His study emphasized CRP as the most powerful predictor of CVD which significantly increases in acute coronary syndromes. It has a prognostic not only in CVD risk assessment, but also in apparently healthy subjects.

The mean plasma fibrinogen observed in the current study was 51% higher in AMI patients compared with controls.Earlier studies conducted by Harkut, et al., (2004) (76), Coppola, et al., (2005) (77), Beg, et al., (2007) (73) and Sivaraman, et al., (2004) (41) reported 25%,55%,61% and 22% rise in plasma fibrinogen in AMI patients. Observations made from the above studies, and supported by the observations of the present study suggest plasma fibrinogen is a predictor and a risk of future CVD if fibrinogen levels are higher in normal subjects.

The mean serum ischemia modified albumin (IMA) levels in MI patients was 19% higher compared to controls and was significant (p<0.001). Earlier study conducted by Chawla, et al., (2006) (78) in MI patients reported 52% higher IMA and was significantly different compared with controls (p<0.001).

Bar-Or. et al., (2001)(79) also observed significantly higher concentration of IMA during transient ischemia which returned to baseline values by 6 hours after percutaneous transluminal angioplasty. The highest peak of IMA concentration obtained by their study was 144.6 (U/ml) in 3-4 hours during ischemia, but in the present study we obtained a maximum IMA levels up to 134.4 (U/ml) in AMI patients in 3 hours after admissions to coronary care unit. The difference in IMA was 7% lower compared to

Bar-Or study. Since cardiac ischemia in clinical setting is not one-event phenomenon and does not stop immediately after the commencement of the treatment in Intensive Coronary Care Unit, it is not expected that all patients to be IMA negative at discharge. A very high- negative predictive value of IMA can help the cardiac emergency room to identify the non-cardiac chest pain cases, who can then be categorized as low risk patients (Auxter, 2003.) (80)

Even though the determination of IMA is promising, the results can only be referred as a prelude to what might prove to be significant change in the approach to hospital admissions and their subsequent treatment plan of Acute Coronary Syndrome subjects. An extensive study with a higher set of patients is thus required which should compare the IMA test with other markers such as the troponins and myoglobin. Whether IMA develops as an independent point-of care or an additional parameter along with troponins to boost the confidence of the clinicians in ruling out the cardiac ischemia is yet to be seen.

The serum mean arylesterase activity in MI patients (29.2%) was significantly lower (p<0.0001) compared with controls in the present study. In studies conducted on CAD patients by Singh, et al., (2007) (81), Ayub et al., (1999) (82) and Sarkar, et al., (2006) (83) observed significantly (p<0.001) lower arylesterase activity in patients compared with controls. On the contrary, study conducted by Azizi, et al., (2002) (84) reported no change in arylesterase activity in AMI patients. They supported their findings based on the concept of inter-ethnic variability and gene polymorphism altering the arylesterase activity. Anothr study conducted (Aviram, et al., 1999) (85) on the preservation of HDL-C functions and HDL-lipid peroxidation, reported the conservation of HDL's antioxidant capacity is maintained by HDL-C arylesterase activity.

Richard, et al., (2000) (86) worked on effect of smoking on arylesterase activity as smoking is considered to be CVD risk for promoting lipid peroxidation. They reported significantly lower arylesterase activity in current smokers compared with non-smokers. They also observed that arylesterase activity returns to normal within 2 years after cessation of smoking.

Jarvik et al., (2002) (87), reported the variation in arylesterase activity by antioxidant vitamins, smoking, and statins. Because arylesterase activity is a better predictor of vascular disease, further studies of the environmental influences on arylesterase activity and additional arylesterase genetic variants are warranted.

References

1. reddy KS. Cardiovascular disease in India. World Health Stat Q 1993; 46:101-7.
2. Reddy KS, Yusuf S. Emerging epidemic of cardiovascular disease in developing countries. Circulation1998; 97:596–601.
3. Bulatao RAO, Stephens PW. Demographic estimates and projections, by region, 1970-2015. In: Jamison DT, Mosley WH, eds. Disease control priorities in developing countries. Washington, DC: World Bank, 1990. (Health sector priorities review no. 13.)
4. Balarajan R. Ethnicity and variations in mortality from coronary heart disease. Health Trends1996; 28:45–51.
5. Chopra V, Wasir H. Implications of lipoprotein abnormalities in Indian patients. Journal Assoc Physicians of India 1998; 46:814-8.

6. Vasisht S, Narula J, Awtade A, Tandon R, Srivastava LM. Lipids and lipoproteins in normal controls and clinically documented coronary heart disease patients. Ann Natl Acad Med Sci (India) 1990; 26:57-66.

7. Malhotra, P., Kumari, S., Singh, S. and Verma, S. Isolated Lipid Abnormalities in Rural and Urban Normotensive and Hypertensive North-West Indians. Journal of Assoc Physicians of India 2003; 51:459-463.

8. Mishra, A., Luthra, K. and Vikram, N.K. Dyspipidemia in Asian Indians: Determminants and Significance. Journal Assoc Physicians India 2005; 52:137-142.

9. Mishra,T.K., Routray, S.N., Patnaik, U.K., Padhi,P.K., Satapathy, C. and Behera, M. Lipoprotein (a) and Lipid Profile in Young Patients with Angiographically Proven Coronary Artery Disease. Indian Heart Journal 2001; 53 :(5) Article No. 60.

10. Ghosh, J., Mishra, T.K., Rao, Y.N. and Aggarwal, S.K.Oxidised LDL, HDL Cholesterol, LDL Cholesterol levels in patients of Coronary Artery Disease. Indian Journal of Clinical Biochemistry 2006; 21(1):181-184.

11. Patil,N., Chavan,V.and Karnik,N.D.Antioxidant Status in Patients with Acute Myocardial Infarction. Indian Journal of Clinical Biochemistry 2007; 22(1):45-51.

12. Rajasekhar D., Srinivasa Rao P.V., Latheef S.A., Saibaba K.S., and Subramanyam G. Association of serum antioxidants and risk of coronary heart disease in South Indian population. Indian J Med Sci 2004; 58(11):465-71.

13. Rani, S.H., Madhavi, G., Ramachandra Rao, V., Sahay, B.K. and Jyothy, A.Risk factors for coronary heart disease in type II diabetes. Indian Journal of Clinical Biochemistry 2005; 20(2):75-80.

14. Gomez, M.A., Anderson, J.L., Karagounis L.A., Muhlestein, J.B. and Mooers, F.B. An emergency medicine based protocol for rapidly ruling out myocardial ischemia reduces hospital time and expense. Results of randomized study (ROMO). J. Am. coll. Cardiol 1996; 28:25-33.

15. Singh S, Venketesh S, Verma JS, Verma M, Lellamma CO, Goel RC. Paraoxonase(PON11) activity in north west Indian Punjabis with coronary artery disease & type II diabetes mellitus. Indian J Med Res 2007; 125:783-7.

16. Berliner JA, Navab M, Fogelman AM, Frank JS, Demer LL, Edwards PA, et al. Atherosclerosis: basic mechanisms. Oxidation. Inflammarion, and genetics. Circulation 1995; 91:2488-96.

17. Frei B, Stocker R, Ames BN. Antioxidant defenses and lipid peroxidation in human blood plasma. Proc Natl Acad Sci USA 1988; 85: 9748-9752.

18. Shrinivas K, Vijaya Bhaskar M, Aruna Kumari M, Nagaraj K, Reddy KK. Antioxidants, lipid peroxidation and lipoproteins in primary hypertension. Indian Heart J 2000; 52:285-88.

19. Maritim AC, Sanders RA, Watkins JB. Diabetes, oxidative stress, and antioxidants: a review. J Biochem Mol Toxicol 2003; 17: 24-38.

20. Executive Summary of The Third Report of The National Cholesterol Education Program (NCEP) Expert panel on Detection, Evalation, and treatment of high Blood Cholesterol in Adults (Adult Treatment Panel III). Expert Panel of Detection, Evaluation, and Treatment of High Blood Cholesterol in Adults. JAMA 2001; 285(19):2486-97.

21. Rose, GA, Blackburn H, Gillum RF, Prineas RJ. Cardiovascular survey methods 2nd Ed. WHO Monograph Series No.56 Geneva. World Health Organisation, 1982.

22. Friedewalds, W.T., Levy, R.I. and Fredrickson, D.S. (1972).Estimation of the concentration of low density lipoprotein cholesterol in plasma without the use of preparative ultracentrifuge. Clin. Chem. 18, 499-502.

23. Perry,B.W., Doumas,B.T. Effect of heparin on albumin determination by use of bromocresol green and bromocresol purple. Clin Chem 1979; 25:1520-1522.

24. Brown, H. J Clin Chem 1945; 158:601.

25. Jendrassik L, Grof B. Biochem Zeit 1938; 297:81 9.

26. Paglia DE, Valentine WN. Studies on quantitative and qualitative characterization of erythrocyte glutathione peroxidase. J Lab Clin Med 1967; 70: 158-69.

27. Sun Y, Oberly LW, Li Y. A simple method for clinical assay of superoxide dismutase. Clin Chem 1988; 34: 497-500.

28. Beutler E. Red Cell Metabolism: A Manual of Biochemical Methods, 3rd edition. New York, Grune and Stratton, 1984; 105.

29. Bernheim S, Bernheim MLC, Wilbur KM. The reaction between thiobarbituric acid and the oxidant product of certain lipids. J Biol Chem 1948; 174: 257-264.

30. Recknagel RO, Glende EA. Spectrophotometric detection of lipid conjugated dienes. Methods Enzymol 1984; 105:331-337.

31. Ravin, H.A.(1961) An improved colorimetric enzymatic assay of caeruloplasmin. J. Lab. Med., 58, 161-168.

32. Libby P. Vascular biology of atherosclerosis: Overview and state of art. Am J Cardiol 2003; 91(suppl): 3A-6A.

33. Roe, J.H., Kuether, C.A.(1943). J. Biol Chem 147:399.

34. Kumar, A., Sivakanesan, R. Does plasma fibrinogens and C-reactive protein predict the incidence of myocardial infarction in patients with normal lipids profile? Pak J Med Sci 2008; 24:336-339.

35. Welborn,T.A., Dhaliwal, S.S. and Bennett, S.A.Waist-hip ratio is the dominant risk factor predicting cardiovascular death in Australia. Med J Aust; 2003; 179:580–5.

36. Heitman, B.L., Frederickson, P. and Lissner, L. Hip Circumference and Cardiovascular Morbidity and Mortality in Men and Women. Obesity Research 2004; 12:482-487.

37. Megnien J.L., Denarie N., and Cocaul M. Predicitve value of Waist-to-hip ratio on Cardiovascular Risk Events. Int J Obes Relat Metab Disord 1999; 23:90-97.

38. Goswami,K.& Bandyopadhyay. Lipid profile in middle class Bengali population of Kolkata. Ind J of Clin Biochem 2003; 18:127-130.

39. Burman, A., Jain, K., Gulati,R., Chopra, V., Agrawal, D.P. & Vaisisht, S. Lipoprotein (a) as a marker of Coronary Artery Disease and its Association with Dietary Fat. J Assoc Physicians India 2004; 52:99-102.

40. Yadhav, A.S., Bhagwat, V.R. & Rathod, I.M. Relationship of Plasma homocysteine with lipid profile parameters in Ischemic Heart disease. Indian Journal of Clinical Biochemistry 2006; 21(1):106-110.

41. Sivaraman, S.K., Zachariah, G., Annamalai, P.T. Evaluation of C - reactive protein and other Inflammatory Markers in Acute Coronary Syndromes. Kuwait Medical Journal 2004; 36(1):35-37.

42. Shinde, S., Kumar, P.& Patil, N. Decreased Levels Of Erythrocyte Glutathione In Patients With Myocardial Infarction. The Internet Journal of Alternative Medicine 2005; 2:1.

43. Kharb,S. Low Glutathione levels in acute myocardial infarction. Ind J Med Sci 2003; 57; Issue8: 335-7.

44. Das,S., Yadav,D., Narang, R. & Das, N. Interrelationship between lipid peroxidation, ascorbic acid and superoxide dismutase in coronary artery disease. Current Science 2002; 83:488-491.

45. Olusi, S.O., Prabha, K. & Sugathan, T.N. Biochemical Risk factors for Myocardial Infarction Among South Asian Immigrants and Arabs. Annals of Saudi Medicine 1999; 19: 147-149.

46. Djousse, L., Rothman, K.J., Cupples, L.A., Levy,D., Ellison, R.C. Effect of serum albumin and bilirubin as a risk factor for Myocardial infarction. Am J Cardiol 2003; 91: 485- 488.

47. Hopkins, Paul.N., Lily,L. Wu., Hunt, Steven, C., James, Brent,C., Vincent, M. G. & Williams, R.R.(1996). Higher Serum Bilirubin Is Associated With Decreased Risk for Early Familial Coronary Artery Disease. Arteriosclerosis, Thrombosis, and Vascular Biology 1996; 16:250-255.

48. Jing, F. & Alderman, M.H. Serum uric acid and cardiovascular mortality. JAMA 2000; 283: 2404-2410.

49. Brand, F.N. Mcgee, D.L., Kannel, W.B., Stokes,J. & Castelli, W.P. Hyperuricemia as a rsik factor of coronary heart disease: The Framingham Study. American Journal of Epidemiology 1985; 121: 11-18.

50. Niskanen, L.K., Laaksonen, D.E., Nyyssonen, K. Alfthan, G., Lakka, H.M., Lakka, T.A.& Salonene, J.T. Uric acid level as a risk factor for cardiovascular and all- cause moratlity in middle-aged men: a prospective study. Arch Intern Med 2004; 164:1546-51.

51. Bruce F. Culleton, Martin G. Larson, William B. Kannel, & Daniel Levy. Serum Uric Acid and Risk for Cardiovascular Disease and Death: The Framingham Heart Study. Annals of Internal Medicine 1999; 131: 7-13.

52. Nyyssonen, K., Markku, T.P., Salonen, R., Tuomilehto, J. & Salonen J.T. Vitamin C deficiency and risk of myocardial infarction: prospective population study of men from eastern Finland. BMJ 1997; 314:634.

53. Bhakuni, P., Chandra, M. & Misra, M.K. Levels of free radical scavengers and antioxidants in post perfused patients of myocardial infarction. Current Science 2005; 89: 168-170.

54. Kurl, S., Tuomainen, T.P., Laukkanen, J.A., Nyyssonen, K., Lakka, T., Sivenius, J.& Salonen, J.T.Plasma Vitamin C Modifies the Association Between Hypertension and Risk of Stroke. Stroke 2002; 33:1568.

55. Aulinskas, T.H., Vander Westhuyzen, D.R. & Coetzee, G.A. Ascorbate increases the number of low density lipoprotein receptors in cultured arterial smooth muscle cells. Atherosclerosis 1983; 47: 159-71.

56. Senthil, S., Veerappan, R.M., Ramakrishna Rao, M. & Pugalendi, K.V. Oxidative stress and antioxidants in patients with cardiogenic shock complicating acute myocardial infarction. Clin Chim Acta 2004; 348 (1-2):131-7.

57. Bhakuni, P., Chandra, M & Misra, M.K. Oxidative stress parameters in erythrocytes of post-reperfused patients with myocardial infarction. J Enzyme Inhib Med Chem 2005; 20(4):337-81.

58. Jain A.P., Mohan A., Gupta O.P.,Jajoo U.N., Kalantri S.P., and Srivastava L.M. Role of oxygen free radicals in causing endothelial damage in acute myocardial infarction. J.Assoc Physicians India 2000; 48(5):478-80.

59. Gupta, M. & Chari, S. Proxidant and Antioxidant status in patients of type II Diabetes Mellitus with IHD. Indian Journal of Clinical Biochemistry 2006; 21(2):118-122.
60. El- Badry, I., Abon, El Noor., Yehia, T. Kishk. & Zakhari, M.M. Free radicals activity in Acute Myocardial Infarction. The Egyptian Heart Journal 1995; 47: 71-78.
61. Chandra,M., Chandra, N., Agarwal, R., Kumar, A., Ghatak, A.& Pandey, V.C. The free radical system in ischemic heart disease. Int J Cardiol 1994; 43(2):121-5.
62. Dusinovic, S., Mijalkovic,D., Saicic, Z.S., Duric, J., Zunic,Z., Niketic, V.& Spasic, M.B.(1998).Antioxidative defense in human myocardial reperfusion injury. J Environ Pathol Toxicol Oncol 1998;17(3-4):281-4.
63. Pandey, N.R., Kaur,G., Chandra, M., Sanwal, G.G.& Mishra, M.K. Enzymatic oxidant and antioxidants of human blood platelets in unstable angina and myocardial infarction. Int J Cardiol 2000; 76(1):33-8.
64. Guha,S.,Chatterjee, S.,Mazumder,R., Sadek Ali,S.K., Guha, S.,Chatterjee,N., Biswas,S. & Bhattacharya,G.C.(2001).Lipoprotein (a), Lipid Tetrad Index and Coronary Artery Disease: A Correlative Study.Indian Heart Journal 53:(5) Article No. 28
65. Bal,B.S., Bhangu, M.S., Chhabra, N., Sandhu, P.S., Mahajan, M. & Batra, K.S. Incidence of Raised Lipoprotein (a) Level in Cases of Angina with
Hyperhomocysteinemia and Normal Lipid Profile. Indian Heart Journal 2001;53:(5) Article No. 47
66. Nascetti, S., D' Addato, S., Pascarelli, N., Sangiorgi, Z., Grippo, M.C. & Gaddi, A. Cardiovascular disease and Lp(a) in the adult population and in the elderly: the Brisighella study. Riv Eur Sci Med Farmacol 1996; 18(5-6):205-12.
67. Grobusch, K.K., Grobbee, D.E., Koster, J.F., Lindemans, J., Boeing, H., Hofman, A., Witteman, Jacqueline, C.M.(1999). Serum caeruloplasmin as a coronary risk factor in the elderly: the Rotterdam Study. British Journal of Nutrition 81:139-144.
68. Awadallah, S.M., Hamad, M., Jbarah, I., Salem, N.M. & Mubarak, M.S. (2006). Autoantibodies against oxidized LDL correlate with serum concentrations of caeruloplasmin in patients with cardiovascular disease. Clin Chim Acta; 365: 330-336.
69. Giurgea, N., Constantinescu, M.I., Stanciu, R., Suciu, S. & Muresan, A. Caeruloplasmin- acute –phase reactant or endogenous antioxidant? The case of cardiovascular disease. Med Sci Monit 2005; 11: RA 48-51.
70. Shukla, N., Maher, J., Masters, J., Angelini, G.D. & Jeremy, J.Y. Does oxidative stress change ceruloplasmin from a protective to a vasculopathic factor? Atherosclerosis 2006; 187: 238-250.
71. Berton, G., Cordiano, R., Palmieri, R., Pianca, S., Pagliara, V. & Palatini, Paolo. C-Reactive Protein in Acute Myocardial Infarction: Association With Heart Failure. Am Heart J 2003; 145(6):1094-1101.
72. Bhagat, S., Gaiha, M., Sharma, V.K. & Anuradha, S. A Comparative Evaluation of C - reactive protein as a Short-Term Prognostic Marker in Severe Unstable Angina- A Preliminary Study. *Journal of Assoc Physicians* 2003; 51:349-354.
73. Beg, M., Nizami, A., Singhal, K.C., Mohammed, J., Gupta,A. & Azfar, S.F. Role of serum fibrinogen in patients of ischemic cerevascular disease. Nepal Med Coll J 2007; 9: 88-92.
74. Kulsoom,B. & Nazrul, S.H. Association of serum C - reactive protein and LDL: HDL with myocardial infarction. J Pak Med Assoc 2006; 56 (7):318-22.
75. Boncler,M., Luzak,B. & Watala, C. Role of C-reactive protein in atherogenesis. Postepy Hig Med Dosw 2006; 60:538-46.
76. Harkut, P.V., Sahashrabhojney,V.S. & Salkar, R.G.(2004).Plasma fibrinogen as a marker of major adverse cardiac events in patients of type 2 Diabetes with unstable angina. Int J Diab Dev Countries 2004; 24: 69-74.
77. Coppola, G., Rizzo, M., Maurizio, G.A., Corrado,E., Alberto, D.G., Braschi,A., Braschi,G. & Novo, S. Fibrinogen as a predictor of mortality after acute myocardial infarction: a forty-two-month follow up study. Ital Heart J 2005; 6:315-322.
78. Chawla, R., Goyal, N., Calton,R., & Goyal, S. Ischemia modified albumin: A novel marker for acute coronary syndrome. Indian Journal of Clinical Biochemistry 2006; 21(1):77-82.
79. Bar-Or,D., Lau,E., Rao,N., Bampos,N., Winkler,J.V. & Curtis,C.G. Reduction in the cobalt binding capacity of human albumin with myocardial ischemia. Ann. Emerg. Med 1999; 34: 556.
80. Auxter, S. Cardiac Ischemia testing: a new era in chest pain evaluation. Clin Lab News 2003; 29, 1-3.
81. Singh, S., Venketesh, S., Verma, J.S., Verma, M., Lellamma, C.O.& Goel, R.C. Paraoxonase(PON1) activity in north west Indian Punjabis with coronary artery disease & type 2 diabetes mellitus. Indian J Med Res 2007; 125: 783-787.
82. Ayub, A., Mackness, M.I., Sharon, A., Mackness, B., Patel, J., Durrington, P.N. Serum Paraoxonase After Myocardial Infarction. Arteriosclerosis, Thrombosis, and Vascular Biology 1999; 19:330-335.
83. Sarkar, P.D., T.M.S. Madhusudhan, B. Association between paraoxonase activity and lipid levels in patients with premature coronary artery disease. Clin Chim Acta 2006; 373:77-81.

84. Azizi, F., Rahmani,M., Raiszadeh, F., Solati, M. & Navab, M. Associations of lipids, lipoproteins, apolipoproteins and paraoxonase enzyme activity with premature coronary artey disease. Coronary Artery Dis 2002; 13(1): 9-16.

85. Aviram, M., Rosenblat, M., Billecke, S., Eroul, J., Sovenson, R.& Bisaier, C.L. Human serum paraoxonase (PON1) is in activated by oxidized low density lipoprotein and preserved by antioxidants. Free Radic Biol Med 1999; 26:892-904.

86. Richard, J.W., Leview, I. & Righetti, A. Smoking Is Associated With Reduced Serum Paraoxonase Activity and Concentration in Patients With Coronary Artery Disease. Circulation 2000; 101:2252.

87. Jarvik, G.P., Tsai, N.T., Mckinstry, L.A., Wani, R., Victoria, H.B., Richter, R.J., Schellenberg,G.D., Heagerty, P.J.,Hatsukami, T.S.& Furlong, C.E. Vitamin C and E Intake Is Associated With Increased Paraoxonase Activity. Arteriosclerosis, Thrombosis, and Vascular Biology2002; 22:1329.

Chapter 7

Smoking Is Associated With Reduced Serum Paraoxonase, Antioxidants and increased Oxidative stress in Normolipidemic Acute Myocardial Infarct Patients

80

Abstract

Background: Paraoxonase is an HDL-associated enzyme that protects lipoproteins from oxidative modifications and to become atherogenic in nature. Smoking is a well known major cardiovascular risk factor that promotes lipid peroxidation. The present study examined the hypothesis that smoking modulated activities of paraoxonase and depletes antioxidants.

Aim: The present study evaluated paraoxonase activity, antioxidant status and lipid peroxidation in smoker and non-smoker normolipidemic AMI patients and results were compared to controls. SETTING & DESIGN: The serum paraoxonase activities, antioxidants and lipid peroxidation were determined in 86 normolipidemic patients diagnosed of AMI and 86 age-sexes matched healthy volunteers served as control.

Material & methods: Serum Paraoxonase activities were measured by enzymatic kit. The glutathione peroxidase, superoxide dismutase, catalase activity was determined by standard methods. Malondialdehyde (MDA) was measured by thiobarbituric acid (TBA) reaction. Conjugated diene (CD) levels by Recknagel and Glende method. Serum uric acid, total bilirubin, serum albumin and lipid profile were analyzed by standard methods.

Statistics: The values were expressed as means ± standard deviation (SD) and data from patients and control was compared using student's 't'-test.

Results and conclusion: Total cholesterol, TC/HDL-C ratio, triglycerides, LDL-cholesterol, LDL/HDL-C ratio and TG/HDL-C ratio were significantly higher and HDL-C were significantly lower in smokers compared to non-smokers AMI patients. The superoxide dismutase, glutathione peroxidase and catalase were significantly higher in non-smokers compared to smokers. Serum albumin, uric acid and bilirubin were higher in control compared to smokers AMI patients. The Malondialdehyde (MDA) and Conjugated dienes (CD) were significantly higher and paraoxonase activities were significantly lower in smokers compared to non-smokers.

Key words: Smoker, Paraoxonase, Normolipidemia, Acute Myocardial Infarction, Antioxidants, Oxidative Stress.

Introduction

Paraoxonase (PON1) is a serum enzyme complexed to high density lipoprotein – cholesterol (HDL-C) [1]. HDL associated Paraoxonase (PON1) enzyme is known to have protective effects on lipid peroxidation and oxidative modifications further delaying the atherogenesis [2]. The verdict is justified by developing PON knockout mouse model that demonstrated greater susceptibility of the lipoproteins to oxidation [3]. In humans PON is an independent, genetic risk factor for coronary artery disease (CAD) [4, 5]. This observation has been confirmed in independent studies [6, 7, 8, 9, 10] although not uniformly [11, 12]. Numerous cohort studies and clinical trials have confirmed the association between a low HDL-cholesterol concentration and increased risk of CHD. High density lipoprotein (HDL) is one of the most important independent protective factors for the arteriosclerosis which underlies coronary heart disease. Though many factors may play a role in its pathogenesis, low PON1 activity could be an independent risk factor [13]. PON1 activity is inversely related to the risk of developing an atherosclerotic lesion, which contains cholesterol-loaded macrophage foam cells. Although experimental studies have demonstrated the reduction in PON1 activity due to oxygen free radicals in ischemia and reperfusion [14], there are controversial data on correlation between PON1 HDL-C and ischemia process. Under oxidative stress not only LDL, but other serum lipids are exposed to oxidation. As it is well established that dyslipidemia is an important contributory factor for AMI and PON1 activity is decreased in dyslipidemia so the present study was undertaken with the objective of studying the PON1 activity in Normolipidemic AMI patients and also to observe whether PON1 activity could be an independent risk factor in this group of patients. Also the study aimed to observe the relationship between smoker, PON1, antioxidants and free radicals in normolipidemic AMI patients.

Smoking is widely known and firmly established major cardiovascular risk factors. Oxidative stress is considered to be the major, pathological mechanism associated with smoking, leading notably to lipid peroxidation [15, 16, 17]. Several studies have demonstrated increased susceptibility of LDL to oxidation and higher levels of oxidized LDL in smokers [18, 19, 20]. This would provide an important causal mechanism that links smoking with vascular disease given the numerous pathological effects of oxidized LDL [21, 22].

Smoking may enhance oxidative stress not only through the production of reactive oxygen radicals in smoke but also through weakening of the antioxidant defense mechanisms. In this context, a recent in vitro study showed that extracts of cigarette smoke inhibited the enzymatic activity of PON [23]. Given its hypothesized, antioxidant role, this could also contribute to the increased oxidation of LDL in smokers. The present study examined the hypothesis that smoking is associated with lower serum PON activity and antioxidants status in normolipidemic AMI patients causing the severity of vascular disease.

Materials and methods

Eighty six patients with AMI and 86 age-sex matched healthy volunteers were taken for this study. The design of this study was pre-approved by the institutional ethical committee board of the Institution and informed consent was obtained from the patients and controls.

Clinical and biochemical parameters like smoking habits, systolic and diastolic blood pressure and family history were recorded after clinical confirmation of AMI.

Diagnostic Criteria of patients: All the patients had their first episode of MI with diagnostic criteria: typical chest pain, specific abnormalities for MI on electrocardiogram, elevated serum creatine phosphokinase (CPK-MB) levels.

Exclusion Criteria: Patients with diabetes mellitus, renal insufficiency, hypertension, hepatic disease or taking lipid lowering drugs or antioxidant vitamin supplements were excluded.

Criteria for Normolipaedemics: Normal lipid profile was defined if LDL was <130mg/dl, HDL ≥ 35 mg/dl, Total cholesterol (TC) <200 mg/dl and Triglycerides (TG) <150 mg/dl [24].

Venous blood was collected after overnight fast of 12-hours and EDTA was added and samples were processed for lipid profiles.

Blood collection and biochemical methods used: 10 ml of blood was collected after overnight fasting in different containers.

Preparation of erythrocytes for antioxidants studies: Five ml of blood was taken. Red cells were washed 3-4 times with ice-cold normal saline and used for estimation of glutathione peroxidase, superoxide dismutase and catalase.

Serum for lipid profile, lipid peroxides, endogenous antioxidants and conjugated dienes measurement: Remaining blood was taken and serum was separated. Serum was used for determination of lipid profile, albumin, uric acid, bilirubin, malondialdehye and conjugated dienes.

For PON1 activity studies blood samples were collected in patients who were admitted in Intensive Care Unit 4-6 hours after AMI. Only Normolipidemic AMI patients were included in the study. Lipid profile (Total cholesterol, triglycerides, and HDL-cholesterol) were analyzed enzymatically using kit obtained from (Randox Laboratories Limited, Crumlin, UK). Plasma LDL-cholesterol was determined from the values of total cholesterol and HDL-cholesterol using the following formulae:

$$LDL\text{-}c = TC - \frac{TG}{5} - HDL\text{-}c \ (mg/dl)$$

For PON1 studies an assay kit manufactured from Zeptometrix Corporation 872 Main street, Buffalo New York 14202 (ZMC catalogue 0801199) [25, 26]. The assay is based on the principle; PON1 catalyzes the cleavage of phenyl acetate resulting in the phenol. The rate of formation of phenol is measured by monitoring the increase in absorbance at 270 nm at 25°C. One unit of arylesterase activity is equal to 1 µM of phenol formed per minute. The activity is expressed in kU/L, based on the extinction coefficient of phenol of 1310 $M^{-1}cm^{-1}$ at 270 nm, pH 8.0, and 25 °C. Blank samples containing water are used to correct for non-enzymatic hydrolysis.

Glutathione Peroxidase (GPx): The glutathione peroxidase activity was determined by the procedure of Paglia and Valentine [27]. Briefly, the oxidized glutathione produced during GPx enzyme reaction was immediately reduced by NADPH and glutathione reductase. Therefore, the rate of NADPH consumption was monitored as a measure of formation of oxidized glutathione. Results were expressed as units of GPx per gram of hemoglobin.

Superoxide dismutase (SOD): Superoxide dismuatse enzyme activity was measured by SOD assay kit using rate of inhibition of 2-(4-indophenyl)-(4-Nitrophenol)-5-phenyltetrazolium chloride (I.N.T) reduction method modified method of Sun Y Oberly [28] using assay Ransod kit SD 125, Randox Lab. One unit of SOD activity was defined as the amount of protein that inhibits the rate of I.N.T. reduction by 50%. Enzyme activity was expressed as unit per gram hemoglobin (U/gHb). Hemoglobin was measured by Drabkin's method.

Catalase: Catalase activity was measured spectrophotometrically as described by Beutler [29, 30]. One unit of enzyme activity was expressed as micromole hydrogen peroxide decomposed per min per gram hemoglobin.

TBARS: Malondialdehyde (MDA) levels were estimated by thiobarbituric acid (TBA) reaction [31]. Using 40% tricholoroacetic acid, proteins were precipitated from 0.5 ml serum, and precipitated proteins were incubated with TBA reagent in a boiling water bath for one hour. After bringing down to room temperature, the colored complex formed was measured using spectrophotometer at 532 nm.1, 1, 2, 3-tetraethoxypropane (1 nmol/l) was used as a standard for MDA estimation. Concentrations were expressed in nmol/l.

Conjugated dienes (CD): CD levels were measured by Recknagel and Glende method [32] with little modification. Briefly, the principle of the assay is based on with the rearrangement of double bonds in polyunsaturated fatty acids leading to the formation of DC, which absorb light at 233 nm. The oxidation index of the lipid sample at 233 nm and 215 nm is computed which reflect the diene content and the extent of peroxidation. The Lipid Peroxidation (LP) products measured in serum were treated with antioxidant Butylated hydroxytoluene (BHT) twice, immediately after obtaining and before adding the test reagents to suppress artefactual changes during handling and assay procedures. The first stage of LP consists of the molecular rearrangement of the double bonds in polyunsaturated fatty acids residues of lipids, which leads to conjugated dienes (CD) formation and conversion of CD in hydroperoxide (LOOH). Serum was chosen to avoid possible influences of substances required for plasma preparation. Serum sample (150 µl) and (150µl) of 0.9% NaCl (reagent blank contains only isotonic saline) were incubated at 37°C for 25 minutes. 0.25% Butylated hydroxyl Toluene (BHT) (150µl) was added and the lipids were extracted by heptane/isopropanol (1:1). Then samples were acidified by 5 mol/L HCl and extracted by cold heptane (1600µl). After centrifugation for 5 minutes at 3000 rpm the absorbance of heptane fraction were measured spectrophotometrically at absorbance maximum between 220 nm and 250 nm. The amount of hydroperoxides produced was calculated using Molar Coefficient of 2.52×10^4 m^{-1}.

Other assays- For estimation of other biochemical parameters standardized reagents and chemicals of analytical grade were obtained from Sigma-Aldrich Company, New

Delhi. Serum uric acid was estimated by the method of Brown based on the development of a blue color due to tungsten blue as phosphotungstic acid is reduced by uric acid in alkaline medium [33] serum total bilirubin was estimated by the method of Jendrassik and Grof [34] and serum albumin by bromocresol green dye binding method [35].

Statistical analysis: Data on lipid profile and PON1 activity was entered in Microsoft excel for windows 2003. The mean ± SD was obtained using excel software. The two-sample-t-test value was obtained between the patients and the control. The distribution of 't'- Probability was calculated depending on 'n' and significance of test was obtained. For p value <0.001 was considered as highly significant.

Result

Total cholesterol, TC/HDL-C ratio, triglycerides, LDL-cholesterol, LDL/HDL-C ratio and TG/HDL-C ratio were higher in smokers AMI patients when compared to non-smokers AMI patients [**Table 1**], (p<0.001). The HDL-C levels were significantly lowered in smokers when compared with non-smokers AMI patients. Also, significant differences were observed in total cholesterol, TC/HDL-C ratio, triglycerides, LDL-cholesterol, LDL/HDL-C ratio and TG/HDL-C ratio in smoker AMI patients when compared with healthy controls but the differences were not significant when compared with non-smokers to healthy controls [**Table 2**], (p<0.001).

The superoxide dismutase, glutathione peroxidase and catalase were significantly higher [**Table 3**], (p<0.001) in non-smokers when compared with the observations among smokers AMI patients. Similar findings were observed in the levels of albumin, uric acid and Bilirubin [Table-3], (p<0.001) when compared with smokers and non-smokers AMI patients. The oxidative stress indicators namely MDA and CD were significantly higher and paraoxonase activity were significantly lower in smokers when compared to non-smokers indicating the extent of free radicals generated in smokers [**Table 3**, **Fig. 1**], (p<0.001).

Table 1. Lipid profile in smoker and non-smoker AMI patients (mean ±SD).

Variables	AMI Patients (n=86)		
	Smokers (n=43)	Non-Smokers (n=43)	P value (95%CI)
Age yrs	62.32 ± 3.35	60.25 ± 2.76	0.0037 (61.61-63.02)
Total Cholesterol †	173.36 ± 11.84	157.67 ± 13.56	<0.001 (170.85 -175.86)
HDL-Cholesterol †	37.87 ± 5.73	53.83 ± 7.89	<0.001 (36.65- 39.08)
TC: HDL-C*	4.55 ± 0.67	2.86 ± 0.47	<0.001 (4.40-4.69)
Triglycerides †	135.47 ± 15.34	117.36 ± 13.53	<0.001(132.22-138.71)
LDL-Cholesterol †	121.46 ± 13.62	81.73 ± 12.61	<0.001(118.58-124.33)
LDL:HDL-C*	3.13 ± 0.72	1.47 ± 0.36	<0.001(2.97-3.28)
TG: HDL-C*	3.53 ± 0.37	2.13 ± 0.53	<0.01(3.45-3.60)

* ratio † (mg %); S=Smokers; NS=Non-Smokers.
All values are Mean ± SD.
Values in the parenthesis indicate the number of subjects.

Table 2. Lipid Profile in smoker and non-smoker AMI patients and healthy controls (mean ±SD).

Variables		AMI Patients (n=86)		
	Control (n=86)	S vs. NS	Mean ± SD	P* value
Total Cholesterol †	155.58 ± 12.16	S (43)	173.36 ± 11.84	0.001
		NS(43)	157.67 ± 13.56	0.067
HDL-Cholesterol †	55.51 ± 6.78	S (43)	37.87 ± 5.73	0.001
		NS(43)	53.83 ± 7.89	0.079
TC: HDL-C*	2.78 ± 0.36	S (43)	4.55 ± 0.67	0.001
		NS(43)	2.86 ± 0.47	0.069
Triglycerides†	114.84 ± 11.51	S (43)	135.47 ± 15.34	0.01
		NS(43)	117.36 ± 13.53	0.037
LDL-Cholesterol †	80.59 ± 11.95	S (43)	121.46 ± 13.62	0.001
		NS(43)	81.73 ± 12.61	0.021
LDL:HDL-C*	1.42 ± 0.31	S (43)	3.13 ± 0.72	0.001
		NS(43)	1.47 ± 0.36	0.137
TG: HDL-C*	2.11 ± 0.35	S (43)	3.53 ± 0.37	0.01
		NS(43)	2.13 ± 0.53	0.073

* ratio † (mg %); S=Smokers; NS=Non-Smokers.
All values are Mean ± SD.
Controls = Healthy subjects.
Values in the parenthesis indicated the number of subjects.
P* = Significance between control and S and NS groups separately.

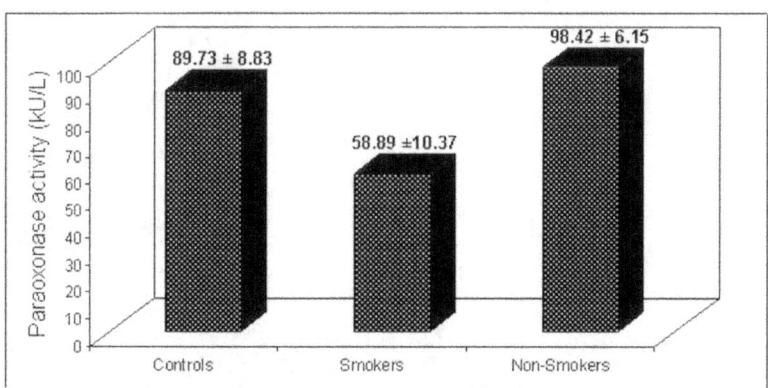

Figure1. PON1 activities in Controls and Smoker and Non-Smoker AMI patients.

P value significant (<0.001) between control and smoker.
P value significant (<0.001) between smoker and non-smoker.
P value not significant (0.087) between control and non-smoker.

Table 3. Antioxidant and Paraoxonase activities in smoker and non-smoker AMI patients (mean ±SD).

Variables	AMI Patients (n=86)		
	S (n=43)	NS (n=43)	P value (95%CI)
Superoxide dismutase (U/gHb)	793.59 ± 78.53	1826.47 ± 31.86	<0.001 (776.98 -810.19)
Glutathione Peroxidase (U/gHb)	35.28 ± 7.92	61.29 ± 3.94	<0.001(33.60-36.95)
Catalase (k/gHb)	174.28 ± 28.73	256.15 ± 26.65	<0.001 (168.20-180.35)
Albumin †	3.98 ± 0.47	4.43 ± 0.31	<0.01(3.88-4.07)
Uric Acid†	4.21 ± 0.83	5.82 ± 1.26	<0.001(4.03-4.38)
Bilirubin†	0.58 ± 0.27	0.77 ± 0.16	<0.01(0.52-0.63)
MDA (nmol/L)	16.98 ± 2.87	5.71 ± 0.97	<0.001(16.37-17.58)
Conjugated diene(µmol/L)	56.93 ± 6.78	31.04 ± 2.68	<0.001(55.49-58.36)
Paraoxonase (kU/L)	58.89 ± 10.37	98.42 ± 6.15	<0.001(56.69-61.08)

† (mg %); S=Smokers; NS=Non-Smokers
All values are Mean ± SD
Values in the parenthesis indicate the number of subjects.

Table 4: Antioxidant and Paraoxonase activities in smoker and non-smoker AMI patients and healthy controls (mean ±SD).

Variables	AMI Patients (n=86)			
	Control (n=86)	S vs. NS	Mean ± SD	P*Value
Superoxide dismutase (U/gHb)	1867.43 ± 97.19	S (43)	793.59 ± 78.53	0.001
		NS(43)	1826.47 ± 31.86	0.089
Glutathione Peroxidase (U/gHb)	66.13 ± 6.36	S (43)	35.28 ± 7.92	0.001
		NS(43)	61.29 ± 3.94	0.124
Catalase (k/gHb)	293.06 ± 35.87	S (43)	174.28 ± 28.73	0.001
		NS(43)	256.15 ± 26.65	0.722
Albumin†	4.61 ± 0.33	S (43)	3.98 ± 0.47	0.01
		NS(43)	4.43 ± 0.31	0.234
Uric Acid†	5.76 ± 0.38	S (43)	4.21 ± 0.83	0.001
		NS(43)	5.82 ± 1.26	0.141
Bilirubin†	0.76 ± 0.23	S (43)	0.58 ± 0.27	0.01
		NS(43)	0.77 ± 0.16	0.031
MDA (nmol/L)	5.67 ± 1.66	S (43)	16.98 ± 2.87	0.001
		NS(43)	5.71 ± 0.97	0.065

Conjugated diene (µmol/L)	28.31 ± 3.43	S (43)	56.93 ± 6.78	0.001
		NS(43)	31.04 ± 2.68	0.253
Paraoxonase (kU/L)	89.73 ± 8.83	S (43)	58.89 ± 10.37	0.001
		NS(43)	98.42 ± 6.15	0.087

† (mg %); S=Smokers; NS=Non-Smokers.
All values are Mean ± SD.
Controls = Healthy subjects.
Values in the parenthesis indicated the number of subjects.
P* = Significance between control and S and NS groups separately.

Although there was statistically significant difference in observations among smokers and non-smokers in the levels of antioxidants and lipid peroxidation along with paraoxonase activity, but when the findings were compared with the healthy controls, the results observed was found to be statistically significant among controls with those of smokers, but not much differences were observed among controls with those of non-smokers AMI patients [**Table 4**, **Fig. 1**], ($p < 0.001$).

Discussion

Cigarette smoking is widely established as a primary risk factor for atherosclerosis and cardiovascular disease. Increased oxidative stress is one of the principal mechanisms by which it may exert its pathological influence [16]. Earlier studies conducted provide supportive arguments for PON as an antioxidant function, [4, 36, 37] which has anti-atherogenic potential. In this context, the results of the current study are agreeable with the hypothesis oxidative modifications due to smoking causes changes in serum PON activity there by accelerating the atherogenic process. Dyslipidaemia and myocardial infarction may also be associated with a lower activity of serum PON, [38] which could be linked to HDL and shows significant correlations with apoA-I concentrations[39,40]. Myocardial infarction are also associated with lower serum levels of HDL concentrations hence could explain alterations in PON activities. Antioxidants and free radicals could conceivably protect PON through augmentation of the overall antioxidant capacity therefore the result of the current study showed significant differences among smokers when compared to non-smokers but the results were not significantly different among non- smokers to those of healthy controls which does not influence the results.

The evident question is whether the observations are of relevance to the occurrence of cardiovascular disease. Smoking has such a powerful impact on the risk of disease that it is difficult to dissociate a risk factor that may interact with it. The rationale was that if serum PON were of relevance, lower levels could be observed in more severe cases of disease. The analysis demonstrated that enzyme activities and concentrations were significantly lower in patients with 3-vessel disease.

More important, perhaps, we demonstrate that differences in PON concentrations, on the order of those observed in the present study, can influence the ability of HDL to protect LDL from oxidation. Thus, incremental increases in HDL PON are associated with incremental decreases in the level of LDL hydroperoxides generated under oxidization conditions.

In vitro studies are providing a wealth of data on the functions of PON, but observations that concern the clinical consequences of modifications to serum PON are less abundant. A limited number of studies have reported lower PON activities in pathologies associated with a higher risk of vascular disease. PON has also been identified as a genetic risk factor for vascular disease. The current study observed the association between smoking, a prooxidant phenomenon with a demonstrated inhibitory effect on PON, and serum PON activities and concentrations and its concentrations remain unaltered in non-smokers. Our data also indicate that lower serum PON levels are associated with increased severity of CAD and reduced capacity to protect LDL from oxidation. They are consistent with the hypothesis that smoking modifies serum PON such that there is an increased risk of CAD, which may be due to a diminished capacity to protect lipoproteins from oxidative stress.

Research into paraoxonases has flourished over the last decade. It seems now evident that PON1 has the ability to degrade lipid peroxides in lipoproteins and in cells, and that plays a protective role against oxidative stress and inflammation, which are key processes involved in the pathophysiology of atherosclerosis, leading to myocardial infarction. In future PON measurement could be included to the battery of routine analyses in clinical chemistry laboratories.

References

1. Singh S, Venketesh S, Verma JS, Verma M, Lellamma CO, Goel RC. Paraoxonase (PON11) activity in northwest Indian Punjabis with coronary artery disease & type II diabetes mellitus. Indian J Med Res 2007; 125:783-787.
2. Berliner JA, Navab M, Fogelman AM, Frank JS, Demer LL, Edwards PA, et al. Atherosclerosis: basic mechanisms. Oxidation, Inflammation, and genetics. Circulation 1995; 91:2488-2496.
3. Steinberg D. Low density lipoprotein oxidation and its pathobiological significance. J Biol Chem 1997; 272:20963–20966.
4. Aviram M, Rosenblat M, Bisgaier CL, et al. Paraoxonase inhibits high-density lipoprotein oxidation and preserves its functions: a possible peroxidative role for paraoxonase. J Clin Invest 1998; 101:1581–1590.
5. Shih DM, Gu L, Xia Y-R, et al. Mice lacking serum paraoxonase are susceptible to organophosphate toxicity and atherosclerosis. Nature 1998; 394: 284–287.
6. Serrato M, Marian AJ. A variant of human paraoxonase/arylesterase (HUMPONA) gene is a risk factor for coronary heart disease. J Clin Invest 1995; 96: 3005–3008.
7. Odawara M, Tachi Y, Yamashita K. Paraoxonase polymorphism (Gln192-Arg) is associated with coronary heart disease in Japanese noninsulin-dependent diabetic patients. J Clin Endocrinol Metab 1997; 82:2257–2260.
8. Sanghera DK, Saha N, Aston CE, et al. Genetic polymorphisms of paraoxonase and the risk of coronary heart disease. Arterioscler Thromb Vasc Biol1997; 17:1067–1073.
9. Zama T, Murata M, Matsubara Y, et al. A [192]Arg variant of the human paraoxonase (HUMPONA) gene polymorphism is associated with an increased risk for coronary artery disease in the Japanese. Arterioscler Thromb Vasc Biol 1997; 17: 3565–3569.
10. Pfohl M, Koch M, Enderle MD, et al. Paraoxonase: Gln/Arg gene polymorphism, coronary artery disease, and myocardial infarction in type 2 diabetes. Diabetes 1999; 192:48:623–627.
11. Antikainen M, Murtomaki S, Syvänne M, et al. The Gln-Arg191 polymorphism of the human paraoxonase gene (HUMPONA) is not associated with risk of coronary artery disease in Finns. J Clin Invest 1996; 98: 883–885.
12. Herrmann S-M, Blanc H, Poirier O, et al. The Gln/Arg polymorphism of human paraoxonase (PON 192) is not related to myocardial infarction in the ECTIM study. Atherosclerosis 1996; 126:299–304.
13. Gur M, Aslan M, Yildiz A, Demirbaq R, Yilmaz R, Selek S, Erel O, Ozdoqru I. Paraoxonase and Arylesterase activities in Coronary Artery disease. Eur J Clin Invest 2006; 36:779-787.
14. Lorentz K, Flatter B, Augustin E. Arylesterase in Serum: Elaboration and Clinical application of a Fixed-Incubation Method. Clin Chem 1979; 25:1714-1720.

15. Scheffler E, Wiest E, Woehrle J, et al. Smoking influences the atherogenic potential of low density lipoprotein. J Clin Invest 992; 70:263–268.
16. Pryor WA, Stone K. Oxidants in cigarette smoke: radicals, hydrogen peroxide, peroxynitrate and peroxynitrite. Ann N Y Acad Sci1993; 686:12–27.
17. Morrow JD, Frei B, Longmire AW, et al. Increases in circulating products of lipid peroxidation (F2-isoprostanes) in smokers: smoking as a cause of oxidative damage. N Engl J Med1995; 332: 1198–1203.
18. Yokode M, Kita T, Arai H, et al. Cholesterol ester accumulation in macrophages incubated with low density lipoprotein pretreated with cigarette smoke extract. Proc Natl Acad Sci USA1988; 85: 2344–2348.
19. Harats D, Ben-Naim M, Dabach Y, et al. Cigarette smoke renders LDL susceptible to peroxidative modification and enhanced metabolism by macrophages. Atherosclerosis 1989; 79:245–252.
20. Heitzer T, Yla-Herttuala S, Luoma J, et al. Cigarette smoking potentiates endothelial dysfunction of forearm resistance vessels in patients with hypercholesterolemia: role of oxidized LDL. Circulation1996; 93:1346–1353.
21. Berliner JA, Navab M, Fogelman AM, et al. Atherosclerosis: basic mechanisms: oxidation, inflammation, and genetics. Circulation 1995; 91:2488–2496.
22. Ross R. Atherosclerosis: an inflammatory disease. N Engl J Med 1999; 340:115–126.
23. Nishio E, Watanabe Y. Cigarette smoke extract inhibits plasma paraoxonase activity by modification of the enzyme's free thiols. Biochem Biophys Res Commun 1997; 236:289–293.
24. National Cholesterol Education Program. Detection, evaluation and treatment of high blood cholesterol in adults (Adult Treatment Panel III). Circulation 2002; 106:3143-3421.
25. Haagen L, Brock A. A new Automated method of Phenotyping Arylesterase (EC 3.1.1.2) Based UPON1 Inhibition of Enzymatic Hydrolysis of 4-Nitrophenol Acetate by Phenyl Acetate. Eur J Clin Chem Clin Biochem 1992; 30:391-395.
26. Tartan Z, Orhan G, Kasikçioglu H, Uyarel H, Unal S, Ozer N, Ozay B, Ciloglu F, Cam N. The role of paraoxonase (PON1) enzyme in the extent and severity of the coronary artery disease in type-2 diabetic patients. Heart Vessels 2007; 22:158-1564.
27. Paglia DE, Valentine WN. Studies on quantitative and qualitative characterization of erythrocyte glutathione peroxidase. J Lab Clin Med 1967;70: 158-69.
28. Sun Y, Oberly LW, Li Y. A simple method for clinical assay of superoxide dismutase. Clin Chem 1988; 34: 497-500.
29. Beutler E. Red Cell Metabolism: A Manual of Biochemical Methods, 3rd edition. New York, Grune and Stratton, 1984; 105.
30. Beutler E, Duron O, Kelly B. An improved method for the determination of blood glutathione. J Lab Clin Med 1963;61: 822-826.
31. Bernheim S, Bernheim MLC, Wilbur KM. The reaction between thiobarbituric acid and the oxidant product of certain lipids. J Biol Chem 1948; 174: 257-264.
32. Recknagel RO, Glende EA. Spectrophotometric detection of lipid conjugated dienes. Methods Enzymol 1984; 105:331-337.
33. Brown H. The determination of uric acid in human blood. Journal of Biological Chemistry, 1945; 158:601-608.
34. Jendrassik, J. & Grof P.Vereinfachte photometrische Methoden Zur Beetimmung des Blutbilirubin. Biochem. Z., 1938;297; 81-89.
35. Perry BW, Doumas BT. Effect of heparin on albumin determination by use of bromocresol green and bromocresol purple. Clin Chem 1979; 25:1520-1522.
36. Mackness MI, Arrol S, Durrington PN. Paraoxonase prevents accumulation of lipoperoxides in low-density lipoprotein. FEBS Lett 1991; 286:152–154.
37. Watson AD, Berliner JA, Hama SY, et al. Protective effect of high density lipoprotein associated paraoxonase: inhibition of the biological activity of minimally oxidised low density lipoprotein. J Clin Invest 1995;96:2882–2891.
38. Abbott CA, Mackness MI, Kumar S, et al. Serum paraoxonase activity, concentration, and phenotype distribution in diabetes mellitus and its relationship to serum lipids and lipoproteins. Arterioscler Thromb Vasc Biol 1995; 15:1812–1818.
39. Blatter Garin M-C, James RW, Dussoix P, et al. Paraoxonase polymorphism Met-Leu54 is associated with modified serum concentrations of the enzyme: a possible link between the paraoxonase gene and increased risk of cardiovascular disease in diabetes. J Clin Invest 1997; 99: 62–66.
40. Blatter Garin M-C, Abbot C, Messmer S, et al. Quantification of human serum paraoxonase by enzyme-linked immunoassay: population differences in protein concentrations. Biochem J 1994; 304:549–554.

Chapter 8

Oxidative Stress and antioxidant status in patients of myocardial infarction with normal lipid profile

Abstract

The objectives of the study were to observe the correlation between oxidative stress and antioxidants in myocardial infarct patients with normal lipid profile. In the present study investigation of lipid peroxidation and antioxidants were done in patients. This study was carried out on 165 AMI patients,(123 males and 42 females). The control group consisted on 165 normal healthy age-sex matched subjects (123 males and 42 females). Levels of Superoxide dismutase, Glutathione Peroxidase, Catalase, Malondialdehyde and Conjugated dienes were measured. The study found Superoxide dismutase, Glutathione Peroxidase, Catalase were significantly lower in activities ($p<0.001$) in AMI patients compared to controls. The markers of lipid peroxidation namely Malondialdehyde and Conjugated dienes were higher in AMI patients as compared to controls ($p<0.001$). The present study is clearly suggestive of increased oxidative stress in AMI patients. Oxidative stress appears as an etiological factor for myocardial infraction as a consequence the free radical scavengers levels are lowered in AMI patient.

Key words: Oxidative stress, Antioxidants, AMI and Normal Lipid Profile.

Introduction

Free radicals contain one or more unpaired electrons. They play an important role in the pathogenesis of tissue damage in many different clinical disorders (1).Oxygen free radicals are produced continuously. Normally there is a balance between tissue oxidant and antioxidant activity (2). The later is achieved by the antioxidant scavenger system which includes enzymes (superoxide dismutase, catalase, glutathione peroxidase) and antioxidant vitamins (C, A, E and other carotenoids (3). Imbalance of this reaction either due to excess free radical formation or insufficient removal by antioxidants leads to oxidative stress (4). Increased generation of OFRs can cause atherosclerosis due to oxidative modification of LDL molecules which is one of the causes of Acute Myocardial Infarction (5). Coronary Heart disease (CHD) is associated with the greatest morbidity and mortality in industrialized countries (6).Due to increased oxidation of

LDL, the formation of malondialdehyde (MDA) and conjugated dienes (CD) takes place with increased lipid peroxidation. The increased concentration of CD and extensive lipid peroxidation could also be due to dyslipidaemias and aberrations of lipid profiles. Literature survey reveals that the risk of heart attacks is particularly in those groups of individuals who have dyslipidemia. Now a latest trend is emerging that even in normolipaedemic subjects the chances of Acute Myocardial Infarction persists.

The present study was planned to evaluate the oxidative stress and antioxidants enzyme status in AMI patients. The present study was undertaken due to lacunae of data available on normal lipidaemic patients with myocardial infarction.

Materials and methods

Setting Design and patients: The study consisted of 165 patients (123 men and 42 women) with AMI, admitted to the Intensive Cardiac Care Unit. The diagnosis of AMI was established according to diagnostic criteria: chest pain, which lasted for up to 3 hours, ECG changes (ST elevation of 2 mm or more in at least two leads) and elevation of serum creatine phosphokinase (CPK-MB) and aspartate aminotransferase enzyme elevation. The control group consisted of 165 age-sex matched healthy volunteers, 123 men and 42 women. The study was conducted for a period of four and half years from April 2002 to August 2006. Informed consent was taken.

Inclusion criteria: Patients with diagnosis of AMI with normal lipid profile.

Exclusion criteria: Patients with diabetes mellitus, renal insufficiency, current and past smokers, hepatic disease or taking lipid lowering drugs or antioxidant vitamin supplements.

Blood collection and biochemical methods used: 10 ml of blood was collected after overnight fasting in different containers.

1. **EDTA vial:** 5.0 ml of blood was taken. Red cells were washed 3-4 times with ice-cold normal saline and used for estimation of glutathione peroxidase, superoxide dismutase and catalase.

2. **Plain vial:** Remaining blood was taken and serum was separated. Serum was used for determination of lipid profile, malondialdehye and conjugated dienes.

Lipid profile (Total cholesterol, triglycerides, and HDL-cholesterol) were analyzed enzymatically using kit obtained from (Randox Laboratories Limited, Crumlin, UK). Plasma LDL-cholesterol was determined from the values of total cholesterol and HDL-cholesterol using the following formulae:

LDL-cholesterol = Total cholesterol - Triglycerides − HDL-cholesterol (mg/dl)

5

All chemicals of analytical grade were obtained from Sigma chemicals, India.

Glutathione Peroxidase (GPx): The glutathione peroxidase activity was determined by the procedure of Paglia and Valentine (7). Briefly, the oxidized glutathione produced during GPx enzyme reaction was immediately reduced by NADPH and glutathione reductase. Therefore, the rate of NADPH consumption was monitored as a measure of formation of oxidized glutathione. Results were expressed as units of GPx per gram of hemoglobin.

Superoxide dismutase (SOD): Superoxide dismuatse enzyme activity was measured by SOD assay kit using rate of inhibition of 2-(4-indophenyl)-(4-Nitrophenol)-5-phenyltetrazolium chloride (I.N.T) reduction method modified method of Sun Y Oberly (8) using assay Ransod kit SD 125, Randox Lab. One uinit of SOD activity was defined as the amount of protein that inhibits the rate of I.N.T. reduction by 50%. Enzyme activity was expressed as unit per gram hemoglobin (U/gHb). Hemoglobin was measured by Drabkin's method.

Catalase: Catalase activity was measured spectrophotometrically as described by Beutler (9, 10). One unit of enzyme activity was expressed as micromole hydrogen peroxide decomposed per min per gram hemoglobin.

MDA Method: MDA levels were estimated by thiobarbituric acid (TBA) reaction (11). Using 40% tricholoroacetic acid, proteins were precipitated from 0.5 ml serum, and precipitated proteins were incubated with TBA reagent in a boiling water bath for one hour. After bringing down to room temperature, the colored complex formed was measured using spectrophotometer at 532 nm. 1, 1, 2, 3-tetraethoxypropane (1 nmol/l) was used as a standard for MDA estimation. Concentrations were expressed in nmol/l.

Conjugated dienes (CD): CD levels were measured by Recknagel and Glende method (12) with little modification. Briefly, the principle of the assay is based on with the rearrangement of double bonds in polyunsaturated fatty acids leading to the formation of DC, which absorb light at 233 nm. The oxidation index of the lipid sample at 233 nm and 215 nm is computed which reflect the diene content and the extent of peroxidation. The Lipid Peroxidation (LP) products measured in serum were treated with antioxidant Butylated hydroxytoluene (BHT) twice, immediately after obtaining and before adding the test reagents to suppress artefactual changes during handling and assay procedures. The first stage of LP consists of the molecular rearrangement of the double bonds in polyunsaturated fatty acids residues of lipids, which leads to conjugated dienes (CD) formation and conversion of CD in hydroperoxide (LOOH). Serum was chosen to avoid possible influences of substances required for plasma preparation. Serum sample (150 μl) and (150μl) of 0.9% NaCl (reagent blank contains only isotonic saline) were incubated at 37°C for 25 minutes. 0.25% Butylated hydroxyl Toluene (BHT) (150μl) was added and the lipids were extracted by heptane/isopropanol (1:1). Then samples were acidified by 5 mol/L HCl and extracted by cold heptane (1600μl). After centrifugation for 5 minutes at 3000 rpm the absorbance of heptane fraction were measured spectrophotometrically at absorbance maximum between 220 nm and 250 nm. The amount of hydroperoxides produced was calculated using Molar Coefficient of 2.52×10^4 m^{-1}.

Statistical analysis: The data from patients and controls were compared using Student's 't'-test. Values were expressed as mean ± standard deviation (SD). Microft excel for windows 2000 was used for statistical analysis. 'P' value of less than 0.05 was considered to indicate statistical significance.

Results

Demographic data of control and AMI patients are shown in **Table 1** and **Table 2**. The differences in age, height and body mass index (BMI) in control and AMI patient are insignificant. The weight and waist circumference were higher in AMI subjects as compared to control (p<0.001) **(Table 1)** and **(Table 2)**. Systolic and diastolic blood

Table 1. Demographic data in Control and AMI patients (mean ±SD).

Variables	Control (n=165)	Case (n=165)
Age	60.55 ± 3.98	61.84 ± 3.80†
Height (cm)	1.63 ± 0.04	1.64 ± 0.05 ‡
Weight (kg)	68.34 ± 3.97	72.01 ± 5.37 §
BMI (kg/m2)	25.40 ± 1.20	26.16 ± 1.45||
Waist Circumference(cm)	93.70 ± 3.63	100.77 ± 6.06 §
Hip Circumference (cm)	100.01 ± 3.16	105.72 ± 5.23 §
Waist: Hip*	0.93 ± 0.01	0.95 ± 0.01 ¶
Systolic blood pressure(mm of Hg)	113 ± 8	136 ± 23 **
Diastolic blood pressure(mm of Hg)	85 ± 7	95 ± 10 **

* ratio † (p=0.0037) ‡ (p=0.2919) § (p<0.001) \|\|(p<0.01) ¶ (p<0.02)** (p<0.05)

Table 2. Demographic data in males and females in Control and AMI patients (mean ± SD).

Variables	Control		Case	
	Male (n=123)	Female (n=42)	Male (n=123)	Female (n=42)
Age	60.68 ± 4.14	60.52 ± 2.93	61.53 ± 3.28 †	62.73 ± 4.97 **
Height (cm)	1.64 ± 0.04	1.61 ± 0.03	1.66 ± 0.05‡	1.59 ± 0.04 ††
Weight (kg)	68.64 ± 3.78	67.47 ± 4.41	71.68 ± 5.28 §	72.45 ± 5.69 §
BMI (kg/m^2)	25.33 ± 1.06	25.63 ± 1.54	26.02 ± 1.34 ||	26.57 ± 1.69 ‡‡
WC (cm)	93.38 ± 3.37	94.64 ± 4.21	100.18 ± 5.69 §	102.50 ± 6.82 §
HC (cm)	99.73 ± 2.89	100.80 ± 3.75	105.28 ± 4.98 ¶	107.00 ± 5.78 §
Waist: Hip*	0.93 ± 0.01	0.93 ± 0.01	0.95 ± 0.01¶	0.95 ± 0.01 §
SBP (mm of Hg)	114 ± 7	118 ± 8	136 ± 13 ¶	132 ± 17 ¶
DBP (mm of Hg)	86 ± 8	87 ± 9	95 ± 15 ¶	94 ± 13 ¶

* ratio †(p=0.0366) ‡(p=0.0081) §(p<0.001) \|\|(p=1.5085) ¶(p<0.05) **(p=0.0356) ††(p=0.0170) ‡‡(p=0.0001)

Table 3. Lipid profile in control and AMI patients (mean ± SD).

Variables	Controls (n=165)	Patients (n=165)
Total Cholesterol §	168.58 ± 12.16	186.44 ± 13.95 †
HDL-Cholesterol §	50.51 ± 6.78	41.27 ± 4.62 †
TC: HDL-C*	3.39 ± 0.36	4.57 ± 0.58 †
Triglycerides §	107.84 ± 11.51	128.96 ± 12.19 †
LDL-Cholesterol §	83.59 ± 11.95	119.37 ± 14.05 †
LDL:HDL-C*	1.90 ± 0.31	2.93 ± 0.51 †
TG: HDL-C*	2.17 ± 0.35	3.16 ± 0.49 ‡

* ratio † (p<0.001) ‡ (p= 1.0008) § (mg%).

pressure was significantly higher in AMI patient compared with controls (p<0.05) (**Table 1**) and (**Table 2**).

The lipid profile are shown in **Table 3** and **Table 4**. Total cholesterol, TC: HDL-C ratio, triglycerides, LDL-cholesterol, LDL: HDL-C ratio were higher in AMI subjects as compared to control (Table-3) (p<0.001). Also, significant differences were seen in HDL-C levels between AMI and controls (p<0.001). Total cholesterol, TC: HDL-C ratio, triglycerides were higher in both genders of AMI subjects as compared to control (**Table 4**) (p<0.001). Significant differences were seen in HDL-C levels between AMI and control only in female (**Table 4**) (p<0.001).LDL-cholesterol, LDL: HDL-C ratio were higher in male AMI subjects compared to control (**Table 4**) (p<0.001)

The antioxidant enzymes status and index of lipid peroxidation are shown in **Table 5** and **Table 6**. All the antioxidant enzymes were significantly decreased (p<0.001) in AMI patients compared to controls. Serum malondialdehye and conjugated dienes were significantly increased in AMI patients compared to controls.

Table 4. Lipid Profile in control and male and female AMI patients (mean ± SD).

Variables	Control (n=165)		Patients (n=165)	
	Male (n=123)	Female (n=42)	Male (n=123)	Female(n=42)
Total Cholesterol **	168.09 ± 12.10	170.00 ± 12.35	183.84 ± 13.65 †	194.03 ± 13.03 †
HDL-Cholesterol **	49.90 ± 7.30	52.31 ± 4.58	41.78 ± 4.88 ‡	39.77 ± 3.37 †
TC: HDL-C*	3.42 ± 0.30	3.28 ± 0.47	4.45 ± 0.58 †	4.96 ± 0.44 †
Triglycerides **	105.02 ± 10.31	116.11 ± 10.96	126.22 ± 11.74 †	136.99 ± 9.81 †
LDL-Cholesterol **	79.88 ± 7.98	94.47 ± 14.81	116.82 ± 13.76 †	126.86 ± 12.22||
LDL:HDL-C*	1.92 ± 0.25	1.83 ± 0.44	2.84 ± 0.52 †	3.21 ± 0.40 ¶
TG:HDL-C*	2.15 ± 0.37	2.23 ± 0.28	3.06 ± 0.47 §	3.47 ± 0.41 †

* ratio † (p<0.001) ‡(p=1.7609) § (p=2.53035) ||(p=1.2743) ¶ (p=1.0255) ** (mg%)

Table 5. Antioxidant Status and Lipid Peroxidation in Control and AMI patients (mean ± SD).

Variables	Control(n=165)	Case(n=165)
Superoxide dismutase (Ug/Hb)	1826.47 ± 31.86	813.95 ± 208.98 *
Glutathione Peroxidase(U/gHb)	61.29 ± 3.94	42.56 ± 6.36 †
Catalase (k/gHb)	256.15 ± 26.65	193.06 ± 35.87 †
TBARS (nmol/L)	5.71 ± 0.97	14.81 ± 1.66 *
Conjugated dienes (μmol/L)	31.04 ± 2.68	48.28 ± 5.50 †

* (p<0.02) † (p<0.001)

Table 6. Antioxidant Status and Lipid Peroxidation in control AMI males and females (mean ± SD).

Variables	Control		Case	
	Male (n=123)	Female (n=42)	Male (n=123)	Female (n=42)
Superoxide dismutase (Ug/Hb)	1825.59 ± 32.23	1829.06 ± 31.00	813.87 ± 212.76*	814.19 ± 199.99*
Glutathione Peroxidase (U/gHb)	61.07 ± 4.12	60.14 ± 3.11	42.24 ± 6.94*	43.52 ± 4.19*
Catalase (k/gHb)	260.10 ± 27.59	244.60 ± 19.81	198.52 ± 36.54*	188.26 ± 32.07*
TBARS (nmol/L)	5.57 ± 1.03	6.11 ± 0.61	14.76 ± 1.81*	14.96 ± 1.14*
Conjugated dienes (µmol/L)	30.24 ± 1.91	33.37 ± 3.20	46.83 ± 5.37*	52.34 ± 3.21†

* ($p<0.001$) † ($p<0.01$)

Discussion

Involvement of oxygen free radicals (OFRs) in the pathophysiology of inflammation, ischemia and in reperfusion damage in a number of organs and tissues have been reported in literature (2, 13). Indirect evidence of OFR generation in patients with AMI has been observed by measuring a variety of by products of lipid peroxidation, such as pentane, conjugated dienes and malondialdehyde (MDA). In the present study, a significant increase in malondialdehyde and conjugated dienes in patients with AMI as compared to controls. The plasma concentration of these substances has been reported to be increased in AMI patients in many studies (14). Reduction in infarct size in animal models of temporary coronary artery occlusion and reperfusion has been reported by means of several different anti-free radical interventions (15). OFRs are generated particularly in early stage of AMI and antioxidants are involved in the reduction of hydrogen peroxide radicals, resulting in a decrease in their activities during that period (15, 16). In the present study, low activities of superoxide dismutase, glutathione peroxidase and catalase were observed in AMI patients as compared to control. Despite data linking OFR generation and reperfusion injury, there are reports that fail to show a beneficial effect of oxygen radical scavengers or other agents on infarct size reduction (17). Thus, the present study is suggestive of imbalance between oxidant and antioxidants in AMI patients which is mainly due to increased oxidative stress. Future research including measurement of parameters of oxidative stress and inflammatory markers should be carried out as the role of inflammatory markers like C-reactive proteins, Caeruloplasmin are emerging which could be possibly be a causative factor for atherosclerosis.

Conclusion

Myocardial Infarction is a multifactorial disease which could be caused even in normo-lipaedemic subjects. The earlier concept of keeping in check with lipid profile has become obsolete as the present study unearths fact. It is advisable to keep a check on serum antioxidant status and peroxidative markers as the present study highlight the fact. Oxidative stress appears to be an etiological factor for myocardial infraction as a consequence the free radical scavengers namely antioxidants levels tends to lower in patients with myocardial infarction.

References

1. Halliwell B, Gutteridge GMC, Corss CE. Free radicals and antioxidants and human disease: where we are now? J Lab Clin Invest 1992; 119: 589-620.
2. Frei B, Stocker R, Ames BN. Antioxidant defenses and lipid peroxidation in human blood plasma. Proc Natl Acad Sci USA 1988; 85: 9748-9752.
3. Shrinivas K, Vijaya Bhaskar M, Aruna Kumari M, Nagaraj K, Reddy KK. Antioxidants, lipid peroxidation and lipoproteins in primary hypertension. Indian Heart J2000; 52:285-88.
4. Maritim AC, Sanders RA, Watkins JB. Diabetes, oxidative stress, and antioxidants: a review. J Biochem Mol Toxicol 2003; 17: 24-38.
5. Boullier A, Bird DA, Chang MK, Dennis EA, Friedman P, Gillotre-Taylor K et al. Scavenger receptors, oxidized LDL, and atherosclerosis. Am NY Acad Sci2001; 947:214-222.
6. Mendis S, Wissler R. A Nutritional experiment to study short term effects of coconut in diet on serum cholesterol and platelet factor 4 in man. Proceedings of the International Congress on Coronary Heart Disease Conference; 1988 Feb 18-21; Bombay, India.
7. Paglia DE, Valentine WN. Studies on quantitative and qualitative characterization of erythrocyte glutathione peroxidase. J Lab Clin Med 1967;70: 158-69.
8. Sun Y, Oberly LW, Li Y. A simple method for clinical assay of superoxide dismutase. Clin Chem 1988; 34: 497-500.
9. Beutler E. Red Cell Metabolism: A Manual of Biochemical Methods, 3rd edition. New York, Grune and Stratton, 1984; 105.
10. Beutler E, Duron O, Kelly B. An improved method for the determination of blood glutathione. J Lab Clin Med 1963;61: 822-826.
11. Bernheim S, Bernheim MLC, Wilbur KM. The reaction between thiobarbituric acid and the oxidant product of certain lipids. J Biol Chem 1948; 174: 257-264.
12. Recknagel RO, Glende EA. Spectrophotometric detection of lipid conjugated dienes. Methods Enzymol 1984; 105:331-337.
13. Uhling S, Wendel A. The physiological consequences of glutathione variations. Life Sci 1992; 51: 1083-94.
14. Dubois-Raade JL, Artiguo JY,Darmon JY. Oxidative stress in patients with unstable angina. Eur Heart J 1994; 15: 179-83.
15. Kocak H, Yekeler I, Basoglu A. The effect of superoxide dismutase and reduced glutathione on cardiac performance after coronary occlusion and reperfusion. In experimental study in dogs. Thorac Cardiovas Surgeon 1992; 40:140-3.
16. Kloner AR, Przyklenk K, Whittaker P. Deleterious effects of oxygen radicals in ischemia/reperfusion: resolved and unresolved issue. Circulation 1989; 80:1115-27.
17. Patch B, Jerudi MO, O'Neil PG. Human superoxide dismutase fails to limit infarct size after 2 h ischemia and reperfusion. Circulation 1988; 78:II-373.

Chapter 9

Serum Paraoxonase Activity in Normolipidemic Patients with Acute Myocardial Infarction

Abstract

Background: Although studies have demonstrated the HDL-C Paraoxonase is involved in the protection from the deleterious effects of oxygen free radicals in ischemia and reperfusion, there are controversial data on the correlation between Paraoxonase activity and ischemia process.

AIM: The present study was planned to evaluate Paraoxonase activity in patients with acute myocardial infarction (AMI) with normal lipid profile.

Setting & design: The serum paraoxonase activities were determined in 165 normolipademic patients diagnosed of AMI and 165 age-sexes matched healthy volunteers served as control.

Material & methods: Serum Paraoxonase activities were measured by using enzymatic kit manufactured from Zeptomatrix Corporation, New York, USA in AMI and control patients. Also lipid profile was analyzed enzymatically in these subjects.

Statistics: The values were expressed as means ± standard deviation (SD) and data from patients and control was compared using student's 't'-test.

Results and conclusion: Serum Paraoxonase activity were significantly decreased in AMI as compared to control (p<0.001). Also total cholesterol, TC: HDL-C ratio, triglycerides, LDL-cholesterol, LDL-C: HDL-C ratio and TG: HDL-C ratio were higher in AMI subjects (p<0.001) and HDL-cholesterol were lower in AMI subjects (p<0.001). No correlation was observed between PON1 activity and HDL-C levels in patients and controls. These findings suggest that decreased Paraoxonase activity could be due to increased oxidative stress in AMI.

Key words: Acute Myocardial Infarction, Normal Lipid Profile, Paraoxonase.

Introduction

With the explosive rise in the incidence of Coronary Artery disease (CAD) it is estimated that this will be the leading cause of morbidity and mortality in the developing world by the year 2015. [1] People hailing from Indian subcontinent had a higher probability of dying due to CAD. It is a multifactorial disease and some predisposing factors are hereditary, hyperlipidemia, obesity, hypertension, environmental factors and life style variables like stress, smoking, alcohol consumption, etc. [2] Diet especially fat plays an important role the development of CAD and the risk further increases in the presence of dyslipidemia. Lipoprotein profile has been investigated extensively in recent years, which is found to be deranged in large proportion of CAD patients; especially Asians showing a mixed picture of dyslipidemia. Low density lipoprotein cholesterol (LDL) is considered as the most important risk factor of CAD. However, a significant proportion of patients have a normal lipid profile. [3] The oxidation of LDL is believed to have a central role in atherogenesis. Subendothelial accumulation of foam cells plays a key role in the initiation of atherosclerosis. These foam cells, which may be generated by the uptake of oxidized LDL by macrophages via scavenger receptors, accumulate in fatty streaks that evolve to more complex fibro fatty or atheromatous plaques.[4] Oxidized LDL may also be involved in atherogenesis by inducing smooth muscle cell proliferation. [5] and smooth muscle foam cell generation. Under oxidative stress not only LDL, but other serum lipids are exposed to oxidation. High density lipoprotein (HDL) is one of the most important independent protective factors for the arteriosclerosis which underlies CHD. HDL associated Paraoxonase (PON1) enzyme is known to have protective effects on lipid peroxidation.[6] Numerous cohort studies and clinical trials have confirmed the association between a low HDL-cholesterol concentration and increased risk of CHD. Though many factors may play a role in its pathogenesis, low PON1 activity could be an independent risk factor.[7] PON1 activity is inversely related to the risk of developing an atherosclerotic lesion, which contains cholesterol-loaded macrophage foam cells. Although experimental studies have demonstrated the reduction in PON1 activity due to oxygen free radicals in ischemia and reperfusion,[8] there are controversial data on correlation between PON1 HDL-C and ischemia process. As it is well established that dyslipidemia is an important contributory factor for AMI and PON1 activity is decreased in dyslipidemia so the present study was undertaken with the objective of studying the PON1 activity in Normolipidemic AMI patients and also to observe whether PON1 activity could be an independent risk factor in this group of subjects.

Materials and methods

One hundred sixty five patients (males 123; females 42) with AMI and 165 age-sex matched healthy volunteers were taken for this study. The study was conducted for a period of four and half years from April 2002 to August 2006. Informed consent was taken. Smoking habits, systolic and diastolic blood pressure and family history of coronary heart diseases were recorded after clinical confirmation of AMI.

Diagnostic Criteria of patients: All the patients had their first episode of MI with diagnostic criteria: typical chest pain, specific abnormalities for MI on electrocardiogram, elevated serum creatine phosphokinase (CP-MB) and aspartate aminotransferase enzyme levels.

Exclusion Criteria: Patients with diabetes mellitus, renal insufficiency, hypertension, current smokers, hepatic disease or taking lipid lowering drugs or antioxidant vitamin supplements were excluded.

Criteria for Normolipaedemics: Normal lipid profile was defined if LDL was <160mg/dl, HDL ≥ 35 mg/dl, Total cholesterol (TC) <200 mg/dl and Triglycerides (TG) <150 mg/dl.[9]

Venous blood was collected after overnight fast and EDTA was added and samples were processed for lipid profiles.

For PON1 activity studies blood samples were collected in patients who were admitted in Intensive Care Unit 4-6 hours after AMI. Only Normolipidemic AMI patients were included in the study. Lipid profile (Total cholesterol, triglycerides, and HDL-cholesterol) were analyzed enzymatically using kit obtained from (Randox Laboratories Limited, Crumlin, UK). Plasma LDL-cholesterol was determined from the values of total cholesterol and HDL-cholesterol using the following formulae:

$$\text{LDL-cholesterol} = \text{Total cholesterol} - \frac{\text{Triglycerides}}{5} - \text{HDL-cholesterol (mg/dl)}$$

For PON1 studies an assay kit manufactured from Zeptometrix Corporation 872 Main street, Buffalo New York 14202 (ZMC catalogue 0801199). [10], [11] The assay is based on the principle; PON1 catalyzes the cleavage of phenyl acetate resulting in the phenol. The rate of formation of phenol is measured by monitoring the increase in absorbance at 270 nm at 25°C. One unit of arylesterase activity is equal to 1 μM of phenol formed per minute. The activity is expressed in kU/L, based on the extinction coefficient of phenol of 1310 $M^{-1}cm^{-1}$ at 270 nm, pH 8.0, and 25 °C. Blank samples containing water are used to correct for non-enzymatic hydrolysis. Statistical analysis: Data on lipid profile and PON1 activity was entered in Microsoft excel for windows 2000. The mean ± SD was obtained using excel software. The two-sample-t-test value was obtained between the patients and the control. The distribution of 't'- Probability was calculated depending on 'n' and significance of test was obtained. For p value <0.001 was considered as highly significant.

Result

PON1 activity was significantly decreased in patients with AMI than in controls [**Table 1**], [**Table 2**] and [**Table 3**] (p<0.001). Total cholesterol, TC: HDL-C ratio, triglycerides, LDL-cholesterol, LDL: HDL-C ratio were higher in AMI subjects as compared to control [**Table 1**], (p<0.001). Also, significant differences were seen in HDL-C levels between AMI and controls (p<0.001). Total cholesterol, TC: HDL-C ratio, triglycerides were higher in both genders of AMI subjects as compared to control [**Table 2**] and [**Table 3**] (p<0.001). Significant differences were seen in HDL-C levels between AMI and control only in female [**Table 3**] (p<0.001). No correlation was observed between PON1 and HDL-C levels in patients and controls. LDL-cholesterol, LDL: HDL-C ratio were higher in male AMI subjects compared to control [**Table 2**] (p<0.001)

Table 1. Paraoxonase activity and lipid profile in patients and healthy controls (mean ±SD).

Variables	Controls (n=165)	Patients (n=165)	P value (95%CI)
Age	60.55 ± 3.98	61.84 ± 3.80	0.0037(61.26-62.42)
Total Cholesterol †	168.58 ± 12.16	186.44 ± 13.95	<0.001(184.31-188.56)
HDL-Cholesterol †	50.51 ± 6.78	41.27 ± 4.62	<0.001(40.56-41.97)
TC: HDL-C*	3.39 ± 0.36	4.57 ± 0.58	<0.001(4.48-4.65)
Triglycerides †	107.84 ± 11.51	128.96 ± 12.19	<0.001(127.10-130.82)
LDL-Cholesterol †	83.59 ± 11.95	119.37 ± 14.05	<0.001(17.22-21.51)
LDL:HDL-C*	1.90 ± 0.31	2.93 ± 0.51	<0.001(2.85-3.00)
TG: HDL-C*	2.17 ± 0.35	3.16 ± 0.49	0.3149(3.086-3.234)
Paraoxonase activity (kU/L)	98.42 ± 6.15	69.66 ± 9.99	<0.001(68.13-71.18)

* ratio † (mg %)

Table 2. Paraoxonase activity and Lipid Profile in Male patients and healthy controls (mean ±SD)

Variables	Control Male (n=123)	Male Patients (n=123)	P value(95%CI)
Age	60.68 ± 4.14	61.53 ± 3.28	0.0366(60.95-62.10)
Total Cholesterol †	168.09 ± 12.10	183.84 ± 13.65	<0.001(182.41-186.25)
HDL-Cholesterol †	49.90 ± 7.30	41.78 ± 4.88	0.0801(40.91-42.64)
TC: HDL-C*	3.42 ± 0.30	4.45 ± 0.58	<0.001(4.34-4.55)
Triglycerides†	105.02 ± 10.31	126.22 ± 11.74	<0.001(124.14-128.29)
LDL-Cholesterol †	79.88 ± 7.98	116.82 ± 13.76	<0.001(114.38-119.25)
LDL:HDL-C*	1.92 ± 0.25	2.84 ± 0.52	<0.001(2.74-2.93)
TG:HDL-C*	2.15 ± 0.37	3.06 ± 0.47	0.0123(2.97-3.14)
Paraoxonase activity(kU/L)	98.00 ± 6.29	69.43 ± 10.20	<0.001(67.61-71.23)

*ratio † (mg %)

Table 3. Paraoxonase activity and Lipid Profile in Female patients and healthy controls (mean ±SD).

Variables	Control Female (n=42)	Patients Female (n=42)	P value(95%CI)
Age	60.52 ± 2.93	62.73 ± 4.97	0.0356(61.22-64.23)
Total Cholesterol †	170.00 ± 12.35	194.03 ± 13.03	<0.001(190.08-197.97)
HDL-Cholesterol †	52.31 ± 4.58	39.77 ± 3.37	<0.001(38.75-40.78)

TC: HDL-C*	3.28 ± 0.47	4.96 ± 0.44	<0.001(4.82-5.09)
Triglycerides †	116.11 ± 10.96	136.99 ± 9.81	<0.001(134.02-139.95)
LDL-Cholesterol †	94.47 ± 14.81	126.86 ± 12.22	0.2044(123.16-130.55)
LDL:HDL-C*	1.83 ± 0.44	3.21 ± 0.40	0.3066(3.08-3.33)
TG:HDL-C*	2.23 ± 0.28	3.47 ± 0.41	<0.001(3.34-3.59)
Paraoxonase activity(kU/L)	100.07 ± 5.45	70.33 ± 9.44	<0.001(67.47-73.18)

*ratio † (mg %)

Discussion: Involvement of oxygen free radicals (OFRs) in the pathophysiology of inflammation, ischemia and in reperfusion damage in a number of organs and tissues have been reported in literature. [12] Indirect evidence of OFR generation in patients with AMI has been observed by measuring the activity of PON1. [13] The activities of PON1 have been reported to decrease in patients with AMI in earlier studies. [14],[15] The decrease in PON1 activity could be due to over production of OFRs at the time of Infarction. Diabetics are more prone to develop AMI as it is one of the conventional risk factors and studies have indicated that serum PON1 activity is decreased in Diabetes Mellitus (DM). The lack of protective effect of PON1 enzyme on OFR's may be a factor in acceleration of Coronary Artery Disease in DM[16] Reduction in infarct size in animal models of temporary coronary artery occlusion and reperfusion has been reported by means of several different anti-free radical interventions.[17] OFRs are generated particularly in early stage of MI and PON1 is involved in the reduction of hydrogen peroxide radicals, resulting in a decrease in PON1 activity during that period.[18] In the present study, low activity of PON1 was observed in patients compared to control. Decreased PON1 activity may be associated with enhanced protective mechanism to oxidative stress in AMI at the time of ischemia or else it due to overwhelming production of toxic free radicals, the efficiency to hydrolyze lipid peroxides is decreased showing a consecutive decrease of PON1 activity as observed in the present study. Despite data linking OFR generation and reperfusion injury, there are reports that fail to show a beneficial effect of oxygen radical scavengers or other agents on infarct size reduction. [19] The present study has its limitations as the study was only on Normolipidemic AMI patients. If the PON1 activity was compared between Normolipidemic and dyslipidemia subjects then, it could have been better to draw a conclusion that the decreased activity of PON1 as an independent risk factor in Normolipidemic patients, and whether there is any significant difference in the PON1 activities in those two groups of patients. The infarction in Normolipidemic patients could not only be due to decreased activity of PON1 but also due to decreased enzymatic antioxidants in them which might be due to increased lipid peroxides. One can even predict that the decreased activity of PON1 could be due to the decrease in HDL levels as PON1 is associated with HDL. The prediction can be over ruled as the study didn't observe any correlation between HDL and PON1 activity. The study concludes, due to overwhelming production of free radicals, there is a decreased activity of PON1, and due to its incapability to scavenge free radicals, AMI patients becomes more prone to infarction. As PON1 is associated with HDL and it breakdown lipid peroxides and free radicals associated with the lipoprotein so its activity must be intact, acting as the first line of defense against the oxidized LDL molecules which is the known cause of atherosclerosis. If PON1 activity could have been normal in these normolipidemia patients of AMI the chances of infarction could be decreased. Future research including measurement of parameters of oxidative stress, enzymatic antioxidants and PON1 activity in both normolipidemia and dyslipidemia patients with AMI and to measure the PON1 activity after two days and few months of infarction is necessary to arrive at final conclusions about the role of PON1 in AMI.

References

1. Reddy KS. Cardiovascular disease in India. World Health Stat Q 1993; 46:101-7.
2. Chopra V, Wasir H. Implications of lipoprotein abnormalities in Indian patients. Journal Assoc Physicians of India 1998; 46:814-8.
3. Vasisht S, Narula J, Awtade A, Tandon R, Srivastava LM. Lipids and lipoproteins in normal controls and clinically documented coronary heart disease patients. Ann Natl Acad Med Sci (India) 1990; 26:57-66.
4. Ross R. The pathogenesis of atherosclerosis: a perspective for the 1990s. Nature 1993; 362:801–809.
5. Paul H, Johan V, Stefaan J, Frans Van de W, Désiré C. Oxidized LDL and Malondialdehyde-Modified LDL in Patients with Acute Coronary Syndromes and Stable Coronary Artery Disease. Circulation 1998; 98:1487-1494.
6. Singh S, Venketesh S, Verma JS, Verma M, Lellamma CO, Goel RC.
7. Paraoxonase(PON11) activity in north west Indian Punjabis with coronary artery disease & type II diabetes mellitus. Indian J Med Res 2007; 125:783-7.
8. Berliner JA, Navab M, Fogelman AM, Frank JS, Demer LL, Edwards PA, et al. Atherosclerosis: basic mechanisms. Oxidation. Inflammarion, and genetics. Circulation 1995; 91:2488-96.
9. Gur M,Aslan M, Yildiz A, Demirbaq R, Yilmaz R, Selek S, Erel O, Ozdoqru I.
10. Paraoxonase and Arylesterase activities in Coronary Artery disease. Eur J Clin Invest 2006; 36:779-87.
11. National Cholesterol Education Programme. Second report of the expert panel on detection,evaluation and treatment of high blood cholesterol in adults (Adult Panel II). 1994.
12. Lorentz K, Flatter B, Augustin E. Arylesterase in Serum: Elaboration and Clinical application of a Fixed-Incubation Method. Clin Chem 1979; 25:1714-1720.
13. Haagen L, Brock A. A new Automated method of Phenotyping Arylesterase (EC 3.1.1.2) Baased UPON1 Inhibition of Enzymatic Hydrolysis of 4-Nitrophenol Acetate by Phenyl Acetate. Eur J Clin Chem Clin Biochem 1992; 30:391-395.
14. Tartan Z, Orhan G, Kasikçioglu H, Uyarel H, Unal S, Ozer N, Ozay B, Ciloglu F, Cam N. The role of paraoxonase (PON1) enzyme in the extent and severity of the coronary artery disease in type-2 diabetic patients. Heart Vessels 2007; 22:158-64.
15. Jaouad L, Milochevitch C, Khalil A. PON11 paraoxonase activity is reduced during HDL oxidation and is an indicator of HDL antioxidant capacity. Free Radic Res 2003; 37:77- 83.
16. Mackness B, Hine D, McElduff P, Mackness M. High C-reactive protein and low paraoxonase1 in diabetes as risk factors for coronary heart disease. Atherosclerosis 2006 ; 186:396-401.
17. Rosenblat M, Karry R, Aviram M. Paraoxonase 1 (PON11) is a more potent antioxidant and stimulant of macrophage cholesterol efflux, when present in HDL than in lipoprotein-deficient serum: relevance to diabetes. Atherosclerosis 2006; 187:74-81.
18. Juretic D, Motejlkova A, Kunovic B, Rekic B, Flegar-Mestric Z, Vujic L, Mesic R, Lukac-Bajalo J, Simeon-Rudolf V. Paraoxonase/arylesterase in serum of patients with type II diabetes mellitus. Acta Pharm 2006; 56:59-68.
19. Kocak H, Yekeler I, Basoglu A. The effect of superoxide dismutase and reduced glutathione on cardiac performance after coronary occlusion and reperfusion. In experimental study in dogs. Thrac Cardiovas Surgeon 1992;40:140-43.
20. Kabaroglu C, Mutaf I, Boydak B, Ozmen D, Habif S, Erdener D, Parildar Z, B ayindir O.Association between serum paraoxonase activity and oxidative stress in acute coronary syndromes. Acta Cardiol 2004; 59:606-11.
21. Patch B, Jerudi MO, O'Neil PG. Human superoxide dismutase fails to limit infarct size after 2h ischemia and reperfusion. Circulation 1988; 78: II-373.

Chapter 10

Effect of Simvastatin on Paraoxonase 1 (PON1) activity and oxidative stress

Abstract

Objective: Paraoxonase has been shown to reduce the oxidation of low density lipoprotein (LDL) and high density lipoprotein (HDL) by hydrolyzing lipid peroxides and using unknown mechanism(s), thus protecting against atherosclerosis. Various factors influence the PON activity including lipid-lowering agents such as simvastatin. So the objectives of the current study was based on the effect of simvastatin treatment on lipid profile and oxidative stress in hypercholesterolaemic Indian population and further determining the effect of simvastatin treatment on the activity of PON.

Methods: In the current study, the effect of simvastatin (10 mg/day) treatment on PON activity and oxidative status in a hypercholesterolaemic Indian population was investigated. The outcomes were analyzed initially before administering any medication and at four months after medication. Lipid and lipoprotein measurement was done by using commercially available enzymatic kits [Randox Diagnostics, Crumlin, UK]. High density lipoprotein (HDL) was determined by the phosphotungstic acid precipitation method and LDL was calculated by using the Friedewald's formula. Lipid peroxidation was measured by three markers namely, conjugated diene, total peroxide, and malondialdehyde. Conjugated diene was assayed by Buege and Aust method. Total peroxide was determined by FOX2 method. Malondialdehyde determination was carried out by Flemming method and total antioxidant status was determined by Ozacan. Paraoxonase activity was determined by measuring the increased in absorbance of p-nitrophenol at 405 nm. Arylesterase activity was calculated from the molar coefficient of 1,310 M^{-1} cm^{-1}.

Results: Simvastatin significantly reduced total cholesterol, triglycerides, LDL, conjugated diene, total peroxide and MDA levels, where as antioxidant status was significantly increased. Interestingly, Simvastatin significantly increased PON1 activity towards paraoxon.

Conclusion: The results from the current study indicated simvastatin may have important antioxidant properties via increasing PON activity.

Key words: Hypercholesterolaemia, Simvastatin, Oxidative stress, India

Introduction

Atherosclerosis is the primary cause of cardiovascular disease (CVD) and coronary heart disease (CHD). It is a leading cause of global morbidity and mortality in the modern world [1]. Atherosclerosis is a complex multi-factorial disease. The oxidative modification theory for atherosclerosis postulates that oxidation of low density lipoprotein (LDL) is the key factor for this pathogenesis [2].

Oxidised LDL acts a chemo attractant for monocyte, transforms macrophage into foam cells. It exerts cytotoxic effects on endothelial cells, increases thrombocyte activation, and stimulates migration and proliferations of smooth muscles cells that lead to formations of atheromatous lesions [2, 3]. Several potentially anti-atherogenic mechanisms have been associated with HDL. These include both the protection of LDL against oxidation and attenuation of the biological activity of Ox-LDL [4, 5, 6]. Antioxidant and anti-atherogenic properties of a HDL are noticed from associated enzyme, paraoxonase1 (PON1). Numerous studies have indicated that PON1 is largely responsible for HDL's anti-oxidative property [7,8,9].

Moreover recent findings of two new PON members, PON2 and PON3 also showed the protective role to oxidative stress in tissues and plasma [10, 11]. Paraoxonase 1(PON1) is a calcium dependent ester hydrolase which is primarily synthesized in liver and associated with HDL in the plasma [12,13,14]. PON1 inhibits LDL and HDL from oxidative modification and also scavenges oxidized phospholipids from LDL [7,8,15]. Moreover, various clinical epidemiological studies demonstrated that PON1 enzyme activity was inversely related to the risk of CHD and CVD [16, 17,18, 19].

On the basis of clinical trial evidence, the most commonly prescribed lipid modifying therapies are the hydroxymethylglutaryl coenzyme A (HMG-CoA) reductase inhibitors, more commonly known as statin. Competitive inhibition of this enzyme by the statin decreases hepatocyte cholesterol synthesis [20]. Statin also shows beneficial effect on other lipid parameters, including increases in HDL and decreases in TG. In general, statin is regarded as a remarkably safe and well tolerated class of drugs. Seven statins are now approved for clinical uses, which are simvastatin, cerivastatin, fluvastatin, lovastatin, pravastatin, atorvastatin and pitavastatin [20]. Though they all have a common function, but differ in term of chemical structures, pharmacokinetic profiles, and lipid modifying efficacy [21]. Simvastatin decreases serum cholesterol by reducing the production and increasing its rate of removal from the body [22]. It also reduces TC, LDL and TG levels and increases HDL levels. Simvastatin acts as an antioxidants, either directly or indirectly and may have beneficial effect on atherosclerosis apart from their effect on serum TC, it also involve in modifying endothelial functions.

The objectives of the present study was:

1. To determine the effect of Simvastatin treatment of lipid profile and oxidative stress in hypercholesterolaemic Indian population.

2. To determine the effect of Simvastatin treatment on the activity of PON in hypercholesterolaemic Indian population.

Materials and Methods

The blood samples were obtained from hypercholesterolaemic subjects with total cholesterol (TC) and low density lipoprotein (LDL) levels >240 mg/dl and >170 mg/

dl, respectively. All subjects were undergone medical check-up at the Department of Cardiology, and were screened for medical history. The anthropometric measurements included weight, height, waist and hip circumference. Blood pressure was also measured. Clinical laboratory investigations included a complete blood cell count, blood urea nitrogen, creatinine, fasting blood sugar, liver function tests, and lipid profile analysis. A pre-tested questionnaire was used to collect information regarding medical history, smoking, and alcohol consumption from the participants.

The study was ethically cleared from the Institutional Ethical Committee. All participants signed the informed consent form before being enrolled for the study.

Study design

Simvastatin 10mg /day was administered, in hypercholesterolaemic subjects having TC >240 mg/dl and LDL >170 mg/dl. After screening visit to determine possible eligibility, participants entered four months active treatment period to receive Simvastatin 10mg /day. The outcomes were analyzed at 0 and 4 months after medication. After 4 months of Simvastatin treatment, hypercholesterolemia subjects were interviewed physically examined, and laboratory investigations including liver function tests (alanine aminotransaminase, ALT and aspartate amino transaminase, AST) were measured for any possible side effects. The drug was discontinued if ALT and AST levels were more than 3 times the normal values.

The study design included screening of hypercholesterolemia subjects with TC>240 mg/dl and LDL>170 mg/dl. Those subjects who entered this inclusion criterion were administered 10 mg simvastatin once daily for a period of four months. A blood sample was collected in the initial stage, and at the end of four months after the completion of completion of drug administration. The parameters analysed from the blood sample initially and after four months were, lipid profile, conjugated diene, malondialdehyde, total antioxidant status, oxidative stress index and paraoxonase activity.

Subjects

Fifty two hypercholesterolaemic volunteers with age's 30-49 y were selected for the study. Simvastatin was administered for four months.

Exclusion criteria: Diabetes, hypertension, hyperthyroidism, liver disease, renal dysfunction, history of myocardial infarction, coronary heart disease, cardiovascular disease, alcoholic, smokers were excluded. Pregnant and lactating women were also excluded. Participants taking hypolipidemic drugs and antioxidants vitamins were also excluded from the study.

Blood Sample collection

All volunteers were properly instructed to fast for 12 hours before the day appointed for venipuncture. Venous blood was collected two times, before and after 4 months of Simvastatin administered. Five ml of blood was collected in a plain tube without anticoagulant and was allowed to clot at room temperature then centrifuged at 3500 X g for 10 mins. Serum was aliquoted for total peroxide, TAS and PON1 activity determinations in microtube without BHT.

Lipid and Lipoprotein measurement

Serum TC and triglycerides (TG) were measured by using commercial available enzymatic kits [Randox Diagnostics, Crumlin, UK]. High density lipoprotein (HDL) was determined by the phosphotungstic acid precipitation method and LDL was calculated by using the Friedewald's formula.

Lipidperoxidation

Lipid peroxidation was measured for by three markers; conjugated diene, total peroxide, and malondialdehyde which corresponded to the extent of lipid peroxidation process.

Determination of conjugated diene (CD)

Conjugated diene was assayed as previously described by Buege and Aust [23]. Lipid was extracted by an organic solvent and evaporated to dryness, then it was dissolved in cyclohexane. A volume of 0.2 ml of serum was diluted with 0.3 ml of water and protein was precipitated by adding 1 ml of methanol. Lipid was extracted by adding 2 ml of chloroform and 3.0 ml of 0.05 M KCl. The mixture was separated and centrifuged at 3,150 X g for 10 minutes then 1 ml of bottom layer was collected and left for air dry at room temperature overnight. Conjugated diene was dissolved in 1.5 ml cyclohexane and measured absorbance at 233 nm by UV spectrophotometer.

Determination of total peroxide

Total peroxide in serum sample was determined by FOX2 method as previously described by Mustafa et al. [24]. Oxidation of ferrous ion to ferric ion by various types of peroxides contained within the serum produced ferric –xylenol orange complex whose absorbance was measured. A 100 µl of serum was mixed with 900 µl of FOX2 reagent. After incubation for 0 min at room temperature, the mixture was centrifuged at 12000 X g for 10 min. Thus peroxide was determined against FOX2 blank at 560 nm by spectrophotometer.

Determination of malondialdehyde (MDA)

Malondialdehyde determination was carried out spectrophotometrically by measuring the levels of thiobarbituric acid reactive substances in serum a previously described by Flemming et al. [25]. Thiobarbituric acid reactive substance formed in serum sample after a calibrated sample pretreatment procedure primarily consist of MDA by a nucleophilic attack involved carbon -5 of TBA onto carbon-1 of MDA, followed by dehydration and a similar reaction of the intermediate MDA-TBA adduct with a second molecule of TBA which formed a red adduct with two molecules of TBA ($MDATBA_2$). A volume of 0.5 ml of serum was mixed with 2.5 mL TCA and incubated 15 min at room temperature. Then 1.5 mL TBA was added and mixed for 30 sec and incubated at 95°C for 30 min. The reaction was stopped by incubating in ice bath for 3 hours. Then 4.0 ml n-butanol was added and mixed vigorously for 3 min. The MDA-TBA adduct was centrifuged at 950 X g for 10 min and absorbance was measured at 532 nm. Tetra methoxy propane was used a standard.

Total antioxidant status (TAS)

Total antioxidant status was determined as previously described by Ozacan [26]. The reduced ABTS molecule is oxidised to ABTS·+ by hydrogen peroxide. Deep green ABTS·+ molecules remains more stable in 30 mM acetate buffer pH 3.6, while it was diluted with a more concentrated acetate buffer at high pH (0.4 M acetate buffer pH 5.8), the color was spontaneously and slowly bleached. Antioxidants present in the serum accelerated the bleaching rate to a degree proportional to their concentrations. The bleaching rate was inversely proportional related with TAS of the serum. The mixture of 1000 μl of reagent 2 was added to determine serum TAS by measuring absorbance at 660 nm after 5 min incubation.

Determination of PON1 activity

PON1 activities were determined by using paraoxon and phenyl acetate as substrates [27,28].

Paraoxon assay

Paraoxonase activity was determined by measuring the increased in absorbance of p-nitrophenol at 405 nm. The activity was measured by adding 20 μl of serum to 1 ml Tris buffer (100 mM, pH 8.0) containing 2 mM $CaCl_2$ and 1.1 mM paraoxon. The rate of hydrolysis of paraoxon was followed by measuring the liberation of p-nitrophenol at 405 nm at 37°C over 50 sec after 1 min lag time with spectrophotometer.

$$\text{Activity} = \frac{(\text{OD/min}) \times \text{assay volume}}{\varepsilon \times \text{sample volume} \times \text{path length}}$$

The enzyme activity was calculated from the molar extinction coefficient (ε) of 18,700 M^{-1} cm^{-1} at 405 nm, pH 8.0. Activity was expressed as catalytic concentration (U/L) which corresponds to the product of 1 μM of p- nitrophenol/min/l of serum.

Arylesterase activity assay

The reaction mixture contained 1.0 mM phenylacetate and 0.9 mM calcium chloride in 10mM Tris-HCl buffer pH 8.0. The reaction was initiated by adding 20 μl serum which was pre diluted 1:20 ratio with 10 mM Tris-buffer pH 7.4. Increase in absorbance of phenol was followed at 270nm at 37°C using spectrophotometer.

$$\text{Activity} = \frac{(\text{OD/min}) \times \text{assay volume}}{\varepsilon \times \text{sample volume} \times \text{path length}}$$

The enzyme activity was calculated from the molar coefficient of 1,310 M^{-1} cm^{-1}. Activity was expressed as catalytic concentration (U/L) which corresponds to the product of 1 mM of phenol per minute per liter of serum.

Total protein estimation

Total protein in monocytes was determined by using Bradford method.

Procedures

Bradford protein assay is a dye binding assay in which a differential color change of dye occurs in response to various concentrations of proteins. A volume of 25 µl sample was mixed with 1 ml of Bradford reagent and incubated at room temperature for 5 min. Total protein was determined at 595 nm by spectrophotometer. Bovine serum albumin was used to make a standard curve.

Results

A total of fifty two hypercholesterolaemic subjects were recruited for the study. Forty-nine of fifty two patients (94.23 %) completed the study. The withdrawal rate in this study was 5.76 % (3/52). Simvastatin treatment was well tolerated and none of the patients experienced serious adverse effects in this study. Three patients discontinued treatment due to loss of follow up.

Demographic characteristics

The demographic characteristics of hypercholesterolaemic subjects are presented in **Table 1**. The mean age was 57.7 years. The study population had a greater proportion of female than male. Out of 52 patients, males were 18 (36.4%) and females were 34 (63.6%). The mean of body mass index (BMI), waist-hip ratio (WHR), systolic blood pressure (SBP), diastolic blood pressure (DBP), fasting blood sugar (FBS) of baseline were 25 ± 3.7 kg/m^2, 0.85 ± 0.1, 132 ± 17.8 mmHg, 80 ± 11.9 mmHg, and 103 ± 9 mg/dl, respectively. As shown in **Table 1**, there were no significant changes in demographic characteristics after 4 months of Simvastatin treatment.

Baseline lipid, Conjugated diene (CD), total peroxide, malondialdehyde (MDA), total antioxidant status (TAS), and oxidative stress index (OSI) levels.

Table 1. Demographic characteristic of study subjects from baseline to four months.

Parameters	Hypercholesterolaemic subjects (n=52)		
	Baseline	3 months	P
Age (years)	57.7 ± 7.4	58.0 ± 7.4	NS
BMI (kg/m2)	25 ± 3.7	26.6 ± 3.4	NS
Waist-hip ratio	0.85 ± 0.1	0.85 ± 0.9	NS
SBP (mmHg)	132 ± 17.8	132 ± 25.4	NS
DBP (mmHg)	80 ± 11.9	74 ± 11.8	NS
FBS (mg/dl)	103 ± 9	108 ± 10	NS

Table 2. Serum lipid parameters at baseline and 4 month after Simvastatin treatment.

Parameters	Hypercholesterolaemic subjects (n=52)		
	Baseline	3 months	P
TC (mg/dl) % Change	254 ± 40	199 ± 36	<0.001 - 24.5%
TG (mg/dl) % Change	185 ± 20	141 ± 15	<0.05 - 24.4%
HDL (mg/dl) % Change	50.1 ± 12.5	50.4 ± 9.2	NS + 3.31%
LDL (mg/dl) % Change	158 ± 32	118 ± 27	<0.001 - 22.4%

Values are shown in mean ± SD.
% change is the mean % change from individual patients.

Table 3. Serum CD, total peroxide, MDA, TAS, and OSI levels at baseline and 4 month after Simvastatin treatment.

Parameters	Hypercholesterolaemic subjects (n= 52)		
	Baseine	3 months	P
CD % Change	0.38 ± 0.06	0.34 ± 0.05	<0.05 - 4.4%
Total peroxide (µmol H2O2/L) % Change	18.4 (13.6-26.6)	15.9 (11.1-24.0)	<0.01 - 13.0%
MDA (mmol/L) % Change	17.6 ± 2.7	14.8 ± 2.9	<0.01 + 27.3%
TAS (mmol Trolox Equiv/L) % Change	0.81 ± 0.14	1.01 ± 0.17	<0.001 + 27.3%
OSI % Change	2.42 ± 0.73	1.79 ± 0.56	<0.001 -24.0%

Values are shown in mean ± SD.
% change is the mean % change from individual patients.

The baseline levels of lipid, lipid peroxidation parameters, TAS, and OSI of the study subjects were summarized in **Table 2** and **Table 3**. The mean levels of total cholesterol (TC), triglycerides (TG), high density lipoprotein (HDL), and low density lipoprotein (LDL) at baseline were 254 ± 40, 185 ± 20, 50.1 ± 12.5 and 158 ± 32 mg/dl, respectively. The mean levels of CD, total peroxide, MDA, TAS, and OSI at baseline were 0.38 ± 0.06, 18.4 (13.6-26.6) µmol H_2O_2/l, 17.6 ± 2.7 mmol/l., 0.81 ± 0.14 mmol/l Trolox equivalent /l and 2.42 ± 0.73, respectively.

Effect of Simvastatin on lipid, Conjugated diene, total peroxide, malondialdehyde, total antioxidant status, and oxidative stress index levels

As shown in **Table 2** and **Table 3**, Simvastatin treatment significantly decreased TC, TG, LDL, CD, total peroxide, MDA, and OSI levels by 24.5%, 24.4%, 22.4%, 4.4%, 13.0%, 15.2% and 24.0%, respectively.

Meanwhile, the mean TAS level significantly increased by 27.3%, however, there was no significant difference in level of HDL at 3 months treatment of Simvastatin (50.4 ± 9.2 mg/dl) when compared with the baseline level (50.1 ± 12.5 mg/dl).

Table 4. PON1 activity at baseline and 4 month after Simvastatin treatment.

Parameters	Hypercholesterolaemic subjects (n= 52)		
PON activity	Baseine	3 months	P
PON 1 levels Paraoxon hydrolysis (µmol/min/ml) % Change	178 ± 77	196 ± 90	<0.05 13.4%
Phenyl acetate hydrolysis (mmol/min/ml) % Change	142 ± 25	145 ± 33	NS 1.35%

The percent (%) change of LDL was positively correlated with % change of TC (R^2=0.63, P>0.05). There was no correlation between % change of TAS and % change of LDL (R^2=0.15, P>0.05). High density lipoprotein level did not increase significantly by Simvastatin treatment and the % change of HDL level was not correlated with change of lipid peroxidation parameter (R^2=0.05).

Basal level of PON1 activity

PON1 activities towards paraoxon and phenylacetate is presented in **Table 4**. The mean levels of PON1 activities towards paraoxon and phenyl acetate were 178 ± 77 µmol/min/ml and 142 ± 25 mmol/min/ml respectively.

Effect of Simvastatin on PON1 activity

As shown in **Table 4** and **Table 5**, there was significant increase in PON1 activity towards paraoxon (+ 13.4%, P<0.05) but PON1 activity towards phenylacetate did not change significantly (+ 1.35%, P>0.05) after 3 month of Simvastatin treatment. How ever, in male slightly significant increase in PON1 activity toward phenyl acetate was observed (P=0.04, **Table 5**). In this study, we found non-significant difference of baseline PON1 activity towards paraoxon between male and female but, PON1 activity towards phenyl acetate was significantly different between male and female (P=0.03, **Table 6**).

The percent change of PON1 activity towards paraoxon was positively correlated with % change of TAS (R^2= 0.30). The very strong positive correlation between % change of PON1 activity towards paraoxon.

Discussion

Oxidative modification of low density lipoprotein is believed to be the underlying cause in pathogenesis of atherosclerosis [2]. With this concept the prevention of atherosclerosis and its consequence could be limited by reducing the ox-LDL levels and oxidative stress. Simvastatin is used as a drug of choice for reducing lipid in hypercholesterolaemic patients. Moreover, Liao and colleague reported that simvastatin exerts beneficial cardiovascular effect independent of their lipid lowering property [29], might be due to its antioxidant properties [30]. In the current study, four months of simvastatin administration on hypercholesterolaemic subjects significantly reduced total cholesterol (TC), triglycerides (TG), and low density lipoprotein (LDL). The reduction of lipid parameters can be explained on the basis of inhibitory effect on hydroxymethylglutaryl coenzyme A (HMG-CoA) reductase by simvastatin, the rate limiting step in *de novo* cholesterol synthesis. This pathway decreases hepatocytes cholesterol synthesis and subsequently clear the LDL from the circulation by LDL receptor of hepatocytes cell surface. The effect of simvastatin in lowering TC, TG, and LDL levels obtained in our study were similar to those described by elsewhere [31,32]. It has been reported that simvastatin also has beneficial effect of raising HDL levels by unknown mechanism(s) [33,34]. However, the present study did not observe any rise in increase in HDL levels by simvastatin as previously reported by others [31,32]. These discrepancies may be partly explained by variations in the participants of the study, such as the severity of dietary control, exercise, genetic effect, patient behavior, and disease state.

Simvastatin exerts beneficial cardiovascular effect independent of their lipid lowering properties [29] and it might be due to its antioxidant effect [30] which is believed to come from HDL-associated enzymes, PON1. There are considerable numbers of potential pharmacological effect of various lipid lowering drugs on PON activity. The increase in serum PON1 activity by statin is still unclear due to the disagreement of results from earlier studies. In this study, simvastatin significantly increased PON1 activity towards paraoxon (P<0.05), however, there was a non-significant trend for the increase in the PON1 activity towards phenyl acetate (P=0.24). Similar results were observed in simvastatin treatment that was studied by Tomas and colleague [35]. PON1 activity has been shown to be substrate dependent and may show varied results for different substrates [36]. Paraoxon is the most commonly used substrate for the determination of PON1 activity and this level of enzyme activity has been shown to reflect the antioxidant capacity of the enzyme [37]. At the baseline, PON1 activity towards paraxon was unaffected by the differences in sex but PON1 activity towards phenyl acetate was significantly higher in male than females (P=004). After four months of simvastatin treatment, PON1 activity towards phenyl acetate significantly increased in male subjects (P=0.03), but did not changed significantly in female subjects (P=0.76). It is rather difficult to explain this finding about mechanism underlying the differences, since the number of participants was less to make a meaningful comparison, which is a draw back of the study. Moreover, most of participants were menopause female and more clinical evidence is required to support the effect of simvastatin on sex differences. The significant increase in PON1 activity in the current study may be due to increased PON1 concentration. Recently, Deakin and colleague had demonstrated that simvastatin increased the nuclear sterol regulating element binding protein-2. This protein binds to the paraoxonase promoter and cause enhanced promoter activity [38]. The current study observed, after four months of simvastatin treatment, percent change in PON1 activity towards paraoxon was positively correlated with percent change of TAS (R^2=0.304), which indicates PON1 reduced the extent of peroxidation and reduces the risk of heart diseases. It is suggested that PON1 inhibits lipid peroxidation by hydrolyzing lipid peroxide and hydrogen peroxide. On the other hand, it possibly reduces oxidative stress and cause a reduction in the inactivation of PON1 and thereby leading to the increase of PON1 activity as observed after 4 months of treatment.

In the present study, simvastatin significantly reduced conjugated diene (CD) (4.4%), total peroxide (13.0%) and malondialdehyde (MDA) (15.2%), whereas, total antioxidant status (TAS) was significantly increased (27.3%). These parameters caused overall significant reduction of oxidative stress index (OSI) (24.0%). The effect of simvastatin in lowering CD, total peroxide, MDA and increasing TAS levels obtained from our study were similar to some previously reported studies [30,34,35]. The reductions of lipid peroxide markers imply that PON functions by hydrolyzing lipid peroxides since the level of lipid peroxidation markers are decreased where as total peroxides and MDA, decreased more than CD. However, the result did not provide enough clear cut evidence to show the precise mechanism since a reduction of lipid peroxidation could partly be due to an effect from the decreased in lipid levels. In this study, the results demonstrated clearly that simvastatin caused a significant reduction of OSI in hypercholesterolaemic subjects. It seems therefore reasonable to postulate that simvastatin exerts beneficial effect on CHD, a mechanism that is beyond its lipid modifying properties. This beneficial effect may have an impact on the prevention of CHD.

In conclusion, the present study shows that simvastatin increased the TAS and PON1 activities and decreased lipid peroxidation and oxidative stress. This might be due to antioxidant or pleiotropic properties of simvastatin. A clear understanding of the effects of lipid lowering drugs on non-lipid risk factors of atherosclerosis will be helpful for selection of optimal treatment according to risk profile of individual patients. The observations from the current study can be applicable to pharmacogenetics and also essential for the development of more effective therapy. However, strong evidence are needed to substantiate the findings of the present study.

Acknowledgements: The research work was self-funded and no institutions or any organization are responsible for any kind of funding and competing interest.

References

1. Lusis A J. Atherosclerosis. Nature 2000; 407:233-241.
2. Roland S and Keaney JF. Role of oxidative modification in atherosclerosis. Physiol Rev 2004; 84:131-1478.
3. Steinberg D. Beyond cholesterol modification of low density lipoprotein that increase its atherogenecity. New Eng J 1889;320: 915-924.
4. Kontush A, John Chapman M. Antiatherogenic small, dense HDL—guardian angel of the arterial wall? Nature Clinical Practice Cardiovascular Medicine 2006; 3: 144-153.
5. Steinberg D. Low Density Lipoprotein Oxidation and Its Pathobiological Significance. J. Biol. Chem 1997; 272: 20963-20966.
6. Nofer JR, Beate K, Manfred F, et al. HDL and atherosclerosis beyond reverse cholesterol transport. Atherosclerosis 2002; 161:1-16.
7. Thomas M. van Himbergena, Yvonne T. van der Schouwb, Hieronymus A.M. Voorbija, Lambertus J.H. van Titsc, Anton F.H. Stalenhoefc, Petra H.M. Peetersb and Mark Roesta. Paraoxonase (PON1) and the risk for coronary heart disease and myocardial infarction in a general population of Dutch women. Atherosclerosis 2008; 199: 408-414.
8. Marta Tomása, Glòria Latorrea, Mariano Sentía, b and Dr Jaume Marrugat. The Antioxidant Function of High Density Lipoproteins: A New Paradigm in Atherosclerosis Revista Espanola de Cardiologia 2004; 57:57-569.
9. Richard W. James, and Sara P. Deakin. The importance of high-density lipoproteins for paraoxonase-1 secretion, stability, and activity. Free Radical Biology and Medicine 2004; 37:1986-1994.
10. Aviram M and Rosenblat M. Paraoxonase 1,2, and 3, oxidative stress and macrophage foam cell formation during atherosclerosis development. Free Rad Bio and Med 2004; 37:1304-1316.
11. Ng CN, Wadleigh DJ, Gangopadhyay A, Hama S, Grijalva VR, Navab M, Fogelman AM and Reddy ST. Paraoxonase-2 is a ubiquitously expressed protein with antioxidant properties and is capable of preventing cell-mediated oxidative modification of low-density lipoprotein. J Biol Chem 2001; 276: 44444-44449.

12. Moren X, S. Deakin, M.-L. Liu, M.-R. Taskinen, and R. W. James. HDL subfraction distribution of paraoxonase-1 and its relevance to enzyme activity and resistance to oxidative stress.J. Lipid Res 2008; 49: 1246 - 1253.

13. Rosenblat M, L. Gaidukov, O. Khersonsky, J. Vaya, R. Oren, D. S. Tawfik, and M. Aviram. The Catalytic Histidine Dyad of High Density Lipoprotein-associated Serum Paraoxonase-1 (PON1) Is Essential for PON1-mediated Inhibition of Low Density Lipoprotein Oxidation and Stimulation of Macrophage Cholesterol Efflux J. Biol. Chem 2006; 281: 7657 - 7665.

14. Ng CJ, Shih DM, Hama AY et al. The paraoxonase gene family and atherosclerosis. Free Radic Biol Med 2004; 38:153-163.

15. Blatter Garin M C, Moren X, and James R W. Paraoxonase-1 and serum concentrations of HDL-cholesterol and apoA-I. J. Lipid Res 2006; 47: 515 - 520.

16. Agrawal S, Tripathi G, Prajnya R, Sinha N, Gilmour A, Bush L and Mastana S. Paraoxonase 1 gene polymorphisms contribute to coronary artery disease risk among north Indians. Ind J Med Sci 2009; 63: 335-344.

17. Robert Superko H. Cardiovascular Event Risk: High-Density Lipoprotein and Paraoxonase. J Am Coll Cardiol 2009; 54:1246-1248.

18. Boemi M, Leviev I, Sirolla C, Pieri C, Marra M, James RW. Serum paraoxonase s reduced in type 1 diabetic patients compared to non-diabetic, first degree relatives: influence on the ability of HDL to protect LDL from oxidation. Atherosclerosis 2001; 155:229-235.

19. Mackness B, Davies GK, Turkie W, Lee E, Roberts DH, Mackness M, Roberts C, Durington P, Mackness MI. Paraoxonase status in coronary heart disease: are activity and concentration more important than genotype? Arterioscler Thromb Vasc Biol 2001;21:1451-1457.

20. Michael S. Chemical, pharmacokinetic and pharmacodynamic properties of statins: an update. Blackwell publishing: Clin Pharma 2004; 19:117-125.

21. Davidson MH. Rosuvastatin: a highly efficacious statin for the treatment of dyslipidemia. Expert Opin Invest Drugs 2002: 11:125-141.

22. Istvan ES, Deisenhofer J. Structural mechanism for statin inhibition of HMG-CoA reductase. Science 2001; 292: 1160-1164.

23. Beuge JA and Aust SD. Microsomal lipid peroxidation. Methods Enzymology 1978; 52: 302-310.

24. Mustafa K, Ozacan E, Eylem S, Sahabettin S. Increased oxidative stress in children exposed to passive smoking. Inter J Cardio 2004; 100:61-64.

25. Flemming N, et al. Plasma malondialdehyde as biomarker for oxidative stress: reference interval and effects of life-style factors. Clin Chem 1997;43:1209-1214.

26. Ozcan E. A novel automated measurement method for total antioxidant capacity using a new generation, more stable ABTS radical cation. Clin Biochem 2004; 37:277-285.

27. Agachan B, Yilmaz H, Ergen A, Karaali ZE and Isbir T. Paraoxonase (PON1) 55 and 192 Polymorphism and Its Effects to Oxidant-Antioxidant System in Turkish Patients with Type 2 Diabetes Mellitus Physiol. Res. 54: 287-293, 2005

28. La Du BN, Billecke S, Hsu C, Halley RW, and Broomfield CA. Serum Paraoxonase (PON1) Isoenzymes: The Quantitative Analysis of Isoenzymes Affecting Individual Sensitivity to Environmental Chemicals. Drug Metabolism and Disposition 2001; 29:566–569.

29. Liao JK. Beyond lipid lowering: the role of statin in vascular protection. Int J Cardiol 2002;86:5-18.

30. Sardo M, Campo S, Bonaiuto M, Bonaiuto A, Saitta C, et al. Antioxidant effect of Simvastatin is independent of PON1 gene T(-107)C, Q 192 R and L55 M polymorphisms in hypercholesterolaemic patients. Curr Medical Res and Opin 2005; 21:777-784.

31. Rosenblat M, Hayek T, Hussein K, Aviram M. Decreased macrophage paraoxonase 2 expressions in patients with hypercholestrolaemia is a result of their increased cellular cholesterol content: effect of Simvastatin therapy. Arterioscler Tromb Vasc Biol 2004; 24:175-180.

32. Paragh G, Torocsik D, Seres I, et al. Effect of short term treatment with simvastatin and Simvastatin on lipids and paraoxonase activity in patients with hyperlipoproteinaemia. Curr Med Res Opin 2004; 20: 1321-1327.

33. Maron DJ, Fazio S, Linton MF. Current perspectives on statins. Circulation 2000;101:207-213.

34. Kural BV, Orem C, Uydu HA, et al. The effects of lipid-lowering therapy on paraoxonase activities and their relationships with the oxidant-antioxidant system in patients with dyslipidemia. Coron Artery Dis 2004;15:277-283.

35. Tomas M, Senti M, Garcia-Faria F. Effect of simvastatin therapy on paraoxonase activity and related lipoproteins in familial hypercholesterolemic patients. Arterioscler Thromb Vasc Biol 2000; 20:2113-2119.

36. Dragomir D, John T, Audrey S, Yoichi O, Roger S and La Du BN. Human paraoxonases (PON1, PON2, and PON3) are lactonases with overlapping and distinct substrate specificities. J lipid Res 2005; 46: 1239-1247.
37. Guxensa M, Marta T, Elosuaa R, Aldasoroe E, Segura A, Fiol M, Sala J, Vilaa J, Fullana M, Sentía M, Vega G, Mónica de la Ricae, Marrugat J, and the IBERICA study research group. Association between Paraoxonase-1 and Paraoxonase-2 Polymorphisms and the Risk of Acute Myocardial Infarction. Revista Española de Cardiología 2008; 61:269-275.
38. Deakin S, Leviv L, Guernier S, James R. Simvastatin modulates expression of the PON1 gene and increases serum paraoxonase: a role for sterol regulatory element-binding protein-2. Arterioscler Thromb Vasc Biol 2003;3:2083-2089.

Chapter 11

Serum TC/HDL-C, TG/
HDL-C and LDL-C/HDL-C
in predicting the risk of
myocardial infarction in
Normolipidemic patients
in South Asia: A case-
control study

Abstract

Background: Dyslipidemia the major cause of atherosclerosis are suggested to act synergistically with non-lipid risk factors to increase atherogenesis. Low-density lipoprotein cholesterol (LDL-C) is the main therapeutic target in the prevention of CVD. Increased triglycerides (TG) and decreased high-density lipoprotein (LDL-C) are considered to be a major risk factor for the development of Insulin resistant and metabolic syndrome. Although the TG/HDL-C ratio has been used in recent studies as a clinical indicator for Insulin resistance, results were inconsistent. The TG/HDL-C ratio is also widely used to assess the lipid atherogenesis. How ever the utility of this rate for predicting coronary heart disease (CHD) risk is not clear. We encountered myocardial infarct patients with normal serum lipid concentration so this study was undertaken to evaluate the usefulness of these lipid ratios in predicting CHD risk in normolipidemic AMI patients and to compare the results with healthy subjects.

AIM: The aim of the present study was to evaluate serum TC/HDL-C, TG/HDL-C and LDL-C/HDL-C in myocardial infarct subjects with normal lipid profile.

Setting & design: Lipid Profile was determined in 165 normolipidemic Acute Myocardial Infarction patients and 165 age/sex-matched controls.

Material & methods: Total Cholesterol, Triglycerides, and HDL-cholesterol were analyzed enzymatically using kits obtained from Randox Laboratories Limited, Crumlin, UK. Plasma LDL-cholesterol was determined from the values of total cholesterol and HDL- cholesterol using the friedwalds formula.

Statistics: The values were expressed as means ± standard deviation (SD) and data from patients and controls was compared using students 't'-test.

Results and conclusion: Total cholesterol, TC: HDL-C ratio, Triglycerides, LDL-cholesterol, LDL: HDL-C ratio were higher in MI patients (p<0.001). HDL-C concentration was significantly lower in MI patients than controls (p<0.001). Higher ratio of TC/HDL-C, TG/HDL-C and LDL-C/HDL-C was observed in AMI patients compared to controls.

Key words: TC/HDL-C, TG/HDL-C, LDL-C/HDL-C, Acute Myocardial Infarction, Normal Lipid Profile.

Introduction

Atherosclerosis begins in early life, especially in children and adolescents with high levels of low density cholesterol (LDL-C) [1]. It is recommended to conduct a full lipid profile on children and adolescents who present with a higher risk family history, including familial hypercholesterolemia, cardiovascular disease (CVD), Diabetes or early heart attack and stroke. Children and adolescents who are also overweight or obese should be screened.[2] Dyslipidemia the major cause of atherosclerosis are suggested to act synergistically with non-lipid risk factors to increase atherogenesis. Low-density lipoprotein cholesterol (LDL-C) is the main therapeutic target in the prevention of CVD. Indeed, more aggressive lowering of LDL-C levels by drugs and LDL-Apheresis is now being practiced in United States [3].

Dyslipidemia characterized by elevated TC, LDL-C and lowered HDL-C, is a conventional risk factor observed in myocardial infarction patients [4, 5, 6, 7, 8, 9, 10, 11]. Increased triglycerides (TG) and decreased high-density lipoprotein (LDL-C) are considered to be a major risk factor for the development of Insulin resistant and metabolic syndrome. Although the TG/HDL-C ratio has been used in recent studies as a clinical indicator for Insulin resistance, results were inconsistent. The TG/HDL-C ratio is also widely used to assess the lipid atherogenesis. How ever the utility of this rate for predicting coronary heart disease (CHD) risk is not clear. Since we have encountered myocardial infarct patients with normal serum lipid concentration, this study was undertaken to evaluate the usefulness of these lipid ratios in predicting CHD risk in normolipidemic AMI patients and to compare the results with healthy subjects.

Materials and Methods

Setting Design and Patients: The study consisted of 165 patients (123 men and 42 women) with AMI, admitted to the Intensive Cardiac Care Unit. The diagnosis of AMI was established according to diagnostic criteria: chest pain, which lasted for ≤ 3 hours, ECG changes (ST elevation of ≥ 2 mm in at least two leads) and elevation in enzymatic activities of serum creatine phosphokinase and aspartate aminotransferase. The control group consisted of 165 age/sex-matched healthy volunteers (123 men and 42 women). The design of this study was pre-approved by the institutional ethical committee board, and informed consent was obtained from the patients and controls.

Inclusion criteria were patients with a diagnosis of AMI with normal lipid profile. Patients with diabetes mellitus, renal insufficiency, current and past smokers, hepatic disease or taking lipid-lowering drugs or antioxidant vitamin supplements were excluded from the study. Normolipidemic subjects was judged by the following criteria: LDL <160 mg/dl, HDL ≥ 35 mg/dl, Total cholesterol (TC), <200 mg/dl; and triglycerides (TG), <150 mg/dl. [12]. Ten milliliters of blood was collected after overnight fasting for lipid profile.

Lipid profile TC, TG, and HDL-cholesterol were analyzed enzymatically using kits obtained from Randox Laboratories Limited, Crumlin, UK. Plasma LDL-cholesterol was determined from the values of total cholesterol and HDL- cholesterol using the following formula [13]:

$$\text{LDL-cholesterol} = \text{TC} - \frac{\text{TG}}{5} - \text{HDL-cholesterol (mg/dl)}$$

Results

Serum parameters in AMI patients and control are shown in **Table 1.** Total cholesterol, its ratio to HDL-cholesterol (TC/HDL-C), LDL-cholesterol, triglycerides was significantly higher in AMI patients compared with control (Table 1-2). Significant difference for HDL-cholesterol between AMI and control was observed (**Table 1**). On the other hand, LDL-cholesterol and its ratio to HDL-cholesterol (LDL-C/HDL-C) were higher in patients compared with controls (**Table 1**). No statistically significant difference was observed in TG/HDL-C ratio among patients with controls. Also, significantly lower HDL-C concentration was observed in AMI patients than in the controls (p<0.001). Lowering of HDL- cholesterol is a known phenomenon in MI subjects [11].

The analysis based on the ratio of TC/HDL-cholesterol, TG/HDL-cholesterol and LDL-cholesterol/HDL-cholesterol is shown in **Table 2.** Higher ratio of TC/HDL-C, TG/HDL-C and LDL-C/HDL-C was observed in AMI patients compared to controls.

Table 1. lipid profile in patients and healthy controls (mean ± SD).

Variables	Controls (n=165)	Patients (n=165)	P-value (95%CI)
Age	60.55 ± 3.98	61.84 ± 3.80	0.0037(61.26-62.42)
Total Cholesterol †	168.58 ± 12.16	186.44 ± 13.95	<0.001(184.31-188.56)
HDL-Cholesterol †	50.51 ± 6.78	41.27 ± 4.62	<0.001(40.56-41.97)
TC: HDL-C*	3.39 ± 0.36	4.57 ± 0.58	<0.001(4.48-4.65)
Triglycerides †	107.84 ± 11.51	128.96 ± 12.19	<0.001(127.10-130.82)
LDL-Cholesterol †	83.59 ± 11.95	119.37 ± 14.05	<0.001(17.22-21.51)
LDL:HDL-C*	1.90 ± 0.31	2.93 ± 0.51	<0.001(2.85-3.00)
TG: HDL-C*	2.17 ± 0.35	3.16 ± 0.49	0.3149(3.086-3.234)

* ratio † (mg %).

Table 2. Distribution pattern of TC/HDL-C, TG/HDL-C and LDL-C/HDL-C ratio in patient and healthy controls (mean ± SD).

Ratio	Controls (n=165)	Patients (n=165)
TC/HDL-C		
2-3	2.90 ± 0.09 (n=28)	-
3-4	3.44 ± 0.25 (n=129)	3.70 ± 0.20 (n=31)
4-5	4.19 ± 0.22 (n=8)	4.53 ± 0.27 (n=90)
5-6	-	5.26 ± 0.23 (n=44)

TG/HDL-C		
1-2	1.77 ± 0.13 (n=56)	-
2-3	2.38 ± 0.23 (n=109)	2.65 ± 0.27 (n=59)
3-4	-	3.42 ± 0.26 (n=99)
4-5	-	4.22 ± 0.19 (n=7)
LDL-C/HDL-C		
1-2	1.71 ± 0.17 (n=106)	1.86 ± 0.15 (n=5)
2-3	2.23 ± 0.21 (n=59)	2.57 ± 0.27 (n=81)
3-4	-	3.32 ± 0.21 (n=74)
4-5	-	4.11 ± 0.12 (n=5)

Discussion

The MI patients for the present study were selected with normal lipid profiles, but their mean serum TC concentration was significantly higher (p<0.001) than the controls (**Table 1**). Goswami, et al., in 2003 [14] conducted a study on lipid profiles of normal individuals in the age group 21-70 years in Kolkata. Their study observed mean TC to be 189.7 mg/dl which was 12.5% higher than controls (168.6 mg/dl) of the present study. Earlier studies conducted [15] on coronary heart disease patients with respect to lipid profiles compared to the controls. The mean serum TC levels observed was 196.6 mg/dl which was 5.3% higher than the present study, but no significant difference was observed.

A retrospective study conducted [6] on the association of modifiable risk factor among patients with CAD, observed higher TC (194.6 mg/dl) compared to controls, which was similar to the findings of the present study.

In a study conducted [16] on the lipid profile pattern in MI patients was 215.7 mg/dl which was 15% higher compared to the present study. Another study conducted [10] on lipid profile parameters in patients of coronary artery disease, observed a higher TC levels (206.2mg/dl) compared to the present study. In another study conducted [17] on lipid profile pattern in CHD patients, showed higher TC compared to the present study. Sivaraman, et al., (2004) [18] evaluated lipid profile in patients of acute coronary syndromes. The study observed higher levels of TC (199.8 mg/dl) as observed in the present study and the differences in lipid profile parameters was significant (p<0.001) when compared to healthy controls.

In another study conducted [4] on lipid profile in young patients with angiographically proven CAD. The aim of their study was to analyze the lipid profile in young patients with CAD. They observed higher mean serum TC levels and the differences was highly significant (P<0.001). The reported findings were coinciding with the findings of the present study.

Study conducted [19] on MI patients, observed lower TC 181 mg/dl compared to the present study. The difference in values was significant (P<0.05).The present study also observed a higher TC levels in MI patients and the differences was highly significant (P<0.0001). In another study [8] determined the lipid profile and their association with CHD in South Indian population. They observed lower TC (179.5 mg/dl) in CHD patients compared to the present study. Kharb [20] studied the lipid profile in AMI patients and observed lower levels of TC (179 mg/dl) compared to the present study. In another study (Das, et al., 2002) [21] determined the lipid profile in CAD patients. Their study observed significantly higher levels of TC (200 mg/dl) in CAD patients compared to the current study. The findings of the present study was also agreeable to the findings of the above mentioned studies where the present study also observed a significantly higher levels of TC in MI patients compared to the healthy controls even the present study all the patients with myocardial infarction were within the normal TC levels.

Observations of Serum High density cholesterol (HDL-C)

The mean serum HDL-C observed in MI patients in the present study was 41.3 mg/dl compared to the controls (50.5 mg/dl) and was significant (p<0.001). Study conducted [14] on lipid profiles of normal individuals in the age group 21-70 years in Kolkata. Their study observed mean serum HDL-C to be 52.9 mg/dl which was 28.1% higher than controls (41.3mg/dl) of the present study. The present study found the results to slightly vary from the observations of Goswami, et al., (2004) [14]. It could be due to differences in sample size as the previous study was conducted on a large population of 1396 subjects and with varied age from 21-70 years compared to present study where 330 subjects including patients and controls. Moreover our subjects had higher range from 48-69 years. Earlier studies conducted [15] on lipid profile pattern in coronary heart disease patients observed mean serum HDL-C was 39.5 mg/dl which was almost similar to the observed values of the present study and no significant difference was observed. A retrospective study conducted [6] on the association of modifiable risk factor among patients with CAD, the mean serum HDL-C observed in patients was 42.11 mg/dl was 2% higher compared to the present study.

The HDL-C levels observed in the present study are similar to those of the earlier studies conducted elsewere [16, 10, 18].

In another study conducted [4] on Lp(a) and lipid profile in young patients with angiographically proven CAD. The aim was to analyze the lipid profile in young patients with CAD. The mean serum HDL-C levels were almost similar to the findings of the current study.

Even the studies conducted [19, 8, 20, 21] also showed lower HDL-C levels in MI patients compared to controls which was similar to present study. The observations made from all the above mentioned studies in MI patients reveals that HDL-C levels is drastically lowered in MI patients which could be an additional risk for patients.

Observations of TC/ HDL-C ratio

In the present the TC/HDL-C ratio observed in MI patients was 35.3% higher compared to controls, showing 4.6 in MI patients and controls showing 3.4. The differences in the ratio between MI patients and the controls was highly significant (P<0.001) (**Table 1**).

Goswami, et al., in 2003 [14] conducted a study on lipid profiles of normal individuals in the age group 21-70 years in Kolkata. They observed the TC/HDL-C ratio 3.6 which was almost similar to the controls of the present study.

Earlier studies conducted [15] on coronary heart disease patients with respect to lipid profiles compared to the controls, the ratio of TC/HDL-C observed was 3.8 in MI patients which were lower than the ratio observed in the present study. A retrospective study conducted [6] on the association of modifiable risk factor among patients with CAD, observed TC/HDL-C ratio 4.6 in patients, which was similar to the findings of the present study. In a study conducted [16] on the relationship of plasma homocysteine and lipid profiles in MI patients, observed TC/HDL-C ratio 5.2 which was higher than the present study. Another study conducted [10] on lipid profile parameters in patients of coronary artery disease, observed TC/HDL-C ratio 4.8 which was almost similar to the ratio observed in the present study. Sivaraman, et al., (2004) [18] evaluated lipid profile in patients of acute coronary syndromes. The study observed TC/HDL-C ratio 5.3 which was higher than the ratio observed in the present study.

Study conducted [19] on MI patients, observed TC/HDL-C ratio 4.7 in patients which was similar to the present study. In another study [8] determined the lipid profile and serum antioxidant levels and their association with CHD in South Indian population. They observed TC/HDL-C ratio 5.1, which was higher than the ratio observed in the present study. Kharb (2003) [20] studied the lipid profile in AMI patients and observed TC/HDL-C ratio 4.6, similar to the observations of the present study. The ratio of TC/HDL-C is crucial in determining the risk of cardiovascular problems as observed from the findings of the above mentioned studies. These observations regarding the HDL-C and TC:HDL-C ratio thus emphasis the fact that despite subjects maintaining normal concentration of total cholesterol, low HDL-C and elevated ratio are more than adequate to increase the risk of developing MI. Thus an individual with normal serum total cholesterol concentration cannot be content of being free of cardiovascular problems.

Observations of Triglycerides (TG)

The Triglycerides (TG) values observed in MI patients was 129 mg/dl which was 21% higher than controls (107.8 mg/dl).Goswami, et al., in 2003 [14] on lipid profiles study in normal individuals in the age group 21-70 years in Kolkata, observed the mean serum TG (132 mg/dl) which was almost similar to the present study. Earlier studies conducted [15] on coronary heart disease patients with respect to lipid profiles compared to the controls. The mean serum TG observed in MI patients was 157.8 mg/dl which was 22.3% higher than the observed TG levels of the present study. In a study conducted [16] on the relationship of plasma homocysteine and lipid profiles in MI patients, the mean serum TG levels observed was 152.8 mg/dl which was 18% higher than the mean serum TG levels observed in the present study.

Sivaraman, et al., (2004) [18] evaluated lipid profile in patients of acute coronary syndromes. The study observed similar TG levels (125.9 mg/dl) compared to the present study. Study conducted [19] on MI patients, observed the mean serum TG in patients was 149 mg/dl which was 15.5% higher than the TG levels observed in the present study. In another study [8] determined the lipid profile and serum antioxidant levels and their association with CHD in South Indian population. The mean serum TG observed in MI patients was 140.5 mg/dl which was 8.5% higher than the TG levels of the present study. Kharb (2003) [20] studied the lipid profile in AMI patients and observed

12.4% higher levels of TG (145 mg/dl) compared to the present study. In all the above mentioned study it was observed that the TG levels were higher in MI patients compared to healthy controls and similar findings was also observed in the present study.

Observations of Low density lipoprotein cholesterol (LDL-C)

The mean serum LDL-C in MI patients was 119.4 mg/dl which was 42.8% higher compared to controls (83.6 mg/dl). Goswami, et al., in 2003 [14] conducted a study on lipid profiles of normal individuals in the age group 21-70 years in Kolkata. The mean serum LDL-C observed in their study was 115.6 mg/dl which was 30.4% higher than the LDL-C levels (83.6mg/dl) observed in the present study. The variations in the fining of the present study could be due to differences in sample size as the previous study [14] was conducted on a large population of 1396 subjects and with varied age from 21-70 years compared to present study where 330 subjects including patients and controls. Moreover our subjects had higher range from 48-69 years. Earlier studies conducted [15] on lipid profile pattern on coronary heart disease patients compared to the controls. The mean serum LDL-C levels observed was 117.2 mg/dl which was similar to the findings of the present study. A retrospective study conducted [6] on the association of modifiable risk factor among patients with CAD, the mean serum LDL-C observed was 130 mg/dl which higher 8.7 % higher than LDL-C levels observed in the present study. In another study conducted [16] on the relationship of plasma homocysteine and lipid profiles in MI patients, observed LDL-C levels to be 110.3 mg/dl which was slightly lower than present study. Another study conducted [10] on lipid profile parameters in patients of coronary artery disease, the mean serum LDL-C observed was 107.7 mg/dl which was also slightly lower than LDL-C levels observed in the present study. Sivaraman, et al., (2004) [18] evaluated lipid profile in patients of acute coronary syndromes also observed 15% higher mean serum LDL-C levels (137.1 mg/dl) compared to the present study. In another study [8] determined the lipid profile and serum antioxidant levels and their association with CHD in South Indian population. The mean serum LDL-C levels observed in their study were 113.1 mg/dl which was similar to the present study. Observations from the above mentioned studies reveal that the LDL-C concentration to be higher in MI patients compared to controls.

Observations of LDL-C/HDL-C ratio

The LDL-C/HDL-C ratio in MI patients was 2.9, which were 52.6% higher than controls (1.9). Goswami, et al., in 2003 [14] conducted a study on lipid profiles of normal individuals in the age group 21-70 years in Kolkata. The LDL-C/HDL-C ratio observed in their study was 2.2 which were 15.8 % higher than the LDL-C/HDL-C observed among the controls of the present study. Earlier studies conducted [15] on lipid profile among coronary heart disease patients compared to the controls, observed LDL-C/HDL-C ratio 3.0 which was almost similar the findings of the present study. A retrospective study conducted [6] on the association of modifiable risk factor among patients with CAD, observed LDL-C/HDL-C ratio 3.1 which was slightly higher than the values observed in the present study. In a study conducted [16] on the relationship of plasma homocysteine and lipid profiles in MI patients, observed LDL-C/HDL-C ratio 2.3 which was 26% higher than the observations of the present study. Another study conducted [10] on lipid profile parameters in patients of coronary artery disease, the LDL-C/HDL-C ratio 2.0 which was 45% lower than the ratio observed in the present study.

In another study [8] determined the lipid profile and serum antioxidant levels and their association with CHD in South Indian population. The LDL-C/HDL-C ratio observed in their study was 3.3 which 13.8% higher than the observed ratio of the present study. In another study [21] determined the antioxidants and lipid profile in CAD patients. The LDL-C/HDL-C ratio observed was 2.6 which was 1.2% lower than observed in the present study. Observations made from the above studies reveal a lower ratio of LDL-C/HDL-C is beneficial and it is indicative of atherogenic lipid profiles. The higher the ratio the higher is the risk of MI or any cardiovascular disease.

Observations of TG/HDL-C ratio

The mean TG/HDL-C ratio in MI patients was 3.2 which were 45.5% higher than controls (2.2).Goswami, et al., in 2003 [14] conducted a study on lipid profiles of normal individuals in the age group 21-70 years in Kolkata. The study observed mean TG/HDL-C ratio 2.5 in controls which was slightly higher than the ratio observed in the present study. The variations could be due to differences in sample size as the previous study was conducted on a large population of 1396 subjects and with varied age from 21-70 years compared to present study where 330 subjects including patients and controls. Moreover our subjects had higher range from 48-69 years. Earlier studies conducted [15] on coronary heart disease patients with respect to Lp(a) and lipid profiles compared to the controls. The mean TG/HDL-C ratio observed in patients was 4.0 which were 25% higher than the ratio observed in the present study. In a study conducted [16] on the relationship of plasma homocysteine and lipid profiles in MI patients, the observed mean TG/HDL-C ratio was 3.6 which was 12.5% higher than the observations of the present study. In another study conducted [17] on lipid profile pattern in CHD patients, the mean TG/HDL-C ratio observed was 3.9 which was 22% higher than the ratio observed in the current study. Sivaraman, et al., (2004) [18] evaluated lipid profile in patients of acute coronary syndromes. The mean TG/HDL-C ratio observed in the study was 3.3 which were almost similar to the present study.

Study conducted [19] on antioxidants and lipid profile pattern in MI patients, the observed mean TG/HDL-C ratio was 3.9 which were 22% higher than the observations of the present study. In another study [8] determined the lipid profile and serum antioxidant levels and their association with CHD in South Indian population. The observed mean TG/HDL-C ratio was 4.0 which were 25% higher than the current study. Kharb (2003) [20] studied the lipid profile in AMI patients; the mean TG/HDL-C ratio observed in their study was 3.7 which was 15.6% higher ratio than observed in the current study. In another study [21] determined the lipid profile in CAD patients, the observed mean TG/HDL-C ratio was 4.2 and it was 31.2% higher than the ratio observed in the present study.

References

1. Libby, P., Palangio, M. Clinical Insights in Lipid Management. Committee of Cardiovascular and Metabolic disease 2008 Vol 1: (12). Online publication released on May 12,2008 www.ccmd.org

2. Larosa, J.C., Chen, Ching-Ling C.Clinical Insights in Lipid Management. Committee of Cardiovascular and Metabolic disease 2008 Vol 1: (11). Online publication released on April 24,2008 www.ccmd.org

3. Moriarty, P.M. www.ldlapersis.org assessed on May 12th 2008

4. Mishra,T.K., Routray, S.N., Patnaik, U.K., Padhi,P.K., Satapathy, C. and Behera, M. Lipoprotein (a) and Lipid Profile in Young Patients with Angiographically Proven Coronary Artery Disease. Indian Heart Journal 2001; 53 :(5) Article No. 60.

5. Malhotra, P., Kumari, S., Singh, S. and Verma, S. Isolated Lipid Abnormalities in Rural and Urban Normotensive and Hypertensive North-West Indians. Journal of Assoc Physicians of India 2003; 51:459-463.

6. Achari,V. and Thakur, A.K. Association of Major Modifiable Risk factors Among Patients with Coronary Artery Disease –A retrospective Analysis. J Assoc Physicians India 2004; 52:103-108.

7. Mishra, A., Luthra, K. and Vikram, N.K. Dyspipidemia in Asian Indians: Determminants and Significance. Journal Assoc Physicians India 2005; 52:137-142.

8. Rajasekhar D., Srinivasa Rao P.V., Latheef S.A., Saibaba K.S., and Subramanyam G. Association of serum antioxidants and risk of coronary heart disease in South Indian population. Indian J Med Sci 2004; 58(11):465-71.

9. Rani, S.H., Madhavi, G., Ramachandra Rao, V., Sahay, B.K. and Jyothy, A. Risk factors for coronary heart disease in type II diabetes. Indian Journal of Clinical Biochemistry 2005; 20(2):75-80.

10. Ghosh, J., Mishra, T.K., Rao, Y.N. and Aggarwal, S.K.Oxidised LDL, HDL Cholesterol, LDL Cholesterol levels in patients of Coronary Artery Disease. Indian Journal of Clinical Biochemistry 2006; 21(1):181-184.

11. Patil,N., Chavan,V.and Karnik,N.D.Antioxidant Status in Patients with Acute Myocardial Infarction. Indian Journal of Clinical Biochemistry 2007; 22(1):45-51.

12. Executive Summary of The Third Report of The National Cholesterol Education Program (NCEP) Expert panel on Detection, Evalation, and treatment of high Blood Cholesterol in Adults (Adult Treatment Panel III). Expert Panel of Detection, Evaluation, and Treatment of High Blood Cholesterol in Adults. JAMA 2001; 285(19):2486-97.

13. Friedewalds, W.T., Levy, R.I. and Fredrickson, D.S. Estimation of the concentration of low density lipoprotein cholesterol in plasma without the use of preparative ultracentrifuge. Clin. Chem 1972;18: 499-502.

14. Goswami,K.& Bandyopadhyay. Lipid profile in middle class Bengali population of Kolkata. Ind J of Clin Biochem 2003; 18:127-130.

15. Burman, A., Jain, K., Gulati,R., Chopra, V., Agrawal, D.P. & Vaisisht, S. Lipoprotein (a) as a marker of Coronary Artery Disease and its Association with Dietary Fat. J Assoc Physicians India 2004; 52:99-102.

16. Yadhav, A.S., Bhagwat, V.R. & Rathod, I.M. Relationship of Plasma homocysteine with lipid profile parameters in Ischemic Heart disease. Indian Journal of Clinical Biochemistry 2006; 21(1):106-110.

17. Sharma, S.B., Dwivedi, S., Parbhu, K.M., Singh, G., Kumar, N. & Lal, M.K. Coronary risk variables in young asymptomatic smokers. Ind Med Res 2005; 122(3): 205-210.

18. Sivaraman, S.K., Zachariah, G., Annamalai, P.T. Evaluation of C - reactive protein and other Inflammatory Markers in Acute Coronary Syndromes. Kuwait Medical Journal 2004; 36(1):35-37.

19. Shinde, S., Kumar, P.& Patil, N. Decreased Levels Of Erythrocyte Glutathione In Patients With Myocardial Infarction. The Internet Journal of Alternative Medicine 2005; 2:1.

20. Simmi,K. Low Glutathione levels in acute myocardial infarction. Ind J Med Sci 2003; 57; Issue8: 335-7.

21. Das,S., Yadav,D., Narang, R. & Das, N. Interrelationship between lipid peroxidation, ascorbic acid and superoxide dismutase in coronary artery disease. Current Science 2002; 83:488-491.

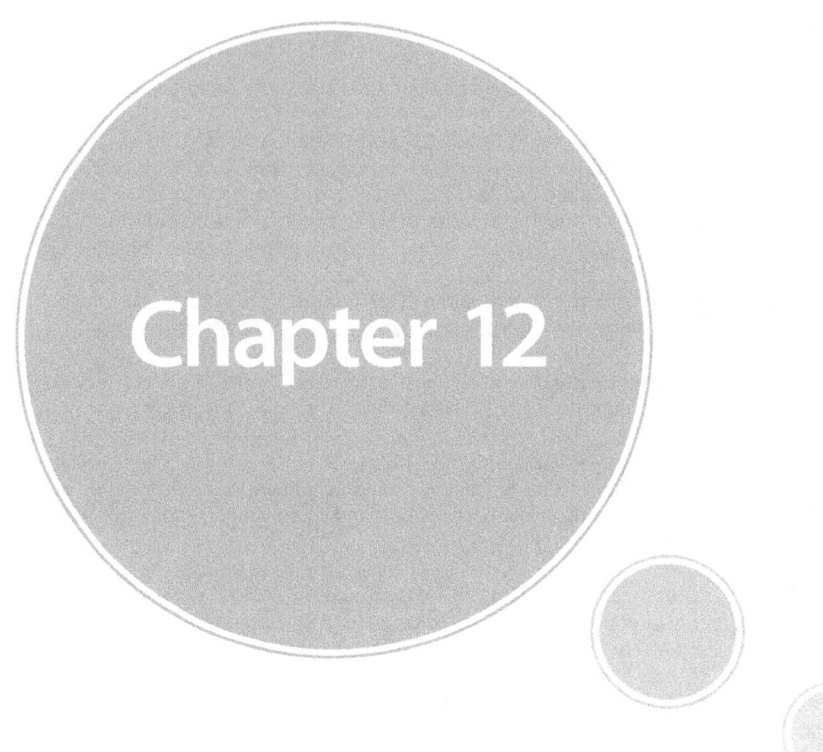

Chapter 12

The clinical utility of lipid profile and positive troponin in predicting future cardiac events

Abstract

Background: Diagnosis of acute coronary syndromes and cardiac events in the early stage of its onset is important in the line of treatment. The invention of highly sensitive and specific immunoassays for myocardial proteins such as cardiac troponin I (cTnI) had made it possible.

However troponin assay indicates the cardiac events only after its onset or after cardiac tissue necrosis has been occurred. Traditionally such high risk patients were earlier identified by using lipid profiles. The future risk and prevention of such coronary syndromes could be more beneficial as it will provide enough time to recover the patients from such irreparable damage.

Aims and Objectives: In this study we proposed to study the usefulness of traditional lipid profile levels in screening subjects who had developed chest pain due to cardiac event as indicated by a positive troponin I test.

Methodology: In this retrospective study data of the 259 patients presented to the emergency department with symptoms of cardiac ischemia who underwent both Troponin and lipid profiles tests were compared with the lipid profiles of 105 normal healthy subjects (controls).

The Troponin was detected qualitatively when a specimen contains troponin I (cTnI) above the 99th percentile (TnI >0.5 ng/ml). The Total cholesterol (TC), High density lipoproteins cholesterol (HDL), Very low density lipoproteins (VLDL), and Triacyl glycerol levels (TG) were also analyzed and low density lipoprotein level (LDL) was calculated using Friedewald's formula.

Results: Patients with chest pain and positive troponin test (with confirmed cardiac event) were found to have significantly elevated levels of TC, TG, LDL and significantly reduced HDL levels when compared to the patients who experienced only chest pain (negative troponin) and healthy controls.

Conclusion: Traditional lipid profile levels is still can be used in screening populations to identify the subjects with high risk of developing cardiac event which is identified by highly sensitive and specific positive troponin test.

Key words: Troponin, Chest pain, Cardiac event, lipid profile,

Introduction

The assessment of patients with acute chest pain of possible cardiac cause continues to be a challenge. The presence of ST segment elevation in the ECG is highly specific (but only about 50% sensitive1) for acute myocardial infarction (MI). However, many patients presenting to coronary care units have chest pain without ST elevation in the ECG. The diagnostic possibilities in these cases include: acute coronary syndrome in evolution, or 'non-ischaemic' chest pain.

The diagnosis of patients with acute chest pain of possible cardiac cause (MI) is challenging and positive diagnosis has psychological, social, and legal implications[1]. The World Health Organization definition, requires the presence of two of the following three features: symptoms of myocardial ischemia, elevation of cardiac marker (protein or enzyme) concentrations in the blood, and a typical electrocardiographic pattern involving the development of Q waves or persistent T wave changes[2]. Further the American Heart Association (AHA) case definition for acute myocardial infarction (AMI) requires an "adequate set" of biomarkers: 2 measurements of the same marker at least 6 h apart [3]

The traditional cardiac enzyme assessments for the detection of MI includes the triad of lactate dehydrogenase (LDH), aspartate transaminase (serum glutamate oxaloacetate transaminase, SGOT), and CK-MB which is of heart origin. However the use of biochemical 'gold-standard' CK-MB levels has limited prognostic power[1]. Hence, many patients occupy CCU beds unnecessarily, and others are discharged only to return with recurrent coronary events[1].

Assessment of proteins with smaller molecular mass such as Myoglobin, Heart fatty acid binding protein (Which is more cardio specific) has been developed. These appear more rapidly in the blood following the onset of necrosis and may have a specific role in the early detection of MI. However, neither of these proteins are considered as cardiac markers in clinical practice[2].

Identification of subjects with small areas of myocardial necrosis has become possible due to the development of specific and highly sensitive immunoassays for myocardial proteins, such as cardiac troponins T and/or I which are components of the thin filaments of the sarcomere[2]. Studies have shown that the magnitude of troponin elevations has correlated consistently with the risk of death and the composite risk of death or non-fatal MI, irrespective of whether the patients had ST elevation or non-ST elevation acute coronary syndromes [2]. Troponin I testing had better sensitivity, specificity and prognostic value than troponin T testing. A positive troponin I result was a strong predictor of cardiac events (death from cardiac causes or MI) in the next 30 days. The predictive value of a negative troponin I result was also high, with a total 30-day event rate of 0.3%, regardless of the admission ECG [1].

The new diagnostic criteria include a characteristic rise and fall in blood concentrations of cardiac troponins and/or creatine kinase (CK)-MB in the context of spontaneous ischemic symptoms or coronary intervention [2]. Cardiac Troponin I and T are highly sensitive and highly specific and may be elevated when CK-MB concentrations are not even mildly elevated. In addition, they may predict recurrent cardiac events in patients with acute coronary syndromes. However, use of troponin testing has been limited by availability of laboratory-based diagnostic techniques and by relatively long processing times [1].

Even minor elevations of troponin concentrations in the blood are indicative of myocyte necrosis and not due to leakage of proteins through the myocyte cell membrane. The current immunoassays assays for troponins T and I reliably detect cardiac (as distinct from skeletal muscle) forms of these proteins[2]. Furthermore, troponins have greater sensitivity and specificity for the diagnosis of MI in acute myocardial ischemia.

However it is important to note that, some patients who were diagnosed of MI did not have elevated troponins or CK values[2]. Some patients had died even much before the cardiac markers reach the threshold for detection[2].

Further troponin concentrations are found to be elevated in tachycardia, percutaneous coronary intervention, pulmonary emboli with right ventricular infarction, cardiac surgery, myocarditis, and renal failure, in which the cause of myocyte necrosis is not known[2].

In this study we proposed to evaluate the association between lipid profile levels of the subjects with chest pain with positive or negative troponin test.

Methods

In this retrospective study, the data of the registry maintained in the department of biochemistry of the Manipal Teaching Hospital, Pokhara, Nepal were analyzed. The WHO case definition [2]was used to retrospectively assign a diagnosis in 259 patients presenting to the emergency department with symptoms of cardiac ischemia. The inclusion criteria was the subjects (n = 259) who were admitted to the Intensive care unit of the hospital complaining severe chest pain and who were requested by the medical staff to get both Troponin and lipid profiles done.

In addition to that, reports of 105 healthy subjects who had got their lipid profiles checked using the Medicare facility were assessed as controls.

The Troponin was detected qualitatively when a specimen contains troponin I (cTnI) above the 99th percentile (TnI >0.5 ng/ml) mehod [4].The Total cholesterol (TC), High density lipoproteins cholesterol (HDL), Very low density lipoproteins (VLDL), and Triacyl glycerol levels (TG) were analyzed, using the kits provided by Human diagnostics and the low density lipoprotein level (LDL) was calculated using Fridewald formula[5]

All the estimations were done using HUMAN 300 semi-auto analyzer and data was analyzed using Epi Info windows version. Significance of the difference of parameters among different groups was analyzed using Z - test.

The reports of the subjects with any of the missing data were excluded. The selection of the reports was done without the prior knowledge of both the subjects and the staff of the intensive care unit, so that healthcare workers and the study subjects were not influenced anyway during the study. Therefore no written consent was obtained from any of the subjects. The ethical clearance was granted by the ethical committee of the Manipal College of Medical Sciences, Pokhara.

Results

Of the 259 subjects with the chest pain and tested for the presence of Troponin in the serum qualitatively, only 38 (14.7 %) subjects were detected positive. The larger proportion of the subjects (85.3 %) with severe chest pain was found to be troponin negative.

Initially, the differences in various lipid parameters among the subjects with chest pain and with or without a troponin were compared (**Table 1**).In addition to that these two groups were compared for the same parameters with those levels of normal healthy subjects(controls)

No significant difference was observed for age among the two groups of subjects (**Table 1**) However except for VLDL all other parameters of the lipid profiles were significantly different in two groups. Among the subjects with chest pain Total cholesterol, Triacylglycerides, low density lipoproteins levels were higher in the subjects with troponin positive than the subjects with a negative troponin Further HDL levels in the subjects with troponin.

The data of the **table** two (**Table 2**) shows the comparison of biochemical data of the subjects with chest pain and with or without a positive test for troponin against the healthy controls.

Of the subjects with chest pain, a significantly (P< 0.001) higher levels of TC, LDL and TG (P<0.05), have been observed in subjects with positive Troponin test, when compared to the healthy subjects (**Table 2**) and the subjects with a negative troponin test (**Table 1**).

Table 1. Comparison of lipid parameters of the subjects with chest pain and with or without a positive troponin test.

Variable	Subjects with Chest Pain (n=259)		
	Troponin –ve (n=221)	Troponin +ve (n = 38)	Significance P value
Age (Yrs)	58.06 ±13.55	56.21 ± 9.94	P = 0.209
Total cholesterol(TC)mg/dl	176 ± 46.17	221 ± 35.80	P = 0.001
Triglycerides(TG) mg/dl	148.20 ± 54.79	163.74 ± 48.22	P = 0.050
Low density lipoprotein (LDL) mg/dl	102.49 ± 44.29	152.26 ± 39.41	P = 0.001
High density lipoprotein (HDL) mg/dl	41.09 ± 5.68	36.82 ± 5.29	P = 0.001
Very low density lipoprotein (VLDL) mg/dl	29.51 ± 10.74	31.47 ± 10.09	P = 0.147

All values are Mean ± SD
Values in the parenthesis indicate the number of subjects.

Table 2. The comparison of lipid profiles of the subjects with chest pain and with and without positive troponin against healthy controls.

Variable	Control (105)	Chest Pain (259) Troponin	Mean ± SD	P* Value
Age yrs	55.84 ±12.61	P (38)	56.21 ± 9.94	0.436
		N (221)	58.9 ± 13.55	0.078
Total cholesterol mg/dl	182.24 ±52.59	P (38)	221.05 ± 5.79	0.001
		N(221)	175.9±46.17	0.134
Triglycerides mg/dl	158.08±58.89	P (38)	163.74±48.22	0.298
		N(221)	148.20±54.79	0.069
LDL mg/dl	105.31 ± 48.26	P (38)	152.26±39.41	0.001
		N(221)	102.50±44.29	0.301
HDL mg/dl	41.56±17.09	P (38)	36.82±5.29	0.047
		N (221)	41.091±5.683	0.356
VLDL mg/dl	31.39±12.09	P (38)	31.47±10.09	0.488
		N(221)	29.51±10.75	0.076

All values are Mean ± SD
Controls = Healthy subjects
Values in the parenthesis indicated the number of subjects.
P = Subjects with chest pain and Troponin positive
N = Subjects with chest pain and Troponin negative
P* = Significance between control and P and N groups separately

Table 3. The effect of sex on the variables in subjects only with chest pain. (when troponin is negative).

Variables	Males (145)	Females (76)	Significance
Age yrs	58.16 ± 13.67	57.88 ± 13.39	NS
TC mg/dl	173.13 ± 42.71	181.2 ± 52.0	NS
TG mg/dl	152.59 ± 60.05	139.8 ± 42.13	0.05
LDL mg/dl	103.58 ± 40.06	100.4 ± 47.00	NS
VLDL mg/dl	30.47 ± 11.77	27.67 ± 8.19	0.03
HDL mg/dl	41.16 ± 6.10	40.96 ± 4.83	NS

Further HDL level of the subjects with chest pain and positive troponin was significantly lower than the HDL levels of controls (**Table 2**)and that of the subjects with a negative troponin test(**Table 1**).

The effect of sex on having only chest pain (when troponin is negative) was evaluated and data are given in the **Table 3**. In the subjects with chest pain which is not due to cardiac event as indicated by negative troponin test a significantly greater levels were observed for TG and for VLDL in males than in females. However all these parameters were within the normal levels. The all other parameters including TC, LDL and HDL levels were the same for both sexes.

The effect of sex of the subjects in having chest pain with a positive Troponin ie chest pain due to cardiac event, was not evaluated as the numbers are not sufficient.

Discussion

In a previous study of subjects with chest pain it was reported that troponin was positive in 160 subjects (31.9%) and negative in 323 (64.3%) subjects[3]. They also reported higher incidence of Acute Myocardial Infarction, Acute heart failure, and death due to cardiac event in the subjects with chest pain and positive troponin confirming that it is a powerful, independent and valuable tool for risk stratification in patients with acute chest pain. Our data indicated that, of the subjects with chest pain (259) only 38 subjects (14.7%) were detected positive and a larger proportion of subjects (85.3%) were detected negative for troponin. Accordingly, those thirty eight subjects with chest pain are at high risk of developing cardiac event though the incidence of cardiac event is lower (14.7%).

It is well known that increased levels of low density lipoproteins (LDL), Triacylglycerides (TG) and total cholesterol (TC) and decreased levels of high density lipoproteins (HDL) are also indicative of increased incidence of cardiac events and are considered as risk factors[6]. Therefore in this retrospective study the relationship between levels of lipid profile parameters and the results of troponin test in predicting cardiac events was evaluated.

The mean TC level of the subjects with positive troponin (221 ± 35.8 (38)) was well above the recommended desirable level (< 200 mg /dl)[6] thus indicating those subjects are susceptible to develop cardiac event. The level of total cholesterol of the subjects with negative troponin test but with chest pain (176 ± 46.17 (221)) was significantly lower than that of the subjects with positive troponin above confirming the importance of maintaining total cholesterol levels below the recommended level[6].

Similarly the mean TG level of the subjects with positive troponin (163.74 ± 48.22 (38)) was well above the both the recommended desirable level[6] (< 150 mg /dl) and the level of TG of the subjects with negative troponin test but with chest pain (148.20 ± 54.79(221)).Further the TG level of the subjects with only chest pain was slightly lower than the recommended safe level.

Increased level of LDL is highly atherogenic as it could get oxidized and initiates the atheroma formation. Thus it is believed that increased level of LDL than the recommended level is a high risk factor in the development of cardiac event.The mean LDL level of the subjects with positive troponin (152.26 ± 39.41 (38)) was well above the recommended desirable level (< 130 mg /dl)[6].

Further the mean LDL level of the subjects with negative troponin test but with chest pain (102.49 ± 44.29 (221)) was well below the recommended level and confirmed the importance of maintaining lower levels of LDL in preventing future cardiac event.

Thus our data indicated that the subjects who developed chest pain due to cardiac event as confirmed by positive troponin test had significantly greater levels of TC.TG, LDL when compared to those levels in subjects without cardiac event as indicated by negative troponin test.

On the other hand lower HDL level (< 40 mg/dl) is also regarded as a cardiac risk factor[6]and the mean HDL level of the subjects with positive troponin (36.82 ± 5.29 (38)) was lower than the recommended safe level. This also indicates that the development of cardiac event was associated with reduced levels of HDL than the recommended level.

Further the subjects with negative troponin test (No cardiac event) had a mean HDL level above the cut off value suggestive of safe levels and that value was (41.09 ± 5.68 (221) significantly (p< 0.001) greater than the mean HDL levels of the subjects who had a cardiac event..

These lipid parameters were also compared with the values of aged matched hundred and five (105) healthy subjects without any known disease condition. All the values of lipid parameters are within the safe levels for healthy subjects indicating they were having a minimum possibility of developing any cardiac event. Only the mean TG level was slightly higher (158.08 ± 58.89(105) than the risk level of 150 mg / dl.

The total cholesterol level and LDL levels of the subjects with positive troponin was significantly (p < 0.001) greater than the healthy subjects and no significant difference was observed for TC between healthy subjects and subjects with a negative troponin test but with chest pain. However no significant differences were observed for TG and VLDL between these groups.

Significantly lower (P< 0.047) mean HDL level was observed in the subjects with positive troponin when compared to healthy subjects and the subjects only with chest pain but with negative troponin test.

These data indicated that the chest pain due to cardiac event as determined by positive troponin test is closely associated with elevated levels of TC, LDL, TG and also with significantly reduced HDL. However the comparison of lipid parameters of males and females in the sub group of negative troponin tests revealed (Table 3) that there were no major significant difference of those parameters due to differences in sex.

Conclusion

Therefore our data clearly shows that patients who developed chest pain due to cardiac event as confirmed by positive troponin test had lipid parameters in the risk levels as suggested by ATP III [6].Therefore the subjects who had lipid profile levels within risk level were at a greater risk of developing chest pain due to cardiac event. Thus it is advisable to screen and identify subjects with risk levels of lipid profile parameters and advise them to control their lipid profiles to maintain within the levels as recommended [6]

Lack of previously published research papers on the relationship between lipid profiles and troponin test for comparison and the fewer number of subjects in our study are the two major limitations in our study. Thus a larger study on this topic should be carried out in the future to extrapolate our observation to the total population.

Acknowledgment

We acknowledged the ethical clearance committee and the CEO and Dean of Manipal college of Medical Sciences for granting us the approval to carry out this study.

References

1. Alp NJ, Bell JA, Shahi M. A rapid troponin-I-based protocol for assessing acute chest pain. Q J Med 2001; 94: 687-694.
2. John KF,Harvey DW. Clinical implications of the new definition of myocardial infarction. Heart; 2004 January; 90(1): 99–106.
3. Macrae AR, Kavsak PA, Lustig V, Bhargava R, Vandersluis R.Palomaki GE, Yerna MJ, Jaffe AS. Assessing the requirement for the 6 hour interval between specimens in the American Heart Association Classification of Myocardial Infarction in Epidemiology and Clinical Research Studies. Clin Chem.2006 May; 52(5):812-8.
4. Alpert JS. Immunochromatographic Rapid Test for the Detection of Human Cardiac Troponin I in whole blood, serum.plasma.J. Am.Coll.Cardiol.2000, 36.959-969.
5. Fridewald WT, Levy RI, Frederickson DS. Estimation of the concentration of low density lipoprotein cholesterol in plasma without use of the preparative ultra centrifuge. Clin Chem. 1972; 18:499-502.
6. National Cholesterol Education Programme (NCEP) Expert panel on Detection, Evaluation, and Treatment of high blood cholesterol in adults (Adult treatment panel III). Third Report of the National Cholesterol Education programme (NCEP).Final Report. Circulation 2002;106:3143-3421.

Chapter 13

Study on lipid profile, oxidation stress and carbonic anhydrase activity in patients with essential hypertension

Abstract

Background of the study: The incidence of cardiovascular diseases (CVDs) is rising and it is predicted to be the largest of death by 2020 in India. Various epidemiological studies have highlighted the increasing incidence of hypertension which is assumed to be one of the major risk factor in CVD. Even though effective treatment measures have been extended against hypertension, still it remains inadequately managed.

Increased level of serum cholesterol, TG, VLDL has been observed in patients with hypertension. Considering the view points and the relationship between hypertension, lipid profile, carbonic anhydrase modulation in diuretic therapy and scanty literature reports in this region, the current study was focused to determine association of lipid profile and carbonic anhydrase activity in essential hypertension patients.

Aims and objectives: The aim of the present study was to determine the serum lipid profile, malondialdehyde levels and carbonic anhydrase activity in known cases of essential hypertensive patients and the results were compared with age-sex matched healthy controls in our community.

Materials and methods: One hundred fifty-six participants (107 males; 49 females) were enrolled for the present study with ages ranging from 32 to 66 years. Seventy patients were hypertensive (42 men and 28 women, 32- 64 yr of age) and 86 normotensive healthy controls (65 men and 21 women, 32-66 yr of age) were recruited for the study. Patients with essential hypertension were included in the study. Smokers, obese and patients on anti-hypertensive drugs for >3 months were excluded from the study. Also patients on lipid lowering drugs and antioxidant vitamin supplements were also excluded. Lipid profile, malondialdehyde levels and carbonic anhydrase activity were analyzed by standard methods in both groups of subjects. The data from patients and controls were compared by Student's *t*-test. Values are expressed as mean

± standard deviation (SD). Microsoft Excel for Windows 2003 was used for statistical analysis. *P*-value <0.05 was considered to indicate statistical significance.

Results: The lipid profile variables were significantly higher when compared to healthy controls. The differences were highly significant in total cholesterol and triglycerides, but not significant in HDL-C, LDL-C and VLDL. The study also observed higher levels of malondialdehyde in hypertensive patients (p<0.005) compared to normotensive controls. The carbonic anhydrase activity in hypertensive patients were also observed to be highly significant (p<0.001) compared to healthy controls.

Conclusion: Lipid profile is bound to alter in essential hypertension along with increased oxidative stress and is associated with increased activities of carbonic anhydrase activities.

Key words: Essential hypertension, Carbonic anhydrase, Malondialdehyde, Lipid profile.

Introduction

according to World Health Report 2002, cardiovascular diseases (CVDs) will be the largest cause of death and disability by 2020 in India [1]. In 2020, 2.6 million Indians are predicted to die due to coronary heart disease which constitutes 54.1 % of all CVD deaths [2]. Nearly half of these deaths are likely to occur in young and middle aged individuals (30-69 years). The contributing factors for the growing burden of CVDs are increasing prevalence of cardiovascular risk factors especially hypertension, dyslipidemia, diabetes, overweight or obesity, physical inactivity and tobacco use. It is an area where major health gains can be made through the implementation of primary care interventions and basic public health measures targeting diet, lifestyles and the environment.

In this area of thrust, one of the earliest study carried out in India, figured 4% prevalence of hypertension (Criteria: >160/95) amongst industrial workers of Kanpur [3].

Subsequently, Indian Council of Medical Research (ICMR) study was conducted in 1994 involving 5537 individuals (3050 urban residents and 2487 rural residents) demonstrated 25% and 29% prevalence of hypertension (Criteria: ≥ 140/90 mm of Hg) among males and females respectively in urban Delhi and 13% and 10% in rural Haryana.

Further, Gupta R [4] from Jaipur, through three serial epidemiological studies (Criteria: ≥ 140/90 mm of Hg) carried out during 1994, 2001 and 2003 demonstrated rising prevalence of hypertension (30%, 36%, and 51% respectively among males and 34%, 38% and 51% among females). In 2002, Hazarika et al [5] reported 61% prevalence among men and women aged >30 years in Assam.

Reports based from the above quoted studies justifies the prevalence of hypertension have been on the rise among Indians. It is known that obesity is a major contributory factor for increasing prevalence and longevity of hypertension. Even though effective treatment measures have been extended against hypertension, still it remains inadequately managed. Essential hypertension is the most prevalent hypertension types, affecting 90–95% of patients suffering from hypertension. Even though no direct cause has been identified itself, factors such as sedentary lifestyle, stress, obesity, hypokalemia, salt sensitivity, alcohol intake, and vitamin D deficiency increases the risk of developing essential hypertension. Risk also increases with aging, some inherited genetic mutations, and having a family history of hypertension. Insulin resistance which is a component of syndrome X, or the metabolic syndrome is also thought to contribute to hypertension. Recent studies have implicated low birth weight as a risk factor for adult essential hypertension.

Currently, gene therapy in the control of hypertension is being practiced. Over expression of vasodilator genes as well as antisense knockdown of vasoconstrictor genes has been successfully used in animal models of hypertension.

Hypertension is also associated with elevated reactive oxygen species and impairment of endogenous antioxidant mechanisms. Increased level of serum cholesterol, TG, VLDL has been observed in patients with hypertension. It has been shown that oxidized lipoprotein inactivates NO and aggravates hypertension. The association of carbonic anhydrase (CA) in hypertension is established and its changes in activities are obvious with altered metabolism, especially in hypertension, diabetes mellitus and hyperlipidemia.

Thiazide diuretic therapy used in hypertension can dose-dependently elevate serum total cholesterol levels, modestly increase low-density lipoprotein cholesterol (LDL-C) levels and raise triacylglycerol (TG) levels, while minimally changing high-density lipoprotein cholesterol (HDL-C) concentrations. All diuretics, including loop diuretics, cause these lipid changes. The mechanisms of diuretic-induced dyslipidemia remain uncertain, but have been related to worsened insulin sensitivity and/or reflex activation of the renin-angiotensin-aldosterone system (RAAS) and sympathetic nervous system in response to volume depletion.

Considering the view points and the relationship between hypertension, lipid profile, carbonic anhydrase modulation in diuretic therapy and scanty literature reports in this region, the current study focused to determine association of lipid profile and carbonic anhydrase activity in essential hypertension patients.

Aim and objective

The aim of the present study was to determine the serum lipid profile and carbonic anhydrase activity in known cases of essential hypertensive patients and the results were compared with age-sex matched healthy controls in our community.

Materials and methods

One hundred fifty-six participants (107 males; 49 females) were enrolled for the present study with ages ranging from 32 to 66 years. Seventy patients were hypertensive (42 men and 28 women, 32- 64 yr of age) and 86 normotensive healthy controls (65 men and 21 women, 32-66 yr of age) were recruited for the study. The study was pre-approved by the Ethical Committee of this Institution Review Board.

Inclusion Criteria: Patients with essential hypertension.

Exclusion Criteria: Subjects who were smokers, obese and on anti-hypertensive drugs for more than three months were excluded from the study. Also patients on lipid lowering drugs and antioxidant vitamin supplements were also excluded.

Sample Collection

Twelve hours fasting blood samples were collected from healthy volunteers and patients with insulin resistance. The patients selected for the study were registered in Out Patients Department (OPD) of College of Medicine & JNM Hospital, Kalyani. Ten ml of blood samples was collected from the participants, of which 5ml of blood was collected in a sterile test tube, allowed to clot and then carefully centrifuged at 3000 r.p.m for 10 minutes. Clear serum were collected and kept in - 4°C until tests were performed. Serum samples obtained were used for analysis of biochemical parameters.

Lipid Profile TC, TG and HDL-cholesterol were analyzed enzymatically using kit obtained from Randox Laboratories Limited, Crumlin, UK. Plasma LDL-cholesterol was determined from the values of total cholesterol and HDL-cholesterol using the following formula [6]:

$$LDL\text{-cholesterol} = TC - \frac{TG}{5} - HDL\text{-cholesterol (mg/dl)}$$

MDA Assay: MDA levels were estimated by thiobarbituric acid (TBA) reaction [7]. Using 40% tricholoroacetic acid, proteins were precipitated from 0.5 ml serum, and precipitated proteins were incubated with TBA reagent in a boiling water bath for one hour. After bringing down to room temperature, the colored complex formed was measured using spectrophotometer at 532 nm.1, 1, 2, 3-tetraethoxypropane (1 nmol/l) was used as a standard for MDA estimation. Concentrations were expressed in nmol/l.

Assay of Carbonic anhydrase activity [8]: The assay system consisted of 100 µl of sample (serum) containing 1.4 ml of 0.05 M Tris-SO4 buffer (pH 7.4) and 1.5 mL of 3mM p-nitrophenyl acetate. The change in absorbance at 348 nm was measured over a period of 3 min., before and after adding the sample. One unit of enzyme activity was expressed as 1 µmol of released p-nitrophenol per minute at room temperature.

All chemicals for carbonic anhydrase activity assay were obtained from Merck chemicals.

Statistical analysis: The data from patients and controls were compared by Student's t-test. Values are expressed as mean ± standard deviation (SD). Microsoft Excel for Windows 2003 was used for statistical analysis. P-value <0.05 was considered to indicate statistical significance.

Results

The findings of the current study based on essential hypertensive patients are summarized in **Table 1.** The difference in both systolic and diastolic blood pressure were highly significant ($p<0.001$) among essential hypertensive patients when compared to normotensive healthy controls. When lipid profile variables were compared, the result was highly significant in total cholesterol and triglycerides, but not significant in HDL-C, LDL-C and VLDL. The study also observed higher levels of malondialdehyde in patients ($p<0.005$) compared to controls. The carbonic anhydrase activity in hypertensive patients were also observed to be highly significant ($p<0.001$) compared to healthy controls.

Table 1. Baseline Variables in Patients and Controls (mean ±SD).

Variable	Normotensive (n=86)	Hypertensive(n=70)
Age (yrs)	42.4 ± 12.5	40.2 ± 7.8 †
Sex (M/F)	65/21	42/28 †
Systolic blood pressure (mmHg)	106.6 ± 13.4	166 ± 18.6‡
Diastolic blood pressure (mmHg)	76.7 ± 7.4	98 ± 8.1‡
Total Cholesterol (mg/dl)	146.6 ± 23.6	208 ± 20.18‡
Triglycerides (mg/dl)	135.2 ± 15.6	194.5 ± 19.3§
HDL-c (mg/dl)	45.4 ± 3.8	36.6 ± 4.8 †
LDL-c (mg/dl)	74.16 ± 4.5	132.5 ± 14.8 †
VLDL (mg/dl)	27.04 ± 5.1	38.9 ± 8.2 †
Malondialdehyde (μmol/ml)	1.83 ± 0.6	5.8 ± 1.8§
Carbonic anhydrase activity (μ mol/l)	4.23 ± 2.5	11.8 ± 3.6 ‡

† NS; ‡ (p <0.001); § (p < 0.005)
p ⃞0.05 considered significant by unpaired, two tailed, student's *t* test

Table 2. Analysis of Variables based on blood pressure (mean ±SD).

Variable	Group I (n=) Systolic (181.4 ± 16.5) Diastolic (109.4 ± 2.5)	Group II (n=) Systolic (156.8 ± 12.1) Diastolic (97.1 ± 2.5)	Group III (n=) Systolic (133.7 ± 19.7) Diastolic (88.5 ± 2.5)
Age (yrs)	42.4 ± 12.5	40.2 ± 7.8 †	40.2 ± 7.8 †
Total Cholesterol (mg/dl)	172.6 ± 7.0	192.1 ± 32.2 ‡	201 ± 30.5 ‡
Triglycerides (mg/dl)	177.5 ± 5.8	191 ± 118.1 §	209.1 ± 96.7 §
HDL-c (mg/dl)	39.8 ± 5.2	36.3 ± 5.3 †	33.6 ± 5.3 †
LDL-c (mg/dl)	100.3 ± 0.65	117.3 ± 3.3 †	125.6 ± 5.8 †
VLDL (mg/dl)	35.5 ± 1.65	38.2 ± 23.26 †	41.82 ± 19.34 †
Malondialdehyde (μmol/ml)	4.6 ± 1.4	5.3 ± 1.2 §	6.7 ± 1.5 §
Carbonic anhydrase activity (μ mol/l)	7.9 ± 9.9	9.3 ± 3.2 ‡	10.8 ± 3.5 ‡

† NS; ‡ (p <0.001); § (p < 0.005);

Figure 1. Carbonic Anhydrase Activity vs. Blood Pressure.

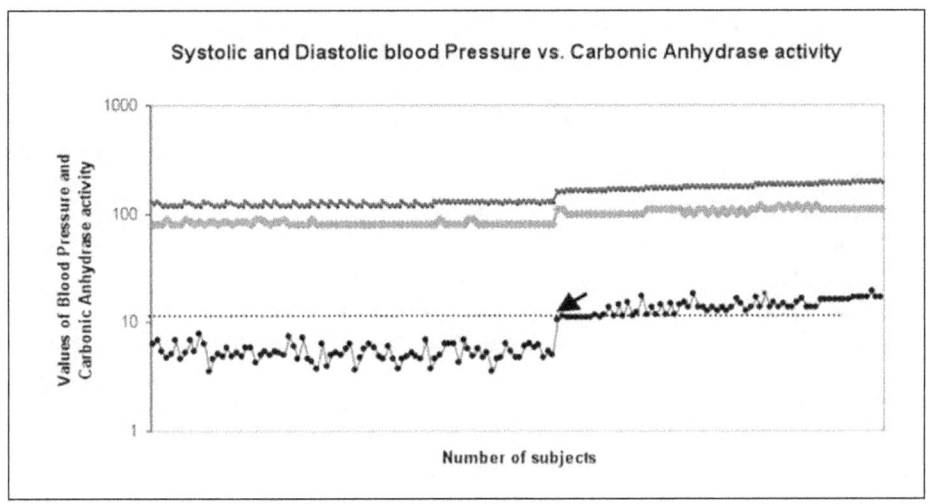

Discussion

The current study was focused to determine the changes in carbonic anhydrase activity and lipid profile accompanied by the measurement of malondialdehyde levels in essential hypertension patients. In the current study, we observed significantly higher ($p<0.001$) levels of total cholesterol and triglycerides ($p<0.005$) with a concomitant increase in serum malondialdehyde concentration ($p<0.005$) and carbonic anhydrase activity ($p<0.001$). It is commonly noticed that hypertension is associated with metabolic abnormalities and oxidative stress as observed in our study. Earlier studies conducted in India [9] also found elevated levels of total cholesterol and triglycerides in hypertensive patients as observed in our study.

Gambhir et al, 2007 also conducted [10] a study to investigate carbonic anhydrase(CA) activity in erythrocytes from normotensive and essential hypertensive subjects reported decreased CA activities in normotensive subjects compared to hypertensive ones, which does not conform the findings of our study where we observed increased carbonic anhydrase activity with increase in blood pressure. Researchers from Bangladesh conducted a prospective study based in the Northern region of Bangladesh, to investigate lipid profile status in hypertensive patients compared to healthy normotensive controls, revealed similar findings of elevated serum total cholesterol, triglyceride and LDL-cholesterol in hypertensive subjects compared to controls as observed in our study [11]. Another comparative prospective study was conducted in patients of type II diabetes mellitus (DM) with and without hypertension revealed a significantly elevated serum total cholesterol, triglyceride and LDL-cholesterol in hypertensive type II DM compared to normotensive type II DM subjects [12].

Another study carried out in Bangladesh to appraise the lipid profile in hypertensive patients also observed the similar findings as observed in our study [13].

Studies strongly associates hypertension and dyslipidaemia and both may add up to increase patients' susceptibility to the development of coronary heart disease.

Study conducted on Nigerian hypertensive patients found significantly higher lipid profile except for HDL-Cholesterol which strongly associates our study [14]. In another retrospective study based on Indians to estimate the prevalence of abnormal lipid profile in hypertensive patients. The medical records of subjects coming for a health check-up were screened for hypertensive subjects, found the prevalence of abnormality in lipid ratios in most (57%) of these subjects attending the regular check up which proves the association of hypertension with lipid profile [15]. Further study conducted in India on type 2 diabetes mellitus (DM) hypertensive males and females to evaluate the lipid profiles in them, observed the mean TC, TG, VLDL-C, HDL-C and LDL-C concentrations, TG/HDL and LDL/HDL ratios were higher in type 2 DM hypertensive patients compared with non-diabetic control subjects. The study also observed hypertensive type 2 diabetic females had significantly higher serum TC than hypertensive non-diabetic males. They suggested that hypertensive type 2 diabetic females are exposed more profoundly to risk factors including atherogenic dyslipidemia compared with males [16]. Another study conducted in Western Nepal on confirmed cases of hypertension to observe their lipid profiles and oxidative stress observed elevated malondialdehyde (MDA) levels and lipid profile compared to control which is in conformity with the findings of our study [17]. In another prospective study conducted in the Northern region of Bangladesh to investigate the serum lipid profile viz the level of total cholesterol (TC), Triglyceride (TG), HDL-cholesterol and LDL-cholesterol of hypertensive patients compared to healthy controls also revealed similar findings as observed in our study [18]. Yet another study conducted based on the objective of evaluating oxidative status, antioxidant activities, and reactive oxygen species byproducts in whole blood and mononuclear peripherals cells and their relationship with blood pressure. Sixty-six hypertensive patients and 16 normotensive volunteers as a control group were studied. In both, whole blood and peripheral mononuclear cells oxidized/reduced glutathione ratio and malondialdehyde was significantly higher, and the activity of superoxide dismutase, catalase, and glutathione peroxidase was significantly lower in hypertensive patients when compared with normal subjects. In our study, we observed malondialdehyde levels to be significantly higher in hypertensive patients compared to healthy controls [19].

In the final analysis it appears that essential hypertension are always associated with an elevated serum TC concentration and other lipid abnormalities. The major concern of this observation is that subjects also have oxidative stress due to abnormalities of lipids and its ratios. Therefore analysis of other risk factors associated with hypertension will be of immense important in the eventual assessment of the risk status as lipid abnormalities and oxidative stress results in future risk of Coronary artery disease.

Conclusion: Lipid profile is bound to alter in essential hypertension along with increased oxidative stress and is associated with increased activities of carbonic anhydrase activities.

What this study adds: The timely assessment of lipid profile in all cases of hypertension is a must as this would further aggravate disorders and risks leading to coronary artery disease. The determination of carbonic anhydrase activities in hypertensive patients is also important as it correlates with the degree of severity of the disorder.

Conflict interests: The author does not have conflict interest from the current study.

References

1. Ahlawat SK, Singh MM, Kumar R, Kumari S, Sharma BK Time trends in the prevalence of hypertension and associated risk factors in Chandigarh. J Indian Med Assoc 2002; 100(9):547-52, 554-5, 572.
2. Kumar A, Nagtilak S, Sivakanesan R, Gunasekera S. Cardiovascular Risk Factors in Elderly Normolipidemic Acute Myocardial Infarct Patients- A Case Controlled Study from India. Southeast Asian J Trop Med Public Health 2009; 40(3): 581-592.
3. Dubey VD. A Study on blood pressure amongst industrial workers of Kanpur. J Indiana State Med Assoc 1954; 23(11):495-498.
4. Gupta R, Gupta VP, Sarna M, Bhatnagar S, Thanvi J, Sharma V, Singh AK, Gupta JB, Kaul V. Prevalence of coronary heart disease and risk factors in an urban Indian population: Jaipur Heart Watch-2. Indian Heart J. 2002; 54(1):59-66.
5. Hazarika NC, Biswas D, Narain K, Kalita HC, Mahanta J Hypertension and its risk factors in tea garden workers of Assam. Natl Med J India. 2002; 15(2):63-8.
6. Friedewalds, WT, Levy RI, Fredrickson DS. Estimation of the concentration of low density lipoprotein cholesterol in plasma without the use of preparative ultracentrifuge. Clin. Chem 1972; 18, 499-502.
7. Bernheim, S,. Bernheim, M.L.C. and Wilbur, K.M. The reaction between thiobarbituric acid and the oxidant product of certain lipids. J Biol Chem. 1948; 174: 257-264.
8. Racker, E., in S. P. Colowick and N. 0. Kaplan (Editors), Methods in Enzymology, Vol. ZZZ, Academic Press, New York, 1963, p. 283.
9. N Lakshmana Kumar, Deepthi J, Rao YN, Deedi Kiran M Study of lipid profile, serum magnesium and blod glucose in hypertension. Biology and Medicine 2010; 2 (1): 6-16.
10. Gambhir, K K., Ornasir, J., Headings, V., & Bonar, A. Decreased total carbonic anhydrase esterase activity and decreased levels of carbonic anhydrase 1 isozyme in erythrocytes of type II diabetic patients. Journal Biochemical Genetics 2007; 45:431-439.
11. M S Saha, N K Sana, Ranajit Kumar Shaha. Serum Lipid Profile of hypertensive patients in the Northern region of Bangladesh. Journal of Bioscience 2006; 14: 93-98.
12. Alam SM, Ali S, Khalil M, Deb K, Ahmed A, Akhter K. Serum lipid profile in hypertensive and normotensive type II diabetes mellitus patients--a comparative study. Mymensingh Med J; 2003 (1):13-16.
13. Sarkar D, Latif SA, Uddin MM, Aich J, Sutradhar SR, Ferdousi S, Ganguly KC, Wahed F. Studies on serum lipid profile in hypertensive patient. Mymensingh Med J. 2007 Jan; 16(1):70-6.
14. Joseph Osagie Idemudia, Emmanuel Ike Ugwuja. Plasma Lipid Profiles in Hypertensive Nigerians. The Internet Journal of Cardiovascular Research™ ISSN: 1540-2592.
15. S J Joglekar, S L Warren, A T Prabhu, S S Kulkarni, A S Nanivadekar. Co-existence of hypertension and abnormal lipid profile: a hospital-based retrospective survey. Indian heart journal
16. Lorenzo Gordon, Dalip Ragoobirsingh, Errol Y St A Morrison, Eric Choo-Kang, Donovan McGrowder, E Martorell. Lipid profile of type 2 diabetic and hypertensive patients in the Jamaican population. Journal of Laboratory Physicians 2010; 2(1): 25-30.
17. Babu Raja Maharjan, J C Jha, P Vishwanath, V M Alurkar, P P Singh. Oxidant–antioxidant Status and Lipid Profile in the Hypertensive Patients. Journal of Nepal Health Research Council, Vol 6, No 2 (2008). doi: doi: 10.3126/jnhrc.v6i2.2185. Journal of Nepal Health Research Council Vol. 6, No. 2, 2008 October Page: 63-68.
18. MS Saha, NK Sana, Ranajit Kumar Shaha. Serum Lipid Profile of Hypertensive Patients in the Northern Region of Bangladesh. Journal of Bio-Science, Vol 14 (2006)
19. Josep Redón; Maria R. Oliva; Carmen Tormos; Vicente Giner; Javier Chaves; Antonio Iradi; Guillermo T. Sáez. Antioxidant Activities and Oxidative Stress Byproducts in Human Hypertension. Hypertension. 2003;41:1096.

Chapter 14

Assessment of lipid profile in patients with Human Immuno Deficiency Virus (HIV/AIDS) without antiretroviral therapy

Abstract

Background: Human immunodeficiency Virus (HIV) infection is pandemic world wide which are often associated with aberration of biochemical parameters like renal profile, liver profile, thyroid profile, thrombocytopenia and severe anemia with high erythrocyte sedimentation rate (ESR). Patients with HIV infection were reported to have hypocholesterolaemia with or without hypertriglyceridemia however the mechanism of decrease in cholesterol levels is not known. Keeping in view of the various biochemical abnormalities associated with lipid metabolism, our research was inclined to assess the lipid profile in HIV positive cases, with an attempt to further elucidate more features of HIV disease which erupts as acquired immunodeficiency syndrome (AIDS) linking any possible involvement of lipid profile in disease progression of AIDS.

Aims and Objectives: The aim of the study was the assess lipid profile in patients with HIV positive infection. The study was also aimed to correlate the variation in lipid profile with the CD4+ and CD8+ cell count and establish the relationship between the variables.

Materials and Methods: Ninety-one participants were enrolled for the present study of which forty seven patients were HIV positive patients and forty four were controls. The study was carried out at College of Medicine & JNM Hospital, Kalyani. Ten ml of blood samples was collected from the participants. The CD4 and CD8 lymphocyte count was estimated by Fluoresence Activated Cell Sorter (FACS) count system (Becton Dickinson). Lipid profiles were analyzed enzymatically using kit obtained from Randox Laboratories Limited, Crumlin, UK.

Results: The changes in total cholesterol (TC), HDL-C, TC/HDL-C and age were not significant when compared between cases and controls. Significantly higher levels of triglycerides, low-density lipoprotein-cholesterol (LDL-C), LDL /HDL-C, TG/HDL-C and CD4/CD8 ratio were observed along with decline in CD-4cells/µL, CD-8cells/µL (p=0.0001). Furthermore there was a strong correlation between CD-4cells/µL and TG, LDL-C. Also triglycerides and LDL-C level increased proportional to the increase in CD-4cells/µL.

Discussion: The current study didn't observed any changes in TC, HDL-C and TC/HDL-C ratio but significantly higher levels of TG, LDL-C, LDL-C/HDL-C and CD4/CD8 ratio with decline in both CD4 and CD8 cell counts in HIV positive patients were observed. Various study conducted elsewhere also observed changes in lipid profile but the changes observed in the current study was not similar to the observations of other studies. It might be said that CD4+ cell count and lipid profile can be a good index of disease progression in HIV infection and AIDS patients.

Conclusion: The changes in lipid profile can be a good index of disease progression in HIV infection.

Key Words: Lipid Profile, CD4 Cell Count, CD8 Cell Count, HIV positive patients and AIDS

Introduction

Human immunodeficiency Virus (HIV) infection is pandemic world wide.[1] Among Indians currently we harbor 3.7 million HIV positive cases which are further predicted to rise in future if successful prevention programs are not implemented.[2] Another factor which makes HIV positive patients ostracized is the social stigma and very often has difficulty in findings physicians who come forward to treat them.[3] Human immunodeficiency virus patients are often associated with aberration of biochemical parameters like renal profile, liver profile, thyroid profile, thrombocytopenia and severe anemia with high erythrocyte sedimentation rate (ESR). Patients with HIV infection were reported to have hypocholesterolaemia with or without hypertriglyceridemia however the mechanism of decrease in cholesterol levels is not known.[4] Studies have observed when HIV patients treated with protease inhibitors; they tend to exhibit hyperlipidaemia with increase in total cholesterol, triglycerides, low-density lipoproteins and concomitant decrease in high-density cholesterol.[5] Infections can increase serum triglycerides levels by decreasing clearance of circulating lipoprotein levels as process seems to inhibit the lipoprotein lipase activity or stimulating hepatic lipid synthesis through increase in either hepatic fatty acid synthesis or reesterification of fatty acids derived from lipolysis.

Keeping in view of the various biochemical abnormalities associated with lipid metabolism, our research was inclined to assess the lipid profile in HIV positive cases, with an attempt to further elucidate more features of HIV disease which erupts as acquired immunodeficiency syndrome (AIDS) linking any possible involvement of lipid profile in disease progression of AIDS. This current study is an attempt to examine whether any changes in lipid profile do take in HIV positive patients and whether those changes which are involved could be linked to the development of clinical AIDS with HIV infection. Thus the current study was undertaken to address whether HIV infection can affect lipid profile status in patients.

Materials and Methods

Ninety-one participants (49 males; 42 females) were enrolled for the present study with ages ranging from 21 to 45 years. Forty seven patients were HIV positive patients (26 men and 21 women, 21- 45 yr of age) and 44 healthy controls (23 men and 21 women, 21-45 yr of age) were recruited for the study. The study was carried out at College of Medicine & JNM Hospital, Kalyani for a period of one year from January 2010 till

December 2010 which was pre-approved by the Ethical Committee of this Institution Review Board. For diagnosis and confirmation of HIV infection we followed the National AIDS control organization (NACO) recommendation for HIV testing (NACO 2003). All the patients were subjected to detail history taking and clinical examination. The informed consent was obtained from the patients before enrolling them for the study.

Inclusion Criteria: Patients with confirmed cases of HIV infection without Anti-retroviral therapy.

Exclusion Criteria: Subjects who were smokers, obese and on anti-hypertensive drugs for more than three months were excluded from the study. Also patients on lipid lowering drugs and antioxidant vitamin supplements were also excluded.

Sample Collection

Twelve hours fasting blood samples were collected from healthy volunteers and patients with insulin resistance. The patients selected for the study were registered in Out Patients Department (OPD) of College of Medicine & JNM Hospital, Kalyani. Ten ml of blood samples was collected from the participants, of which 5ml of blood was collected in a sterile test tube, allowed to clot and then carefully centrifuged at 3000 r.p.m for 10 minutes. Serum samples obtained were used for analysis of lipid profile.

Cell count: The CD4 and CD8 lymphocyte count was estimated by Fluoresence Activated Cell Sorter (FACS) count system (Becton Dickinson)

Lipid Profile Total Cholesterol, Triglycerides and High density lioprotein-cholesterol were analyzed enzymatically using kit obtained from Randox Laboratories Limited, Crumlin, UK. Plasma Low density-cholesterol was determined from the values of total cholesterol and HDL-cholesterol using the following formula: [6]

$$\text{LDL-cholesterol} = TC - \frac{TG}{5} - \text{HDL-cholesterol (mg/dl)}$$

Statistical analysis: The data from patients and controls were compared by Student's t-test. Values are expressed as mean ± standard deviation (SD). Microsoft Excel for Windows 2003 was used for statistical analysis. P-value <0.05 was considered to indicate statistical significance.

Results: The changes in total cholesterol (TC), HDL-C, TC/HDL-C and age were not significant when compared between cases and controls. Significantly higher levels of triglycerides, low-density lipoproteins, LDL/HDL-C, TG/HDL-C and CD4/CD8 ratio were observed along with decline in CD-4cells/µL, CD-8cells/µ (p=0.0001). Furthermore there was a strong correlation between CD-4cells/µL and TG, LDL-C. Also triglycerides and LDL-C level increased proportional to the increase in CD-4cells/µL.

	Cases	N	Mean±SD	P Value
TC	controls	44	171.50±10.672	
	HIV	47	168.55±23.179	0.4
TG	controls	44	135.89±26.099	
	HIV	47	225.43±29.802	0.00001**

HDL-C	controls	44	51.59± 6.475	
	HIV	47	51.45±5.912	0.9
LDL-C	controls	44	107.80± 26.135	0.00001**
	HIV	47	145.30±23.888	
TC/HDL-C	controls	44	3.38±0.48	
	HIV	47	3.33±0.65	0.7
LDL/HDL-c	controls	44	2.13±0.61	
	HIV	47	2.87±0.60	0.00001**
TG/HDL-C	controls	44	2.67±0.58	0.00001**
	HIV	47	4.43±0.76	
CD-4cells/µL	controls	44	840.27±62.92	
	HIV	47	139.38±38.19	0.00001**
CD-8cells/µL	controls	44	547.23±47.77	
	HIV	47	66.55±17.15	0.00001**
CD4/CD8 ratio	controls	44	1.54±0.10	
	HIV	47	2.10±0.30	0.00001**
Age	controls	44	31.41±4.73	
	HIV	47	31.38±5.63	0.9

** Statistically Significant

Table 1 depicts that TC, HDL-C, TC/HDL-C and age were not having significant difference in comparison between cases and controls. But TG, LDL-C, LDL/HDL-C, TG/HDL-C, L and CD4/CD8 ratio had a significant elevation along with declination in CD-4cells/µL, CD-8cells/µ (p=0.0001). Further we analysed the data with correlation and regression. We found there is a strong correlation between CD-4cells/µL and TG, LDL-C.

Graph 1 shows that TG level increases proportional to the increase in CD-4cells/µL) and one unit increase in CD-4cells/µL ratio will result in 0.45 (Confidence Interval0. 26 to 0.64) units increase in TG level (R^2=0.34, p=0.0001).

Graph 2 shows that LDL-C level increases proportional to the increase in CD-4cells/µL and one unit increase in CD-4cells/µL will result in 0.54 (Confidence Interval 0.44 to 0.64) units increase in LDL-C level (R^2= 0.744, p=0.0001).

Discussion

This study included data on 47 HIV positive patients and 44 HIV negative controls. The study observed no changes in total cholesterol (TC), HDL-C and TC/HDL-C ratio. Significantly higher levels of triglycerides (TG), low density lipoprotein (LDL-C), LDL-C/HDL-C and CD4/CD8 ratio with decline in CD4 and CD8 cells in HIV positive patients were observed. Further more the TG and LDL-C levels increased proportional to the increase in CD4 cells.

Study conducted by Pashupati et al [7]observed significant reduction of CD4+ cells in HIV/AIDS compared to controls. Their study observed significantly decreased levels of

Graph 1. Correlation and regression analysis for CD-4cells/µL and TG.

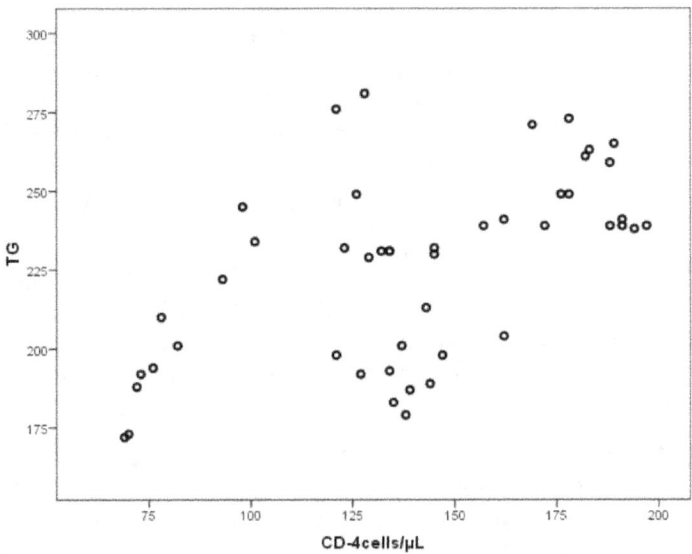

Graph 2. Correlation and regression analysis for CD-4cells/µL and LDL-C.

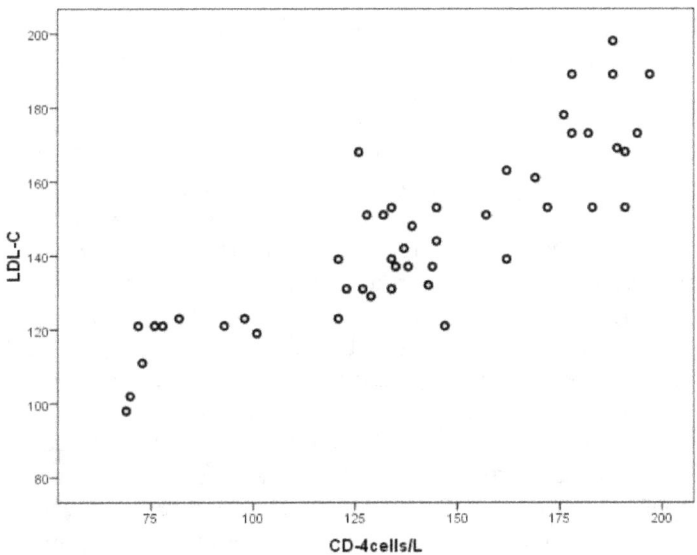

TC, HDL-C and LDL-C in AIDS cases compared to controls which does not conforms with the findings of the current study as we observed no changes in TC, HDL-C but significantly higher levels of LDL-C compared to controls.

Further study conducted (Khiangte et al., 2007)[8] on correlation between the changes in lipid profile and the progression of HIV infection also observed significant decrease in TC, HDL-C, LDL-C with concomitant increase in VLDL-C along with significant reduction in CD4+ cell count as the disease progressed gradually. The serum level of TG was found to be lastly affected. The observations made in this study do not conforms with our study as we observed no changes in TC and HDL-C levels in cases when compared to controls.

Study conducted (Adewole et al., 2010) [9] on the effect of antiretroviral therapy on lipid profile in HIV patients in Nigeria, observed significantly higher levels of LDL-C and lower levels of HDL-C in patients compared to controls, when the patients were on antiretroviral therapy. This conform the changes in lipid profile on administration of antiretroviral therapy.

Contrary to this report, study based on evaluation of lipid profile in AIDS patients with and without HAART therapy [10] observed mean TC, HDL-C and TG were significantly higher in HAART group compared to no-HAART group subjects. Another study conducted [11] on lipid profile assessment in Thai adult with HIV infection receiving protease inhibitors. They observed mean serum TC, LDL-C, TC/HDL-C and TG levels higher and lower HDL-C levels in cases when compared to controls.

In another study conducted (Obirikorang C, et al, 2010) [12], serum TG showed significant increase in the subjects compared to control group, serum total cholesterol (p<0.001), HDL-C (p<0.001) and HDL-C (p<0.001) and LDL-C (p<0.001) showed significant decreases compared to the control group. HDL-C in subjects' with CD4 cells between 200-499 mm^3 and CD4≥ 500 showed no statistically significant difference in comparison to control group.

Yet another study conducted on assessment of lipid profile in Switzerland (Young, et al., 2005) [13] on HIV patients subjected to anti-retroviral therapies and comparing their efficacies and advantages, also observed a better lipid profiles after commencement of protease inhibitors. They observed drastic increase in HDL-C levels and decline in TG levels with increasing exposure to NNRTI-based therapy, whereas triglyceride levels increase with increasing exposure to PI-based therapy. In another study focused on determination of the effect of HIV infection on lipid metabolism in Cameroon (Nguemaïm et.al., 2010) [14] also observed HIV patients with CD4 counts <50 cells/μl had significantly lower TC (P<0.0001) and LDL-C (P<0.0001) but significantly higher triglyceride (TG) values (P<0.001) and a higher atherogenicity index for TC/HDL-C (P<0.01) and HDL-C/LDL-C (P=0.02); patients with CD4 counts of 50–199 cells/μl had significantly lower TC (P<0.001) and significantly higher TG values (P<0.001); patients with CD4 counts of 200–350 cells/μl had significantly higher TG (P=0.003) and a higher atherogenicity index for TC/HDLC (P<0.0002) and HDLC/LDLC (P=0.04); and those with CD4 counts >350 cells/μl had a higher atherogenicity index for TC/HDL-C (P<0.0001) and HDL-C/LDL-C (P<0.001). HDL-C was significantly lower in HIV-positive patients irrespective of the CD4 cell count. Lipid parameters were also influenced by the presence of opportunistic infections (OIs) and concluded HIV Infection is associated with dyslipidaemia, and becomes increasingly debilitating as immunodeficiency progresses. HDL-C was found to be lower than in controls in the early stages of HIV infection, while TG and the atherogenicity index increased and TC and LDL-C decreased in the advanced stages of immunodeficiency. In another study conducted to evaluate the lipid profile of asymptomatic and untreated HIV patients, also observed significant differences in means (controls vs. cases) were found in: HDL-cholesterol (52 mg/dl vs. 38 mg/dl, p>0,0002); LDL-triglycerides (41 mg/dl vs. 63 mg/dl, p>0,012); total cholesterol / HDL-cholesterol (3.4 vs. 4.5 p>0,006); apoA (158 mg/dl vs. 127 mg/dl, p>0,0001); apoB100 (96 mg/dl vs. 86 mg/dl, p>0,05), haematocrit (45% vs. 42%, p>0,05) and total lymphocytes (2450/ml vs. 1668/ml, p>0,004). In the case group LDL-cholesterol correlated to immune activation markers (beta-2-microglobulin, p>0.05 and viral load, p>0.01). Their study concluded HIV-positive patients have a significant lower serum HDL-C and a change in LDL composition pattern, with lower cholesterol and apoB100 content and higher triglyceride content, suggestive of altered synthesis of LDL in the liver. In a study conducted (Palaniswamy, et al., 2008)[7] to establish the changes in CD4+ cell count and lipid profile in HIV infection and AIDS patients. The study observed a significant reduction in CD4+ cell count in HIV/AIDS patients when compared to control subjects. Serum levels of total cholesterol, high-density lipoprotein cholesterol (HDL-C) and low-density lipoprotein cholesterol (LDL-C) were found to be decreased significantly in HIV/AIDS patients when compared with normal counterparts. On the other hand, the levels of triglyceride (TG) and very low-density lipoprotein cholesterol (VLDL-C) were markedly elevated in HIV/AIDS patients compared to normal subjects. Hence, it may be justified that CD4+ cell count and lipid profile can be a good index of disease progression in HIV infection and AIDS patients.

Conclusion

The changes in lipid profile can be a good index of disease progression in HIV infection.

Limitations of the study: The study is limited by low participation rate of HIV positive patients thus lowering the sample size of the study.

Future directions of the study: In future a multicentre study should be carried out encouraging HIV positive patients to participate in the study so that concrete findings would come up pertaining to lipid profile in HIV patients without antiretroviral therapy and explaining the basis of alternations in lipid profile.

What this study contributes: The study could predict the stage of HIV Infection by measuring the changes in lipid profile as the current study observed changes in lipid profile in these HIV positive patients. Further we can establish the association of lipid profile with HIV infection.

Conflict interest: The authors do not have any conflict interest from this study.

References

1. UNAIDS report on global HIV/AIDS epidemic: HIV infection rates decreasing in several countries but global number of people living with HIV continues to rise. Geneva, 2005. (s)
2. Lamptey P., Wigley M., Carr D and Colloymore Y. Facing the HIV/AIDS Pandemic. Population Bulletin, 2002; Vol 57, No: 3. http://www.nhrc.nic.in/report_hiv-aids.htm (Accessed January 15,2011) Adult AIDS Clinical Trials Metabolic Guides: Lipid Disturbances. Available online at aactg.s-3.com/metabolic/default.htm

3. Schmidt HH, Behrens G, Genschel J, Stoll M, Dejam A, Haas R, Manns MP, Schmidt RE. Lipid evaluation in HIV-1-positive patients treated with protease inhibitors. Antivir Ther. 1999; 4(3):163-170. Executive Summary of the Third Report of The National Cholesterol Education Program (NCEP) Expert Panel on Detection, Evaluation, and Treatment of High Blood Cholesterol in Adults (Adult Treatment Panel III). Expert Panel of Detection, Evaluation, and Treatment of High Blood Cholesterol in Adults. JAMA 2001; 285(19):2486-97.

4. Pasupathi P., Bakthavathsalam G., SaravananG., Devaraj A. Changes in CD4+ cell count, lipid profile and liver enzymes in HIV infection and AIDS patients. Journal of Applied Biomedicine 2008; 6(3):139-145.

5. Khiangte L., Vidyabati RK.,Singh MK., Bilasini Devi S., Rajan Singh T., Gyaneshwar Singh W. Study of serum lipid profile in human immunodeficiency virus(HIV) infected patients. Journal, Indian Academy of Clinical Medicine 2007; 8:307-311.

6. Adewole OO, Eze S, Betiku Ye, Anteyi E, Wada I, Ajuwon Z, Erhabor G. Lipid profile in HIV/AIDS patients in Nigeria. African Health Sciences 2010; 10(2):144-149.

7. Silva EF, Bassichetto KC, Lewi DS. Lipid profile, cardiovascular risk factors and metabolic syndrome in a group of AIDS patients. Arq Bras Cardiol 2009; 93(2):113-118.

8. Hiransuthikul N, Hiransuthikul P and Kanasook Y. Lipid Profiles of Thai Adult HIV-Infected Patients Receiving Protease Inhibitors. Southeast Asian J Trop Med Public Health 2007; 38(1): 69-77.

9. Obirikorang C, Yeboah F, Quaye L. Serum Lipid Profiling In Highly Active Antiretroviral Therapy-naive HIV Positive Patients In Ghana; Any Potential Risk?. Webmed Central INFECTIOUS DISEASES 2010;1(10):WMC00987.

10. Young J, Weber R, Rickenbach M, Furrer H, Bernasconi E, Hirschel B, Philip E Tarr, Vernazza P, Battegay M, Heiner C Bucher and the Swiss HIV Cohort Study. Lipid Profiles for antiretroviral-naive patients starting PI- and NNRTI-based therapy in the Swiss HIV Cohort Study Antiviral Therapy 2005; 10:585-591.

12. Nguemaïm Nf, Mbuagbaw J, Nkoa T, Alemnji G, Této1 G, Fanhi1 Tc, Asonganyi T, Samé-Ekobo1 A. Serum lipid profile in highly active antiretroviral therapy-naïve HIV-infected patients in Cameroon: a case–control study. HIV Medicine 2010; 11(6):353–359.

Chapter 15

Socio economic status, life style and behavioral pattern of elderly normolipidemic myocardial infarct subjects- A Case Control study from South Asia

Abstract

Introduction: Emerging epidemics of cardiovascular disease (CVD) have attracted attention as major causes of global disability and mortality [1]. In 1990, it was estimated that 15 of 52 million deaths worldwide were attributable to CVD, and 63% of those deaths occurred in developing countries. CVD (mainly heart disease and stroke) was responsible for approximately half of noncommunicable disease (NCD) mortality and one quarter of the NCD morbidity rate in 1999; low- and middle-income countries were most affected (3). Ischemic heart disease and stroke are projected to be first- and fourth-ranking contributors to global disability

adjusted life-years lost by 2020, and developing countries will experience most of the increase. The disease pattern is increasing drastically among Indians compared to the Westerners [2, 3]. The CAD rates in India are almost four folds compared to United States which were once similar in 1968, and it is expected to be the largest killer by 2015 [4]. Even Indians have less conventional risk factors still we are susceptible to the claws of this disease [5, 6]. The rapid urbanization, life style modifications, blue collar jobs prospects and switching on to more sedentary life due to high profile jobs along with no time for exercise have advanced us towards the risk of Coronary Artery Disease. It is also observed that low socio-economic status (SES) group have higher mortality rates as indicated by educational level, occupation class or income level. It is general observation that only part of the socio gradient in cardiovascular disease mortality can be explained by a higher prevalence of classical risk factors like smoking, serum cholesterol and hypertension [7]. The rates of CAD in metro cities like New Delhi (10%) [8], Chennai (11%) [9] and in state like Kerala where the largest death (13%, Urban and 7%, Rural) occurs due to CAD [10,11]. In Sri Lanka, way back in 1980 the rates of CAD increased and now it is almost similar to India [12]. In India, the rates of hospitalization in Intensive Coronary Care Units (ICCU) due to acute ischemic syndromes are four folds higher compared to the United States and Japanese and almost six times higher than Chinese, even the highest number of smokers exists in China and Japan compared to rest part of the world [13,14,15]. Before we are in the claws of CAD, we should modify our total life style changes and modifications so that at least we can prolong ourselves from the clutches of the dreaded disease. The current study on life style and behavioral pattern among acute myocardial infarction (AMI) subjects were studied in those subjects who were admitted to Intensive Coronary Care Unit due to episode of AMI and those parameters were compared with normal healthy subjects to compare the changes in life style pattern.

Materials and Methods

The study was conducted in Faculty of Medicine, University of Peradeniya, Sri Lanka. The study comprised of 165 normolipidemic AMI patients, male to female ratio was 3:1, with ages ranged from 48-69 years, mean ± SD (61.8 ± 3.8 y). One hundred sixty five age-sex matched subjects, with similar ratio of male: female as in patients were recruited as controls. Their ages ranged from 48-69 years, mean ± SD (60.55 ± 3.98 y). The AMI cases were diagnosed as per diagnostic criteria: chest pain lasting for ≥ 3 hours, ECG changes (ST elevation of 2 mm or more in at least two leads), increased creatine phosphokinase (CPK-MB) and aspartate aminotransferase enzyme. Informed consent was obtained from patients and controls recruited for the study and the study were approved by the ethical committee of the Institution.

Exclusion Criteria: Patients with diabetes mellitus, hyperlipidemia, renal insufficiency, current and past smokers, hepatic disease or taking lipid lowering drugs or antioxidant vitamin supplements.

Inclusion Criteria: Normolipidemic AMI patients as per the NCEP ATP -111 guidelines.

Criteria for Normolipidaemia: Normal lipid profile was defined when total cholesterol was <200 mg/dl, LDL-C<130 mg/dl, HDL-C $\geq$ 35mg/dl and TG < 200 mg/dl (NCEP, Adult Treatment Panel-III) [16].

Criteria for Dyslipidaemia: Subjects with total cholesterol $\geq$200mg/dl, low-density lipoprotein cholesterol $\geq$130mg/dl, high-density lipoprotein <40mg/dl, and triglycerides $\geq$150mg/dl were considered to be dyslipidaemic according to American National cholesterol education Program III guidelines reported [17].

Demographic data: This included various life style factors such as education, socio-economic status, income and type of job. Details of major cardiovascular risk factors such as smoking, diabetes, obesity and hypertension were obtained using a questionnaire.

Blood Pressure: The blood pressure was measured using standard mercury manometer. At least two readings at 5 minutes intervals as per World Health Organization guidelines were recorded. If high blood pressure ($\geq$140/90 mmHg) was noted a third reading was taken after 30 minutes. The lowest of the three readings was taken as blood pressure [18].

Electrocardiogram: Electrocardiogram (12 lead) was performed on all persons using proper standardization.

Criteria of Smoking: Smokers in India consume tobacco in various forms- rolled tobacco leaves (beedi), Indian pipe (chillum, hookah), cigarettes and tobacco chewing and more than one form is used by many making it difficult to accurately measure the amount of tobacco consumed. Therefore, users of all types of tobacco products and present and past smokers were considered as smokers.

Criteria for Hypertension and Obesity: Hypertension was diagnosed when systolic blood pressure was ≥140 mmHg and /or diastolic blood pressure ≥90 mmHg. Body Mass Index (Weight in kg/height in meters²) was calculated and obesity was defined as BMI≥25kg/m². Truncal obesity was established when waist-hip ratio was >0.9 in male and >0.8 in female.

Anthropometric data: Height, weight, biceps skin fold thickness, triceps skin fold thickness and waist-hip ratio were recorded. Height was measured in centimeters using standiometer with an accuracy of 0.01 cm and weight in kilograms using calibrated spring balance. Supine waist girth was measured at the level of umbilicus with a person breathing silently and standing hip girth was measured at inter-trochanteric level. Mid arm circumference was measured half way between the acromion process of the scapula and the tip of the elbow. Triceps skin fold thickness (TSFT) was measured at a point over the triceps muscle mid way between the acromion and olecranon process on the posterior aspect of the arm. For biceps skin fold thickness the same procedure as TSFT was adopted, but with the measurement done in the midline of the anterior part of the upper arm.

Blood (5 ml) was collected for serum lipid profile, within 10 hours once the patients were admitted to intensive coronary care unit.

Total cholesterol, triglycerides, and HDL-cholesterol were estimated by enzymatic methods using the kits obtained from Randox Laboratories Limited, Crumlin, UK. Plasma LDL-cholesterol was determined from the values of total cholesterol and HDL-cholesterol using the following formulae [19]:

$$LDL\text{-}c = TC - \frac{TG}{5} - HDL\text{-}c \ (mg/dl)$$

Statistical Analysis: The data from patients and controls were compared using Student's 't'-test. Values were expressed as mean ± standard deviation (SD). Microsoft Excel for windows 2000 was used for statistical analysis. 'P' value of less than 0.05 was considered to indicate statistical significance.

Results

Anthropometric variables

The age and anthropometric measurements of the control subjects and myocardial infarct (MI) patients are summarized in **Table 1.** The mean height recorded in patients was similar to the controls (**Table 1**). The mean body mass index (BMI) of both controls and patients was > 25 (**Table 1**) and the difference between the 2 groups was significant (p<0.01). Among the control, 66.7% of males and 78.6% of females had body mass index >25.

Even though the mean BMI of the controls and MI patients significantly differed (**Table 1**) analysis of the data gender-wise revealed otherwise (data not shown). It was further noticed that 50 control subjects and 30 AMI patients had BMI values ≤25 while 115 controls and 135 AMI patients had a BMI ≥25. Chi square analysis revealed that the proportion of the AMI patients with BMI values ≥25 was significantly (p<0.01) higher than that of the controls.

Table 1. Anthropometric data of Control subjects and Myocardial Infarct patients.

	Control (n=165)	MI patients (n=165)	p value (95% CI)
Age (years) Range (years)	60.5 ± 3.4 (48-69)	61.8 ± 3.8 (48-69)	0.0037 (61.26-62.42)
Height (m)	1.63 ± 0.04	1.64 ± 0.59	<0.1(1.63-1.64)
Weight (kg)	68.34 ± 3.97	72.01 ± 5.37	<0.001 (71.19-72.82)
BMI (kg/m^2)	25.40 ± 1.20	26.16 ± 1.45	<0.01 (25.93-26.38)
Waist Circumference (cm)	93.70 ± 3.63	100.77 ± 6.06	<0.001 (99.84-101.69)
Hip Circumference (cm)	100.01 ± 3.16	105.72 ± 5.23	<0.001 (104.92-106.51)
Waist-Hip ratio	0.93 ± 0.01	0.95 ± 0.01	<0.02 (0.94-0.95)
Mid Arm Circumference (cm)	29.70 ± 1.47	30.63 ± 1.87	<0.05 (30.34-30.91)
Biceps skin fold thickness (mm)	6.95 ± 1.05	7.5 ± 1.38	<0.001 (7.29-7.70)
Triceps skin fold thickness (mm)	11.97 ± 1.27	12.89 ± 1.69	<0.001 (13.63-14.14)
Systolic blood pressure (mmHg)	121.06 ± 4.19	134.32 ± 11.65	<0.001 (132.54-136.09)
Diastolic blood pressure (mmHg)	79.90 ± 3.64	86.04 ± 4.25	<0.001 (85.39-86.68)

Values are in Mean ± SD.

Eighty percent of the MI patients and 69.7% of the controls were overweight and the difference in the frequency was statistically significant (p<0.001).

The mean waist/hip ratio were significantly (p<0.001) higher in MI patients compared to the controls (**Table 1**). Only 16.3% of controls had their waist/hip ratio >0.95 compared to 69.9% of MI patients. All the female MI patients had a waist: hip ratio ≥0.90 and 64.2% of the males had a ratio ≥0.95. Among the controls, all the females had a waist/hip ratio ≥0.90 but only 6.5% of males had waist: hip ratio ≥0.95.

The mean mid-arm circumference of MI patients was higher than that of controls (Table 1) The biceps and triceps skin fold thickness of the MI patients was significantly higher than that of the controls (p<0.001) (Table1), In summary body weight, waist circumference, hip circumference, waist/hip ratio, mid arm circumference, biceps skin fold thickness and triceps skin fold thickness were significantly higher in MI patients compared to controls. Therefore body weight, waist circumference, hip circumference, waist/hip ratio and mid arm circumference, which reflect the body fat content may be considered as predictive factors in the development of myocardial infarction despite the patients having a normal lipid profile. This observation is significant in view of a great deal of reliance placed on lipid profile to assess the risk of getting MI, at present. Further more the waist/hip ratio is a reliable index than BMI for assessing the risk of subjects who are prone to develop MI since the study revealed that statistically significant difference was observed only in waist/hip ratio and not in body mass index. This parameter should be examined in patients who posses the conventional risk factor.

Lipid Profile pattern

Serum lipid profile parameters in AMI patients and control are shown in **Table 2**. Total cholesterol, its ratio to HDL-cholesterol (TC/HDL-C), LDL-cholesterol, triglycerides was significantly higher in AMI patients compared with control (**Table 2**). Significant difference for HDL-cholesterol between AMI and control was observed (**Table 2**). On the other hand, LDL-cholesterol and its ratio to HDL-cholesterol (LDL-C/HDL-C) were higher in patients compared with controls **(Table 2)**. No statistically significant difference was observed in TG/HDL-C ratio among patients with controls. Also, significantly lower HDL-C concentration was observed in AMI patients than in the controls ($p<0.0001$). Total cholesterol, triglycerides, LDL-cholesterol were higher in AMI subjects as compared to control ($p<0.0001$). Also, significant differences were seen in HDL-C levels between AMI and controls ($p<0.0001$).

Demographic characteristics

The socio economic status and life style characteristics of the control and MI patients are shown in **Table 3** and **4**. The subjects were classified into lower, middle and higher class depending on monthly income of the family. Subjects whose monthly income was ≤ Rs. 5000/month, Rs. 5000-15000 /month and ≥ Rs. 15000/month respectively were

Table 2. Lipid Profile and biochemical parameters in Control subjects and MI patients.

	Control (n=165)	MI patients (n=165)	p value (95%CI)
Total cholesterol (mg/dl)	168.6 ± 12.2	186.4 ± 13.9	<0.001 (184.31-188.56)
HDL-cholesterol (mg/dl)	50.5 ± 6.8	41.3 ± 4.6	<0.001 (40.56-41.97)
Total cholesterol/ HDL-C ratio	3.4 ± 0.4	4.6 ± 0.6	<0.001 (4.48-4.65)
Triglycerides (mg/dl)	107.8 ± 11.5	129.0 ± 12.2	<0.001(127.10-130.82)
LDL-cholesterol (mg/dl)	83.6 ± 12.0	119.4 ± 14.1	<0.001 (117.2-121.50)
LDL-C/HDL-C ratio	1.9 ± 0.3	2.9 ± 0.5	<0.001 (2.85-3.00)
TG/HDL-C ratio	2.2 ± 0.4	3.2 ± 0.5	0.3149 (3.086-3.234)

Values are in Mean ± SD
Lipid profiles were determined in serum.

Table 3. Socio Economic and life style characteristics of Study and Control Subjects.

		Control Group (n=165)	Study Group (n=165)
Age (years)		60.5 ± 3.4	61.8 ± 3.8
Range (years)		(48-69)	(48-69)
	Lower Class	19 (11.51)	12 (7.27)
Civil Status	Middle Class	131 (79.39)	117 (70.90)
	Higher Class	15 (9.09)	34 (20.60)
Type of family	Split	64 (38.78)	20 (12.12)
	Joint	101 (61.21)	145 (87.87)
	Below Matriculate	-	4 (2.42)
	Matriculate	12 (7.27)	8 (4.84)
Education	Higher Secondary	15 (9.09)	13 (7.87)
	Graduate	132 (80.0)	101 (61.21)
	Post Graduate	6 (3.63)	39 (31.70)
	Mild	58 (35.15)	82 (49.69)
Type of Work	Moderate	100 (60.60)	83 (50.30)
	Heavy	7 (5.69)	-
Walking (Brisk)	≤ 180 mins /wk ≥ 180 mins /wk	43 (26.06)	142 (86.06)
		122 (73.93)	23 (13.93)
Hours of Sleep	≤ 7 hours /day ≥ 7hours /day	106 (64.24)	77 (46.66)
		59 (35.75)	88 (53.33)
Smoking	≤ 10 Sticks/day ≥ 10 Sticks/day	29 (17.57)	9 (5.45)
		-	36 (21.81)

Numbers in parentheses are percent unless mentioned otherwise

Table 4. Behavioral pattern of subjects in case and control.

		Control Group	Study Group
Hyperactive	Yes	39 (23.63)	68 (41.21)
	No	126 (76.36)	97 (58.78)
Triffle thinker	Yes	30 (18.18)	99 (60.00)
	No	135 (81.81)	66 (40.00)
Irrelevant thinker	Yes	50 (30.30)	106 (64.24)
	No	115 (69.69)	59 (35.75)

Numbers in parentheses are percent unless mentioned otherwise.

categorized as lower, middle and higher class. It was observed that most of the control subjects (79.4%) and MI patients (70.9%) belonged to the middle class with 85 male (69.1%) and 32 female (76.2%) of AMI were in this category. Further 101 (61.2%) control and 145 (87.9%) patients belonged to joint family, where all the member of the family lived together even after marriage.

The subjects were grouped according to the educational status based on the highest degree they possessed (**Table 3**). It was observed that majority of the subjects in both groups were graduates. The educational qualification reflected their type of job profile.

The percentages of male MI patients engaged in mild and moderated physical activity were 82% and 83% respectively compared to control. Most of the female patients (67.4%) were involved in household jobs (data not shown).

Smoking was recorded only in the males of both groups. Depending on the number of cigarettes they smoked/day the subjects were categorized into 2 groups. Among MI patients 36 males (29.3%) smoked ≥ 10 cigarettes/ day, and 9 (7.3%) ≤ 10 cigarettes/ day compared to 29 (17.6%) in control.

Discussion

The present study was a hospital based study and was conducted in patients who were admitted to intensive coronary care unit after developing symptoms of myocardial infarction (MI). Though it is widely known dyslipidemic subjects are at higher risk of MI [20,21,22], so in order to elucidate the other risks apart from the conventional risk factors, we isolated those patients who had MI but their lipid profiles were within normal reference range as recommended by governing body (NCEP-ATP-III) [16].

In the current study significantly higher values of lipid profile were observed (**Table 2**) among patients when compared with age-sex matched healthy control although patients were within normal range.

The present study has revealed a substantially high rate of prevalence of some of the behavioral and conventional risk factors among myocardial infarct patients compared to controls especially the habit of smoking among men, physical inactivity, stress, insufficient sleep, obesity, dyslipidemia and hypertension.

The findings clearly indicate that the patients mostly belonged to middle class socio economic strata and were from joint family.

We found that CVD mortality rates decreased considerably among educated people compared with those without formal education, even after adjusting for other independent variables such as sex, age, and economic status. This finding is similar to the findings of numerous studies that showed an inverse socioeconomic gradient in CVD mortality in developed (15-18) and developing countries (19).

Likewise, education was an important factor for health among men and among women, particularly in rural areas, because we found that education is usually associated with increased knowledge about health matters and consequent reduction in risky health behaviors. Explanations for the differences in education levels we observed among those who died from CVD include differences in risk factors such as blood pressure, blood cholesterol, smoking, and obesity. Indeed, available evidence from other studies in the Bavi district support the observation that people with lower education levels smoke more (20) and have more hypertension (14).

A strong correlation between old age (50 years and older) and education was also found in relation to CVD mortality. Even though the risk of dying from CVD associated with lower education level was similar for men and women, the effects of women's education are particularly noteworthy. Given the results, together with the relatively higher proportion of women aged 50 years and older (30% of women aged 20 years and older), of whom 55% had no formal education, better education for women may substantially reduce CVD mortality. Better education likely leads to healthier lifestyles (e.g., lower rates of smoking, drinking, physical inactivity) and is likely to improve access to health care.

We found that CVD mortality rates decreased considerably among educated people compared with those without formal education, even after adjusting for other independent variables such as sex, age, and economic status. This finding is similar to the findings of numerous studies that showed an inverse socioeconomic gradient in CVD mortality in developed (15-18) and developing countries (19).

Likewise, education was an important factor for health among men and among women, particularly in rural areas, because we found that education is usually associated with increased knowledge about health matters and consequent reduction in risky health behaviors. Explanations for the differences in education levels we observed among those who died from CVD include differences in risk factors such as blood pressure, blood cholesterol, smoking, and obesity. Indeed, available evidence from other studies in the Bavi district support the observation that people with lower education levels smoke more (20) and have more hypertension (14).

In western countries, twenty per cent of deaths among males and eight per cent among females were attributable to smoking [23]. Since the incubation period of smoking is very long (two or more decades), the resultant impact of smoking in terms of morbid condition may take a long time. However, the high prevalence of this risk factor points to a definite likelihood of high morbidity burden occurring in future year.

The inadequate physical activity, sleep, hyperactivity, truncal obesity (increased waist/hip ratio) among the patients in the present study is likely to impact adversely on the future morbidity burden, especially in the absence of adequate physical activities observed due to increased job tension, blue color jobs, sedentary life style. Physical activities are of prime importance for lowering the levels of cholesterol and blood pressure. Combinations of unhealthy behavioral risk factors are more predictive to describe the lifestyle determinants on chronic diseases and its mortality [24].

It has been observed that some of the behavioral risk factors are potentially modifiable [25]. Cardiovascular diseases, the leading cause of deaths in developed countries, were mainly caused by cigarette smoking, lack of physical activity, obesity, stress, hypertension, etc [26], which is supported by the findings of the current study. The higher prevalence of such risk factors observed in the present study also suggest a high potential for acquiring high morbidity burden for non communicable diseases, especially cardiovascular diseases.

With further ageing of the population, the health problem would become more and more acute, both in terms of morbidity burden as well as its burden on increased medical cost [15], stated that India is widely believed to be heading towards an epidemic of coronary heart disease.

Studies have also demonstrated that intensive (and positive) lifestyle changes or promotion of healthy lifestyle has resulted in the reduction of diseases associated with high risk life style behaviors [27, 28, 29]. Various behavioral risk factors in midlife and late adulthood are predictors of subsequent disability on account of chronic diseases. Not only do persons with better health habits survive longer, but also in such persons, disability is postponed and compressed into fewer years at the end of life [30].

In conclusion, our findings indicated a high prevalence of various behavioral risk factors among the myocardial infarct patients. Public health remedial measures will therefore be urgently needed in order to minimize future morbidity burden, thereby minimizing medical expenditure. Regarding smoking, a strict public policy in restricting its use and its distribution may be considered, besides improving the awareness of its ill effects among the masses, especially the high risk groups, mainly the lower social status groups.

References

1. Reddy KS, Yusuf S. Emerging epidemic of cardiovascular disease in developing countries. Circulation 1998; 97:596-601.
2. Enas EA, Jacob S. Decline of CAD in developed countries: Lessons for India. In: Sethi K, ed. Coronary Artery Disease in Indians - A Global Perspective. Mumbai: Cardiological Society of India, 1998:98 -113.
3. Goyal A, Yusuf S. The burden of cardiovascular disease in the Indian subcontinent. Indian J Med Res 2006; 124:235-244.
4. Reddy KS, Yusuf S. Emerging epidemic of cardiovascular disease in developing countries. Circulation 1998; 97:596–601.
5. Yagalla MV, Hoerr S, Song W, Enas E, Garg A. Relationship of diet, abdominal obesity, and physical activity to plasma lipoprotein levels in Asian Indian physicians residing in the United States. J Am Dietetic Assoc 1996; 96:257-261.
6. Reddy KS. Cardiovascular disease in India. World Health Stat Q 1993; 46:101-7.
7. Enas EA. Management of coronary risk factors: Role of lifestyle modification. Cardiology Today 1998; 2:17-29.
8. Chaddha SL, Radhakrishan S, Ramachandran K. Epidemiological study of coronary heart disease in urban population of New Delhi. Ind J Med Res 1990; 92 (B):424-430.
9. Mohan V, Deepa R, Shanthi Rani S, Premalatha G. Prevalence of coronary artery disease and its relationship to lipids in a selected population in South India. The Chennai Urban Population Study (CUPS No. 5). J Am Coll Cardiol 2001; 38:682-687.
10. Raman Kutty V, Balakrishnan K, Jayasree A, et al. Prevalence of coronary heart disease in the rural population of Thiruvananthapuram district, Kerala, India. Int J Cardiol 1993; 39:59-70.
11. Joseph A, Kutty VR, Soman CR. High risk for coronary heart disease in Thiruvananthapuram City: A study of serum lipids and other risk factors. Indian Heart J 2000;52:29-35.
12. Mendis S. Cardiovascular disease in Sri Lanka.: Ministry of Health, Sri Lanka, 1998:1-36.
13. Yuan JM, Ross R, Wanh X, Gao Y, Henderson B, Yu M. Morbidity and mortality in relation to cigarette smoking in Shanghai, China: A prospective male cohort study. JAMA 1996; 275:1646-1650.
14. Hughes K, Ong CN. Homocysteine, folate, vitamin B12, and cardiovascular risk in Indians, Malays, and Chinese in Singapore. J Epidemiol Community Health 2000; 54:31-34.
15. Ghaffar A, Reddy KS. Burden of non-communicable diseases in South Asia. BMJ 2004; 528: 807-810.
16. W. E. Feeman, Laura Ryan Caldwell, Douglas Iliff, Paul J. Rosch, Bruce L. Ring, Scott M. Grundy, and James I. Cleeman. Executive Summary of The Third Report of The National Cholesterol Education Program (NCEP) Expert panel on Detection, Evalation, and treatment of high Blood Cholesterol in Adults (Adult Treatment Panel III). Expert Panel of Detection, Evaluation, and Treatment of High Blood Cholesterol in Adults. The Journal of the American Medical Association 2001; 285(19):2486-2497.
17. Caudill, S. P., Cooper, G.R., Jaysmith, S. & Myers, G.L.(1998). Assessment of current National Cholesterol Education Program Guidelines for total cholesterol, triglycerides, HDL-cholesterol and LDL-cholesterol measurements. *Clinical Chemistry*, 44:1650-1658

18. Rose GA, Blackburn H, Gillum RF, Prineas RJ. *Cardiovascular survey methods* 2nd Ed. WHO Monograph Series No.56 Geneva. World Health Organisation 1982.
19. Friedewalds, W.T., Levy, R.I. and Fredrickson, D.S. Estimation of the concentration of low density lipoprotein cholesterol in plasma without the use of preparative ultracentrifuge. Clin. Chem 1972;18: 499-502.
20. Achari,V. and Thakur, A.K. Association of Major Modifiable Risk factors Among Patients with Coronary Artery Disease -A retrospective Analysis. J Assoc Physicians India 2004; 52:103-108.
21. Rani SH, Madhavi G, Ramachandra RV, Sahay BK, Jyothy A. Risk factors for coronary heart disease in type II diabetes. Indian Journal of Clinical Biochemistry 2005; 20(2):75-80.
22. Shrinivas K, Vijaya Bhaskar M, Aruna Kumari M, Nagaraj K, Reddy KK. Antioxidants, lipid peroxidation and lipoproteins in primary hypertension. Indian Heart J 2000; 52:285-88.
23. Ezzati M, Lopez A. Estimates of global mortality attributable to smoking in 2000. Lancet 2003; 362: 847-852.
24. Luoto R, Prattala R, Uutela A, Puska P. Impact of unhealthy behaviors on cardiovascular mortality in Finland. Prev Med 1998; 27: 93-100.
25. Coleman CA, Friedman AG, Burright RG. The relationship of daily stress and health related behaviors to adolescents' cholesterol levels. Adolescence 1998; 33 : 447-60.
26. Fuster V, Voute J, Hunn M, Smith SC Jr. Low priority of cardiovascular and chronic diseases on the Global Health Agenda. A case for concern. Circulation 2007; 776: 1966-1970.
27. Ornish D, Scherwitz LW, Billings JH, Brown SE, Gould KL, Merrit TA, et al. Intensive lifestyle changes for reversal of coronary heart disease. JAMA 1998; 280: 2001-2007.
28. Richmond R, Wodak A, Bourne S, Heather N. Screening for unhealthy lifestyle factors in the workplace. Aust NZ J Public Health 1998; 22 : 324-31.
29. Goetzel RZ, Anderson DR, Whitmer RW, Ozminkowski RJ, Dunn RL, Wasserman J. The relationship between modifiable health risks and health care expenditures. An analysis of the multi-employer HERO health risk and cost database. The Health Enhancement research Organization (HERO) Research Committee. JOEM 1998; 40: 843-854.
30. Vita AJ, Terry RB, Hubert HB, Fries JF. Aging, health risks, and cumulative disability. N Engl J Med 1998: 338 : 1035-1041.

Chapter 16

Lipid parameters in predicting the risk of myocardial infarction in elderly Normolipidemic patients in South Asia: a multi centered study from India, Nepal and Sri Lanka

Abstract

Background: The major cause of atherosclerosis, dyslipidaemic, acts synergistically with non-lipid risk factors resulting increase in atherogenesis. Increased (TG) and decreased high-density lipoprotein (HDL-C) and the increased TG/HDL-C ratio are considered as major risk factors in the development of Insulin resistance and metabolic syndrome. The accuracy of TG/HDL-C ratio stands crucial in predicting coronary heart disease (CHD) risk.

AIM: This multi-centered study was undertaken to evaluate the usefulness of lipid ratios TC/HDL-C, TG/HDL-C and LDL/HDL-C in predicting CHD risk in Normolipidemic myocardial infarct patients and compare the findings with healthy controls.

Setting & design: Lipid profile was determined in 1021 Normolipidemic myocardial infarct patients and compared them with 1021 age/sex-matched controls.

Material & methods: Total Cholesterol, Triglycerides, and HDL-cholesterol were analyzed enzymatically using kits obtained from Randox Laboratories Limited, Crumlin, UK. Plasma LDL-cholesterol was determined from the values of total cholesterol and HDL- cholesterol using the friedwald's formula.

Statistics: The values were expressed as means ± standard deviation (SD) and data from patients and controls was compared using students 't'-test.

Results and conclusion: Total cholesterol, TC/HDL-C ratio, Triglycerides, LDL-cholesterol, LDL-C/HDL-C ratio were higher in MI patients (p<0.001). HDL-C concentration was significantly lower in MI patients than controls (p<0.001). Higher ratio of TC/HDL-C, TG/HDL-C and LDL-C/HDL-C was observed in AMI patients compared to controls.

Key words: TC/HDL-C, TG/HDL-C, LDL-C/HDL-C, Acute Myocardial Infarction, Normal Lipid Profile, India, Nepal and Sri Lanka.

Introduction

Atherosclerosis begins in early life, especially in children and adolescents with high levels of low density cholesterol (LDL-C) [1]. It is recommended to conduct a full lipid profile on children and adolescents who present with a higher risk of family history, including familial hypercholesterolemia, cardiovascular disease (CVD), diabetes or early heart attack and stroke. Children and adolescents who are also overweight or obese should be screened.[2] Dyslipidemia characterized by elevated TC, LDL-C and lowered HDL-C, is a conventional risk factor observed in myocardial infarction patients [3, 4, 5, 6, 7, 8, 9, 10] and is the major cause of atherosclerosis are suggested to act synergistically with non-lipid risk factors to increase atherogenesis. Low-density lipoprotein cholesterol (LDL-C) is the main therapeutic target in the prevention of CVD. Indeed, more aggressive lowering of LDL-C levels by statins and LDL-Apheresis is now being practiced in United States [11].

Increased triglycerides (TG) and decreased high-density lipoprotein (HDL-C) are considered to be a major risk factor for the development of Insulin resistant and metabolic syndrome in South Asians. Although the TG/HDL-C ratio has been used as a clinical indicator for Insulin resistance, results were inconsistent. The TG/HDL-C ratio is also widely used to assess atherogenic lipid. How ever the utility of this ratio for predicting coronary heart disease (CHD) risk still needs to be established. Since we have encountered myocardial infarct patients with normal serum lipid profile, this study was undertaken to evaluate the usefulness of these lipid ratios in predicting CHD risk in Normolipidemic AMI patients and to compare the results with healthy subjects.

Materials and Methods Setting Design and Patients: The study consisted of 1021 elderly patients between 47-71 years (754 men and 267 women) with AMI, admitted to the Intensive Coronary Care Unit in Corporate hospitals in India, Nepal and Sri Lanka. The diagnosis of AMI was established according to diagnostic criteria: chest pain, which lasted for $\leq$ 3 hours, ECG changes (ST elevation of $\geq$ 2 mm in at least two leads) and elevation in enzymatic activities of serum creatine phosphokinase and aspartate aminotransferase. The control group consisted of 1021 age/sex-matched healthy volunteers (754 men and 267 women). The design of this study was approved by the institutional ethical committee board of the hospital, and informed consent was obtained from the patients and controls.

Inclusion criteria were patients with a diagnosis of AMI with normal lipid profile. Patients with diabetes mellitus, renal insufficiency, current and past smokers, hepatic disease or taking lipid-lowering drugs or antioxidant vitamin supplements were excluded from the study. Normolipidemic subjects were judged by the following criteria: LDL <130 mg/dl, HDL $\geq$ 35 mg/dl, Total cholesterol (TC), <200 mg/dl; and triglycerides (TG), <150 mg/dl. [12]. Ten milliliters of blood was collected after overnight fasting for lipid profile.

Lipid profile TC, TG, and HDL-cholesterol were analyzed enzymatically using kits obtained from Randox Laboratories Limited, Crumlin, UK. Plasma LDL-cholesterol was determined from the values of total cholesterol and HDL- cholesterol using the following formula [13]:

$$\text{LDL-cholesterol} = \text{TC} - \frac{\text{TG}}{5} - \text{HDL-cholesterol (mg/dl)}$$

Results

Serum parameters in AMI patients and control are shown in **Table 1.** Total cholesterol, its ratio to HDL-cholesterol (TC/HDL-C), LDL-cholesterol, triglycerides was significantly higher in AMI patients compared with control (**Table 1, 2**). Significant difference for HDL-cholesterol between AMI and control was observed (Table-1). On the other hand, LDL-cholesterol and its ratio to HDL-cholesterol (LDL-C/HDL-C) were higher in patients compared with controls (**Table 1, 2**). No statistically significant difference was observed in TG/HDL-C ratio among patients with controls. Also, significantly lower HDL-C concentration was observed in AMI patients than in the controls (p<0.001).

The analysis based on the ratio of TC/HDL-cholesterol, TG/HDL-cholesterol and LDL-cholesterol/HDL-cholesterol is shown in **Table 3.** Higher ratio of TC/HDL-C, TG/HDL-C and LDL-C/HDL-C was observed in AMI patients compared to controls (**Table 2, 3**).

Table 1. Lipid profile in patients and healthy controls (mean ± SD).

Variables	Controls (n=1021)	Patients (n=1021)	P-value (95%CI)
Age	62.13 ± 2.56	61.84 ± 3.80	0.0039 (61.67-62.00)
Height (m)	1.57 ± 0.28	1.64 ± 0.59	0.0031 (1.61-1.66)
Weight (kg)	67.84 ± 3.26	72.01 ± 5.37	<0.01 (71.77-72.24)
BMI (kg/m2)	26.35 ± 1.98	26.16 ± 1.45	<0.01 (26.09-26.22)
Total Cholesterol †	177.53 ± 47.52	180.94 ± 47.69	<0.001 (178.86-183.01)
HDL-Cholesterol †	41.92 ± 9.88	42.83 ± 10.73	<0.001 (42.36-43.29)
Triglycerides †	148.43 ± 59.66	146.87 ± 59.66	<0.001 (144.26-149.97)
LDL-Cholesterol †	105.64 ± 60.14	105.98 ± 41.97	<0.001 (110.05-111.90)

* ratio † (mg %)

Table 2. TC/HDL-C, LDL-C/HDL-C and TG/HDL-C ratio in patients and healthy controls (mean ± SD).

Variables	Controls (n=1021)	Patients (n=1021)	P-value (95%CI)
TC: HDL-C*	3.24 ± 2.36	4.40 ± 2.72	<0.001(4.28- 4.51)
LDL:HDL-C*	1.78 ± 0.98	2.66 ± 1.45	<0.001(2.59 -2.72)
TG: HDL-C*	2.87 ± 1.26	4.16 ± 1.56	<0.01(4.09 -4.32)

* ratio † (mg %)

Table 3. Distribution pattern of TC/HDL-C, TG/HDL-C and LDL-C/HDL-C ratio in patients and healthy controls (mean ± SD).

Ratio	Controls (n=1021)	Patients (n=1021)
TC/HDL-C		
2-3	2.67 ± 0.35 (n=229)	-
3-4	3.67 ± 0.27 (n=1248)	3.97 ± 0.29 (n=423)
4-5	4.39 ± 0.26 (n=544)	4.94 ± 0.26 (n=896)
5-6	-	5.67 ± 0.13 (n=702)
TG/HDL-C		
1-2	1.36 ± 0.24 (n=859)	-
2-3	2.18 ± 0.16 (n=1162)	2.75 ± 0.23 (n=259)
3-4	-	3.62 ± 0.16 (n=1357)
4-5	-	4.82 ± 0.19 (n=405)
LDL-C/HDL-C		
1-2	1.52 ± 0.13 (n=1452)	1.84 ± 0.15 (n=43)
2-3	2.33 ± 0.24 (n=569)	2.87 ± 0.19 (n=278)
3-4	-	3.58 ± 0.21 (n=1285)
4-5	-	4.51 ± 0.22 (n=415)

Discussion

Observations of Total Cholesterol

The lipid profile pattern in Normolipidemic patients with AMI and normal healthy control were studied and the variation in patterns was compared. The mean TC level of the control subjects compared with AMI (186.44 ± 13.95 mg/dl) was significantly (p<0.001) greater than that of subjects without AMI (168.58 ± 12.16 mg/dl).

A previous study have observed a greater value (189.70 mg/dl) for TC than the controls of the present study (Goswami, et al., 2003) [14]. In a study of MI patients [15] a mean TC level of (196.60 mg/dl) was reported and it was 5.3% higher than the TC of MI patients of the present study.

Higher values for TC (196.60 mg/dl) [15] and (215.70 mg/dl) [16] have been reported by previous studies in AMI patients than the subjects without AMI. These values were 5.3% and 15% greater than the values reported in the present study for MI patients.

The TC levels observed (199.80 mg/dl) were slightly higher than the present study have been reported by Sivaraman et al., 2004 [17] in patients with acute coronary syndrome. They also reported a significant higher values (p<0.001) when compared to the controls in their study.

Similarly, significant differences (p<0.001) were observed in young CAD patients compared with control [3]. The result of the present study was in agreement with their observation.

Lower levels of TC (181mg/dl) in MI patients than observed in the present study have been reported by Shindhe, et al., 2005 [18], Rajashekhar, et al., 2004 [7] and Kharb, et al., 2003 [19] in studies on Indian population.

Though the TC levels of the subjects selected in the present study were within the normal lipid profile, the mean levels of TC in MI subjects was greater in the present study and it was in agreement with the observations of the previous studies though they have reported greater or lower levels of TC in subjects with MI than the TC levels in the present study.

Observations of High Density Lipoprotein-Cholesterol

The mean serum HDL-C level observed in patients with MI in the present study (41.3 mg/dl) was significantly lower (p<0.001) than the values observed in controls (50.5mg/dl). In a study on Normolipidemic subjects in the age group 21-70 years it has been reported mean HDL-C levels of 52.9 mg/dl, which is 28.1% higher than the observations of the present study [14].

HDL-C levels similar to the present study have been reported (39.5mg/dl) [15] (42.11mg/dl) [6] in patients with heart disease. Similar levels of HDL-C was reported in many studies [4, 10, 16, 18]. Therefore, most of the research evidences supported drastic lowering of HDL-C levels in AMI patients.

Observations of Triglycerides

Triglyceride (TG) values observed in MI patients was (129mg/dl) significantly higher when compared with controls (107.8mg/dl). A similar level of TG have been reported [14, 18] in Normolipidemic AMI patients as observed in the present study. However 22.3% and 18% higher levels of HDL-C in MI patients was observed and reported by coworkers [15, 16] respectively.

Furthermore, significantly higher levels of TG (149 mg/dl) (15.5%) [19] and (140.5 mg/dl) 8.5% [8] have been observed compared with the observations of the present study.

The findings of the above data confirms that elevated TG levels are associated with the incidence of heart diseases in Normolipidemic AMI patients with body mass index (BMI) positively correlated with serum triglycerides.

Observations of Low Density Lipoprotein-Cholesterol

The mean serum level of LDL-C in the patients was (119.4mg/dl) significantly greater than control (83.6 mg/dl). In a study of healthy subjects with age group of 21-70 years, significantly higher value was reported and it was very much similar to the LDL-C level of the MI patients of the present study [14].

In the studies of patients with a history of MI, greater values were reported by several researchers [6, 18] where as some have reported [10] lower values of LDL-C than the present study. However similar levels of LDL-C in MI patients were also reported in several studies [8, 15, 16]

Observations of TC/HDL-C ratio

The TC/HDL-C ratio in MI patients (4.6) was significantly (p<0.001) higher compared with controls (3.4). Similar TC/HDL-C ratio (3.6) has been observed in Normolipidemic subjects of the age group 21-70 years by Goswami, et al., 2003 [14]. Lower ratio of TC/HDL-C were observed in AMI patients in study conducted elsewhere [15].

Similar ratio (4.6) was reported in MI patients by study conducted elsewhere [10, 16, 19, 20]. Higher ratio compared to the present study has been reported in MI patients [8, 16, 18]. A cut of level of 3.3 has been suggested [12].

These data indicate though the TC levels were within the normal level; the TC/HDL-C ratio was elevated significantly in MI patients indicating the importance of assessing TC/HDL-C ratio even in Normolipidemic subjects.

Observations of LDL-C/HDL-C ratio

Increased LDL-C and reduced HDL-C are considered to be highly atherogenic. Thus the increased level of LDL-C/HDL-C would indicate an increased risk of developing atherosclerosis. A cut of level of 1.6 has been suggested [12].

The present study observed significantly higher ratio (2.9) in AMI patients compared with control (1.9).

Results reported on the ratio were inconsistent, as some studies reported higher ratios [6, 15], similar ratio [15] and lower ratios [21] of LDL-C/HDL-C compared to the present study.

Observations of TG/HDL-C ratio

Increased TG and decreased HDL-C are also thought to be atherogenic and thus increased ratio of TG/HDL-C would indicate an increased atherogenic risk. The present study observed significantly (p<0.001) higher ratio (3.2) in MI patients compared with control (2.2). A slightly higher ratio (2.5) has been reported in healthy subjects earlier [14]. The data reported in previous studies in MI patients were inconsistent to the present study. Some studies have reported higher ratios [8, 15, 16, 17, 19, 21] whereas some reported similar ratios as observed in our study [18]. As per NCEP ATP-111 a cut of level of 2.5 has been suggested [12].

The present study concludes the importance of assessing the lipid ratios even in a normal individual as it is one of the atherogenic factors for development of myocardial infarction and other coronary complications. The practice of computing the ratio should be practiced even in a normal health check up packages.

References

1. Libby, P., Palangio, M. Clinical Insights in Lipid Management. Committee of Cardiovascular and Metabolic disease 2008 Vol 1: (12). Online publication released on May 12,2008 www.ccmd.org
2. Larosa, J.C., Chen, Ching-Ling C.Clinical Insights in Lipid Management. Committee of Cardiovascular and Metabolic disease 2008 Vol 1: (11). Online publication released on April 24,2008 www.ccmd.org
3. Mishra,T.K., Routray, S.N., Patnaik, U.K., Padhi,P.K., Satapathy, C. and Behera, M. Lipoprotein (a) and Lipid Profile in Young Patients with Angiographically Proven Coronary Artery Disease. Indian Heart Journal 2001; 53 :(5) Article No. 60.
4. Malhotra, P., Kumari, S., Singh, S. and Verma, S. Isolated Lipid Abnormalities in Rural and Urban Normotensive and Hypertensive North-West Indians. Journal of Assoc Physicians of India 2003; 51:459-463.
5. Achari,V. and Thakur, A.K. Association of Major Modifiable Risk factors Among Patients with Coronary Artery Disease –A retrospective Analysis. J Assoc Physicians India 2004; 52:103-108.
6. Mishra, A., Luthra, K. and Vikram, N.K. Dyspipidemia in Asian Indians: Determminants and Significance. Journal Assoc Physicians India 2005; 52:137-142.
7. Rajasekhar D., Srinivasa Rao P.V., Latheef S.A., Saibaba K.S., and Subramanyam G. Association of serum antioxidants and risk of coronary heart disease in South Indian population. Indian J Med Sci 2004; 58(11):465-71.
8. Rani, S.H., Madhavi, G., Ramachandra Rao, V., Sahay, B.K. and Jyothy, A. Risk factors for coronary heart disease in type II diabetes. Indian Journal of Clinical Biochemistry 2005; 20(2):75-80.
9. Ghosh, J., Mishra, T.K., Rao, Y.N. and Aggarwal, S.K.Oxidised LDL, HDL Cholesterol, LDL Cholesterol levels in patients of Coronary Artery Disease. Indian Journal of Clinical Biochemistry 2006; 21(1):181-184.
10. Patil,N., Chavan,V.and Karnik,N.D.Antioxidant Status in Patients with Acute Myocardial Infarction. Indian Journal of Clinical Biochemistry 2007; 22(1):45- 51.
11. Moriarty, P.M. www.ldlapersis.org assessed on May 12th 2008
12. Executive Summary of The Third Report of The National Cholesterol Education Program (NCEP) Expert panel on Detection, Evalation, and treatment of high Blood Cholesterol in Adults (Adult Treatment Panel III). Expert Panel of Detection, Evaluation, and Treatment of High Blood Cholesterol in Adults. JAMA 2001; 285(19):2486-97.
13. Friedewalds, W.T., Levy, R.I. and Fredrickson, D.S. Estimation of the concentration of low density lipoprotein cholesterol in plasma without the use of preparative ultracentrifuge. Clin. Chem 1972;18: 499-502.
14. Goswami,K.& Bandyopadhyay. Lipid profile in middle class Bengali population of Kolkata. Ind J of Clin Biochem 2003; 18:127-130.
15. Burman, A., Jain, K., Gulati,R., Chopra, V., Agrawal, D.P. & Vaisisht, S. Lipoprotein (a) as a marker of Coronary Artery Disease and its Association with Dietary Fat. J Assoc Physicians India 2004; 52:99-102.
16. Yadhav, A.S., Bhagwat, V.R. & Rathod, I.M. Relationship of Plasma homocysteine with lipid profile parameters in Ischemic Heart disease. Indian Journal of Clinical Biochemistry 2006; 21(1):106-110.
17. Sivaraman, S.K., Zachariah, G., Annamalai, P.T. Evaluation of C - reactive protein and other Inflammatory Markers in Acute Coronary Syndromes. Kuwait Medical Journal 2004; 36(1):35-37.
18. Shinde, S., Kumar, P.& Patil, N. Decreased Levels Of Erythrocyte Glutathione In Patients With Myocardial Infarction. The Internet Journal of Alternative Medicine 2005; 2:1.
19. Kharb,S. Low Glutathione levels in acute myocardial infarction. Ind J Med Sci 2003; 57; Issue8: 335-7.
20. Das,S., Yadav,D., Narang, R. & Das, N. Interrelationship between lipid peroxidation, ascorbic acid and superoxide dismutase in coronary artery disease. Current Science 2002; 83:488-491.

Chapter 17

Cardiovascular risk factors in Elderly Normolipidemic Acute Myocardial Infarct Patients- A Case Controlled study from India

Abstract

Myocardial Infarction (MI) is a leading cause of death in India. Cardiovascular risk factor varies with regions and individuals. Early detection and identification could reduce the cost effectiveness of high coronary care costs. Only few studies have addressed the cardiovascular risk factors among Indians. The goal of the present study was to address the various risk factors associated in Normolipidemic AMI patients admitted in Intensive Coronary care unit (ICCU) after heart attack. The study evaluated serum lipid profile, lipid peroxidation markers, antioxidants both endogenous and enzymes and inflammatory markers among the two groups consisting of acute myocardial infarction (AMI) patients and age/sex- matched controls.

Lipid profile, lipid peroxidation, enzyme antioxidants, endogenous antioxidants, ischemia modified-albumin (IscMA), caeruloplasmin, C-reactive protein (CRP), fibrinogen, Lipoprotein (a) and paraoxonase -1 activities were analyzed in 330 subjects, 165 acute myocardial infarction (AMI) patients and 165 age/sex-matched controls. We observed significantly higher (p<0.0001) lipid profile but lower high-density lipoprotein-cholesterol (HDL-C) in patients. The Lipoprotein (a), caeruloplasmin, C-reactive protein, fibrinogen were higher while bilirubin, ascorbic acid, uric acid, albumin, superoxide dismutase, catalase, glutathione peroxidase and paraoxonase-1 activities were lower in patients as compared to controls. The malondialdehyde (MDA) and conjugated diene (CD) were significantly increased (p<0.0001) in patients. Cardiovascular risk factor varies in Normolipidemic acute myocardial infarction (AMI) patients.

Introduction

With the explosive rise in the incidence of Coronary Artery disease (CAD) it is projected to be the leading cause of morbidity and mortality among Indians by the year 2015 (Reddy,1993). The World Health Organization (WHO) predicts that deaths due to circulatory system diseases are projected to double between 1985 and 2015 (Reddy and Yusuf, 1998; Bulatao and Stephens, 1990). Indians living abroad indicates a 40% higher risk of ischemic heart disease (IHD) mortality than that for Europeans (Balarajan, 1996).

It is a multi-factorial disease associated with factors like hereditary, hyperlipidemia, obesity, hypertension, environmental and life style variables like stress, smoking, alcohol consumption, etc (Chopra and Wasir 1998). Lipoprotein profile has been investigated extensively in recent years, which is deranged in large proportion of coronary artery disease (CAD) patients; especially Asians showing a mixed picture of dyslipidemia (Vasisht et al, 1990). Literature survey reveals dyslipidaemic subjects are more prone to myocardial infarction, due to increased free radical generation and ischemia as it is a conventional risk factor. (Malhotra et al, 2003; Mishra et al, 2005; Ghosh et al, 2006; Patil et al, 2007; Rajasekhar et al, 2004; Rani et al, 2005; Gomez et al,1996). Lowering of high density lipoprotein- cholesterol (HDL-C) is a common phenomenon observed in MI patients supported by previous studies (Malhotra et al, 2003; Mishra et al, 2005; Ghosh et al, 2006; Patil et al, 2007; Rajasekhar et al, 2004; Rani et al, 2005). High density lipoprotein- cholesterol (HDL-c) is the most important independent protective factor for arteriosclerosis which underlies coronary heart disease (CHD). High density lipoprotein- cholesterol (HDL-c) associated paraoxonase-1 (PON1) enzyme is protective against lipid peroxidation (Singh et al, 2007). Numerous cohort studies and clinical trials have confirmed the association between a low high density lipoprotein- cholesterol (HDL-c) and increased risk of coronary heart disease (CHD). Low density lipoprotein-cholesterol (LDL-C) is considered as the most important risk factor of coronary artery disease (CAD). Its oxidized form promotes foam cells formation which initiates the process of atherosclerosis by accumulating in sub-endothelium cells leading to fatty streaks and complex fibro fatty or atheromatous plaques formation (Berliner et al, 1995). The oxidation of low-density lipoprotein (LDL) can be limited by antioxidant enzyme system, including superoxide dismutase, catalase, glutathione peroxidase and antioxidant vitamins C, A, E and other carotenoids. Among the endogenous antioxidant system, includes albumin, uric acid, and total bilirubin. Imbalance of this reaction either due to excess free radical formation or insufficient removal by antioxidants leads to oxidative stress (Frei et al, 1998; Shrinivas et al, 2000; Maritim et al, 2003).

Various other risk factors have been identified apart from dyslipidemia are caeruloplasmin, C-reactive proteins, Lipoprotein (a), plasma fibrinogen, etc. Since we have encountered myocardial infarct patients with normal serum lipid concentration, we conducted a prospective case-control study to evaluate the concentration of antioxidant enzymes, degree of lipid peroxidation and other risk factors associated with acute myocardial infarction.

Materials and methods

The prospective case-control study consisted of 165 patients (123 men and 42 women) with AMI, admitted to the Intensive Cardiac Care Unit. The diagnosis of AMI was established according to diagnostic criteria: chest pain lasting for ≤ 3 hours, electrocardiographic (ECG) changes (ST elevation ≥ 2 mm in at least two leads) and elevation in enzymatic activities of serum creatine phosphokinase (CPK) and aspartate aminotransferase (AST). The control group consisted of 165 age/sex-matched healthy volunteers (123 men and 42 women). The design of this study was pre-approved by the institutional ethical committee board and informed consent was obtained from the patients and controls. Inclusion criteria were patients with a diagnosis of acute myocardial infarction (AMI) with normal lipid profile. Patients with diabetes mellitus, renal insufficiency, current and past smokers, hepatic disease or taking lipid lowering drugs or antioxidant vitamin supplements were excluded from the study. Normolipidemic status was judged by the following criteria: LDL≤160 mg/dl; HDL, ≥35 mg/dl; total cholesterol (TC), <200 mg/dl; and triglycerides (TG), <150 mg/dl (NCEP, ATP-III, 2001). Ten milliliters of blood was collected after overnight fasting for lipid profile assay. For ischemia-modified albumin (IscMA) analysis, 2 ml of blood was collected from the patients immediately after admission to intensive care unit.

Lipid Profile Total cholesterol (TC), triglyceride (TG) and high density lipoprotein-cholesterol (HDL-c) were analyzed enzymatically using kit obtained from Randox Laboratories Limited, Crumlin, UK. Plasma low density lipoprotein -cholesterol was determined from the values of total cholesterol and high density lipoprotein-cholesterol using the following formula:

$$\text{LDL-cholesterol} = TC - \frac{TG}{5} - \text{HDL-cholesterol (mg/dl)}$$

Other assays - Serum albumin was measured by Bromocresol green binding method (Perry *et al*, 1979). Serum uric acid was estimated by the method of Brown based on the development of a blue color due to tungsten blue as phosphotungstic acid is reduced by uric acid in alkaline medium (Brown,1945). Serum total bilirubin was estimated by the method of Jendrassik and Grof (Jendrassik and Grof, 1938).

The glutathione peroxidase (GPx) activity was determined by the procedure of Paglia and Valentine (Paglia and Valentine,1967). Superoxide dismutase (SOD) enzyme activity was measured by SOD assay kit using rate of inhibition of 2-(4-indophenyl)-(4-Nitrophenol)-5-phenyltetrazolium chloride (I.N.T) reduction method modified by Sun et al (Sun *et al*, 1988). Catalase activity was measured spectrophotometrically as described by Beutler (Beutler, 1984). MDA levels were estimated by thiobarbituric acid (TBA) reaction (Bernheim *et al*, 1948).Conjugated diene (CD) levels were measured by Recknagel and Glende method (Recknagel and Glende, 1984) with little modification. Caeruloplasmin assay was done by *p*-phenylene diamine method (Ravin, 1961). Ischemia-modified albumin (IscMA) concentration was determined by addition of a known amount of cobalt (II) to a serum sample and measurement of the unbound cobalt (II) by the intensity of colored complex formed after reacting with dithiothreitol (DTT) by colorimeter (Libby,2003). Lipoprotein (a), levels were determined by Latex-Enhanced turbidimetric method. Serum paraoxonase was estimated using Zeptometrix Assay Kit obtained from Zeptometrix Corp, New York, 14202 based on the cleavage of phenyl acetate resulting in phenol formation. The rate of formation of phenol is measured by monitoring the increase in absorbance at 270 nm at 25°C.

Estimation of ascorbic acid was carried out by Roe and Kuether method (Roe and Kuether, 1943). The C-reactive protein were determined using high sensitivity enzyme Immunoassay kit manufactured by Life Diagnostics,inc., Catalog Number: 2210. The principle of the assay was based on a solid phase enzyme-linked immunosorbent assay (Kumar and Sivakanesan, 2008). The plasma fibrinogen was determined using kit which was obtained from TEClot Fib Kit 10 Catalog No: 050-500, manufactured by TECO GmbH, Dieselstr. 1, 84088 Neufahrn NB Germany (Kumar and Sivakanesan, 2008).

All chemicals of analytical grade were obtained from Sigma-Aldrich Company, New Delhi.

Results

Anthropometric parameters in acute myocardial infarction (AMI) patients and control are shown in **Table 1.** Total cholesterol, its ratio to high density lipoprotein -cholesterol (TC/HDL-C) and triglyceride were significantly higher in both sexes of patients compared with control (**Table 2 and 3**). The low density lipoprotein –cholesterol (LDL-c) and its ratio to high density lipoprotein –cholesterol (LDL-c) (LDL-C/HDL-C) were higher in acute myocardial infarction (AMI) subjects than in control (Table-3). The behavioral pattern and familial history of cardiovascular disease is presented in **Table 4.** The distribution of risk factors and relative risk according to potential risk factors among cases and controls are presented in **Table 5** and **Table 6**. The status of antioxidants and lipid peroxidation are shown in **Table 7**. All antioxidants were significantly decreased in patients compared with controls. In agreement with this serum malondialdehyde (MDA) and conjugated diene (CD) were more abundant in patients compared with controls. Ischemia-modified albumin (IscMA) levels were also greater in both male and female patients compared with control (**Table 7**).Serum fibrinogen, caeruloplasmin, ischemia- modified albumin and C-reactive protein were significantly higher where as arylesterase activity were significantly lowered in cases compared with controls (**Table 8**).

Table 1. Anthropometric data of control and patients (mean ± SD).

	Control (n=165)	MI patients (n=165)	P- value (95%CI)
Age (years) Range (years)	60.5 ± 3.4 (48-69)	61.8 ± 3.8 (48-69)	0.0037 (61.26- 62.33)
Height (m)	1.63 ± 0.04	1.64 ± 0.59	0.2919 (1.55-1.72)
Weight (kg)	68.34 ± 3.97	72.01 ± 5.37	<0.01 (71.25-72.76)
BMI (kg/m^2)	25.40 ± 1.20	26.16 ± 1.45	<0.01 (25.95-26.36)
Waist Circumference (cm)	93.70 ± 3.63	100.77 ± 6.06	<0.01 (99.91-101.62)
Hip Circumference (cm)	100.01 ± 3.16	105.72 ± 5.23	<0.01 (104.82-106.45)
Waist-Hip ratio	0.93 ± 0.01	0.95 ± 0.01	<0.001 (0.94-0.95)
MAC (cm)	29.70 ± 1.47	30.63 ± 1.87	<0.01 (30.36-30.89)
BSFT(mm)	6.95 ± 1.05	7.5 ± 1.38	<0.001 (7.30-7.69)
TSFT (mm)	11.97 ± 1.27	12.89 ± 1.69	<0.001 (12.65-13.12)
SBP (mmHg)	121.06 ± 4.19	134.32 ± 11.65	<0.05 (132.67-135.96)
DBP (mmHg)	79.90 ± 3.64	86.04 ± 4.25	<0.05 (85.44-86.63)

Table 2. Lipid profile in patients and healthy controls (mean ± SD).

Variables	Controls (n=165)	Patients (n=165)	P-value (95%CI)
Age	60.55 ± 3.98	61.84 ± 3.80	0.0037(61.26-62.42)
Total Cholesterol (mg/dl)	168.58 ± 12.16	186.44 ± 13.95	<0.001(184.31-188.56)
HDL-Cholesterol (mg/dl)	50.51 ± 6.78	41.27 ± 4.62	<0.001(40.56-41.97)
Triglycerides (mg/dl)	107.84 ± 11.51	128.96 ± 12.19	<0.001(127.10-130.82)
LDL-Cholesterol (mg/dl)	83.59 ± 11.95	119.37 ± 14.05	<0.001(17.22-21.51)
TC: HDL-C	3.39 ± 0.36	4.57 ± 0.58	<0.001(4.48-4.65)
LDL:HDL-C	1.90 ± 0.31	2.93 ± 0.51	<0.001(2.85-3.00)
TG: HDL-C	2.17 ± 0.35	3.16 ± 0.49	0.3149(3.086-3.234)

Table 3. Distribution of Lipid ratios in patients and healthy controls (mean ± SD).

Ratio	Controls (n=165)	Patients (n=165)
TC/HDL-C		
2-3	2.90 ± 0.09 (n=28)	-
3-4	3.44 ± 0.25 (n=129)	3.70 ± 0.20 (n=31)
4-5	4.19 ± 0.22 (n=8)	4.53 ± 0.27 (n=90)
5-6	-	5.26 ± 0.23 (n=44)
TG/HDL-C		
1-2	1.77 ± 0.13 (n=56)	-
2-3	2.38 ± 0.23 (n=109)	2.65 ± 0.27 (n=59)
3-4	-	3.42 ± 0.26 (n=99)
4-5	-	4.22 ± 0.19 (n=7)
LDL-C/HDL-C		
1-2	1.71 ± 0.17 (n=106)	1.86 ± 0.15 (n=5)
2-3	2.23 ± 0.21 (n=59)	2.57 ± 0.27 (n=81)
3-4	-	3.32 ± 0.21 (n=74)
4-5	-	4.11 ± 0.12 (n=5)

Table 4. Behavioral Pattern in AMI patients and control.

	Control Group	Study Group
Hyperactive		
Yes	39 (23.63)	68 (41.21)
no	126 (76.36)	97 (58.78)
Triffle thinker *		
yes	30 (18.18)	99 (60.00)
no	135 (81.81)	66 (40.00)
Irrelevant thinker		
yes	50 (30.30)	106 (64.24)
No	115 (69.69)	59 (35.75)

Numbers in parentheses are percent unless mentioned otherwise
*Triffle thinker: subjects who thinks and worries on unnecessary small things

Table 5. Distribution of risk factors among AMI patients and control.

	AMI Cases (n=165)	Controls (n= 165)
Age (y)	61.84 ± 3.80	60.55 ± 3.98
BMI (kg/m^2)	26.16 ± 1.45	25.40 ± 1.20
Waist-to-hip ratio	0.95 ± 0.11	0.93 ± 0.08[a]
Alcohol intake (servings/d)	0.36 ± 0.68	0.15 ± 0.34[a]
Physical activity (MET-min/d)	56.23 ± 123.8	97.83 ± 174.8[a]
Current cigarette smokers (%)	14.45	3.6[b]
Current bidi smokers (%)	23.67	12.31[c]
Family history of MI (%)	37.57	8.48[d]
Hypertension (%)	49.09	1.8[e]
Alcoholics (%)	47.87	20.60[f]

Values are in Mean ± SD
[a,b,c,d,e,f] Significantly different from cases (*t* test for matched data): [a,b,c] $P \leq 0.001$, [d,e] $P \leq 0.0001$, [f] $P \leq 0.003$

Table 6. Relative risk (RR) of Acute Myocardial Infarction (AMI) according to potential risk factors[a]

	No. of cases N	No. of controls N	Age- and sex-adjusted RR (95% CI)[b]	Multivariate RR (95% CI)[c]
Cigarette smoking				
Never smoker	120	136	1.0	1.0
>10 cigarettes/d	36	6	7.8 (4.9, 13.5)	7.4 (4.3, 15.2)
Bidi smoking*				
Never smoker	120	136	1.0	1.0
> 10 bidis/d	49	8	8.2 (5.2, 14.2)	6.5 (3.9, 12.9)
BMI (kg/m2)				
20-24.9	30	51	1.0	1.0
≥ 25	135	114	2.7 (1.8,4.1)	2.9 (1.6, 5.1)
Waist –to-hip ratio				
≤ 0.95	52	137	1.0	1.0
> 1.0	113	28	3.9 (2.1, 6.3)	2.8 (1.6, 5.7)
Family history of MI				
No	97	151	1.0	1.0
Yes	62	14	2.1(1.6, 2.7)	2.7 (1.8, 3.8)
History of Hypertension				
No	136	142	1.0	1.0
Yes	29	23	2.1 (1.7, 3.2)	1.9 (1.4, 2.9)
Education level				
Highest level of education	25	27	1.0	1.0
None	101	132	3.1 (1.3, 5.1)	3.6 (1.0, 6.2)
Type of Family				
Split	20	64	1.0	1.0
Joint	145	101	4.5 (1.5- 2.9)	3.9(1.2-2.6)
Civil Status				
Lower Class	10	19	1.0	1.0
Middle Class	119	131	3.4 (4.3, 6.7)	2.8 (3.7, 5.9)
Higher Class	36	15	4.7 (4.9, 7.2)	3.8 (3.1, 4.7)
Leisure –time exercise				
Non-exerciser	82	58	1.0	1.0
≥ 145 MET-min/d	83	107	0.76 (0.4, 0.8)	0.68 (0.4, 0.7)
Household income				
>10 000 rupees/month	155	146	1.0	1.0

<5000 rupees/month	10	19	1.8 (1.2, 2.7)	1.7 (1.0, 3.1)
Hindu religion				
No	33	12	1.0	1.0
Yes	132	153	0.8 (0.6, 1.1)	0.9 (0.7, 1.3)

a MET, metabolic equivalent. RR estimates were obtained by using conditional logistic regression analysis controlled for the matching factors (age, sex, and hospital) and then additional potential risk factors.

b Also adjusted for hospital.

c Covariates controlled for in the multivariate model were as follows: age; sex; hospital; cigarette smoking [never, current (≤10 cigarettes/d, >10 cigarettes/d)]; bidi smoking [never, current (≤10 bidis/d, >10 bidis/d)]; BMI, in kg/m² (20-24.9, ≥25); waist-to-hip ratio (≤0.95, >1.0); leisure time physical exercise (none, < 145 MET-min/d, ≤145 MET-min/d); history of hypertension (no, yes); history of diabetes (no, yes); history of high cholesterol (no, yes); family history of IHD (no, yes); education (none, primary school, middle, secondary, higher secondary, college, graduate or professional); household income (<5000, 5000-10000, 10000-15000,>10000 rupees/mo); and Hindu religion (no, yes).

* Bidis (pronounced bee-dees) are small hand-rolled cigarettes manufactured in India and other southeast Asian countries. They are exported to as many as 122 countries, according to one bidi manufacturer. Bidi cigarettes are made of tobacco wrapped in tendu or temburni leaf *(Diospyros melanxylon)*.

Table 7. Antioxidant status and Lipid Peroxidation in Control and AMI patients (mean ± SD).

	Control (n=165)	AMI patients (n=165)	P value (95%CI)
Serum albumin (g/dl)	4.4 ± 0.3	4.2 ± 0.3	<0.001(4.17-4.28)
Serum uric acid (mg/dl)	5.8 ± 1.2	4.3 ± 0.9	<0.01(4.18-4.45)
Serum ascorbic acid (mg/dl)	5.3 ± 1.2	2.8 ± 0.7	<0.0001(2.70-2.89)
Serum Total bilirubin (mg/dl)	0.8 ± 0.2	0.7 ± 0.2	<0.001(0.62-0.69)
Serum superoxide dismutase (U/gHb)	1826.5 ± 31.9	813.9 ± 208.9	<0.02 (784.42-843.37)
Serum glutathione peroxidase(U/gHb)	61.3 ± 3.9	42.6 ± 6.3	<0.001(41.71- 43.48)
Serum catalase (k/gHb)	256.2 ± 26.7	193.1 ± 35.9	<0.001(188.03-198.16)
Serum Lipoprotein (a) (mg/dl)	3.0 ± 1.1	10.9 ± 2.2	<0.0001 (10.58-11.21)
Serum malondialdehyde (nmol/L)	5.7 ± 1.0	14.8 ± 1.7	<0.02(11.55-15.06)
Serum conjugated dienes (μmol/L)	31.0 ± 2.7	48.3 ± 5.5	<0.001(47.44-49.11)

TABLE 8. Other Biochemical parameters in Control and AMI patients (mean ± SD).

	Control (n=165)	AMI patients (n=165)	P value (95% CI)
Plasma fibrinogen (mg/dl)	237.5 ± 17.4	357.8 ± 23.2	<0.0001 (354.52 -361.07
Serum caeruloplasmin (mg/dl)	20.4 ± 2.3	51.5 ± 2.4	<0.0001 (51.16-51.83)
Serum Arylesterase activity (kU/L)	98.4 ± 6.2	69.7 ± 10.0	<0.0001(68.28-71.11)
Serum Ischemia modified albumin (U/ml)	81.9 ± 3.9	97.5 ± 11.7	<0.001(95.84-99.15)
Serum C-reactive protein (mg/dl)	1.1 ± 0.3	3.0 ± 1.1	<0.0001(2.84-3.15)

Dicussion

Coronary artery disease (CAD) remains the major cause of morbidity and mortality in all developed and developing countries in the world including India (Reddy and Yusuf, 1998). Dyslipidemia is one of the major modifiable risk factors for CAD (Chopra *et al*, 1998; Vasisht *et al*, 2000; Malhotra *et al*, 2003).

The coronary artery disease (CAD) risk factors do not predict the occurrence of acute myocardial infarction (AMI) as variation in risk factors is observed in South Asian population due to varied dietary habits and life style (Mishra *et al*, 2005). The search for various conventional risk factors among Asians could be helpful in recognizing the future events of stroke. These curiosities prompted us to identify the newer risk factors, with respect to Indian population.

The search for the newer risk factors continues and researchers are investigating the role of inflammatory markers and other potential risks factors which could link with acute myocardial infarction (AMI).

In this prospective case-control study in India, only Normolipidemic acute myocardial infarction (AMI) patients were selected. The study was designed to identify and evaluate potential risk factors in Normolipidemic acute myocardial infarction (AMI) patients. The subjects selected for the study comprised of 165 controls, 48-69 y and 165 acute MI patients, 48-69 y.

Anthropometric variables in acute myocardial infarction (AMI) patients showed highly significant differences in waist/hip ratio and biceps skin fold thickness. Study reported (Heitman *et al*, 2004) that waist /hip ratio is a dominant, independent and predictive variable of cardiovascular disease and coronary heart disease deaths in Australian men and women. Megnien *et al*, 1999 also reported high hip circumference relative to weight and waist circumference is a better predictor of low incidence of cardiovascular disease and coronary heart disease. The present study is in good agreement with the observations of the above studies. Among Indians the cardiovascular risk is high even the prevalence of obesity is minimal (Megnien *et al*, 1999). In the present study the mean body mass index and waist /hip ratio in all subjects was 26.56 and 0.96 respectively, showing a significantly higher body mass index and weight /hip ratio in patients compared with control.

Based on the observations of the aforementioned studies and further supported by the present study it could be concluded that weight/hip ratio is a better predictor of cardiovascular disease (CVD) than body mass index. So it is better tool for indentifying the future risk of acute myocardial infarction (AMI) in subjects by non-invasive procedures.

Observations of lipid profile

The mean total cholesterol level of the controls compared with acute myocardial infarction patients (186.44 ± 13.95 mg/dl) was significantly (p<0.001) higher compared with controls (168.58 ± 12.16 mg/dl). The mean high density lipoprotein-cholesterol level in the patients was significantly lower (p<0.001) compared with controls. Triglyceride (TG) values observed in acute myocardial infarction (AMI) patients was (129mg/dl) significantly higher than controls (107.8mg/dl). The mean low density lipoprotein-cholesterol (LDL-c) levels in patients was (119.4mg/dl) significantly higher than controls (83.6 mg/dl). The total cholesterol / high density lipoprotein – cholesterol ratio in acute myocardial infarct patients (4.6) was significantly (p<0.001) higher compared with controls (3.4). The present study observed significantly higher ratio (2.9) in acute myocardial infarction patients compared with control (1.9).

Earlier studies in lipid profile analysis conducted on acute myocardial infarction patients (Mishra *et al*, 2001; Das *et al*, 2002; Goswami *et al*, 2003; Kharb *et al*, 2003; Malhotra *et al*, 2003; Burman *et al*, 2004; Rajashekhar *et al*, 2004; Sivaraman *et al*, 2004; Rani *et al*, 2005; Shindhe, *et al*, 2005; Yadhav *et al*, 2006; Patil *et al*, 2007) observed higher total cholesterol, triglyceride, low-density lipoprotein –cholesterol and lower levels of high-density lipoprotein-cholesterol in patients compared to controls.

Also higher ratio of total cholesterol to high density lipoprotein-cholesterol, low-density lipoprotein-cholesterol to high-density cholesterol-lipoprotein and higher triglyceride to high-density cholesterol-lipoprotein was observed in the present study. The present study concludes the importance of assessing the lipid ratios even in Normolipidemic subjects as it is one of the atherogenic factors for development of myocardial infarction and other coronary complications. The practice of computing the ratio should be implemented even in a normal health check up packages. In the final analysis it appears that myocardial infarction and coronary artery disease are not always associated with an elevated serum total cholesterol concentration. The major concern of this observation is that subjects who maintain desirable total cholesterol concentration also are targets for myocardial infarction (MI) and coronary artery disease (CAD) and therefore analysis of other risk factors that are non-conventional and newly emerging will be of immense important in the eventual assessment of the risk status. The existing literature and the results of the present study all point out that acute myocardial infarction and coronary artery disease patients have significantly higher total cholesterol concentration whether the values are in the desirable range or elevated.

Antioxidant status

The serum endogenous antioxidants were decreased in acute myocardial infarction compared to controls. Similarly the enzyme antioxidants were also significantly lowered in patients.

Study conducted (Olusi *et al*, 1999; Djousse *et al* 2003) in acute myocardial infarction patients, reported significantly lower (p<0.0001) albumin and bilirubin (p<0.0001), where as lower levels of uric acid (Jing *et al*, 2000; Brand *et al*, 1985; Niskanen *et al*, 2004) and ascorbic acid (Nyossen *et al*, 1997; Bhakuni *et al*, 2006; Das *et al*, 2002; Kurl *et al*, 2002) in acute myocardial infarct patients were reported.

The aforementioned studies suggested the expected risk of acute myocardial infarction is increased where these endogenous antioxidants are lowered due to enhanced utilization during oxidative stress in patients. Though, uric acid is well established antioxidant, but at times it can also act as a pro-oxidant, which might increase the risk of myocardial infarction. Aulinskas et al, (1983) established the role of ascorbic acid as up regulator of low density –lipoprotein (LDL) receptors, facilitating the clearance of low density –lipoprotein (LDL). The low levels of ascorbic acid in acute myocardial infarction (AMI) patients in the present study might be due to enhanced utilization of ascorbic acid during oxidative stress in patients.

The enzymatic antioxidants namely superoxide dismutase, catalase and glutathione peroxidase are also lowered in patients compared with controls. The findings of the present study concurs to earlier studies (Senthil et al, 2004; Bhakuni et al, 2006; Jain et al, 2000; Rajashekhar et al, 2004; Das et al, 2002; Gupta et al, 2006; Patil et al, 2007) where lower activities of superoxide dismutase, catalase and glutathione peroxidase. Studies conducted (Senthil et al, 2004; Shindhe et al, 2005; Rajasekhar et al, 2004; El-Badry et al, 1995; Gupta et al, 2006 and Kharb 2003) also reported reduced activities of glutathione peroxidase in patients compared with controls. These studies are based on the hypothesis of decreased antioxidants due to oxidative insult in myocardial infarct patients. Thus it is indicative that low levels of both endogenous and enzyme antioxidants in circulation may be due to its increased utilization to scavenge toxic lipid peroxides.

Lipoprotein (a) and lipid peroxidation

The mean serum Lipoprotein (a) malondialdehyde (MDA) and conjugated diene (CD) levels in MI patients were higher compared with controls. Earlier studies conducted (Burman et al, 2004; Guha et al, 2001; Bal et al, 2001; Rajashekhar et al, 2004) also observed higher Lipoprotein (a) in AMI patients where as Nascetti et al, (1996) did not observed any change in Lipoprotein (a) levels in cardiovascular disease (CVD) patients and concluded lipoprotein (a) not to be considered as an independent risk factor in cardiovascular disease (CVD) patients.

Studies conducted (Senthil et al, 2004; Das et al, 2002; Kharb 2003; Bhakuni et al, 2006; Shindhe et al, 2005; Gupta et al, 2006) reported higher levels of malondialdehyde (MDA) in myocardial infarct patients.

Other biochemical parameters

The levels of caeruloplasmin, C-reactive protein, fibrinogen, ischemia-modified albumin were higher and arylesterase activities were lowered in patients. Studies conducted (Grobusch et al, 1999; El-Badry et al, 1995; Giurgie, 2005; Awadallah et al, 2006) observed significantly higher (p<0.001) levels of caeruloplasmin where as (Berton et al, 2003; Bhagat et al, 2003; Sivaraman et al, 2004; Kulsoom et al, 2006; Boncler et al, 2006) observed higher levels of C-reactive protein in patients. Shukla et al, (2006) stated elevated levels of caeruloplasmin as a risk factor for acute myocardial infarct patients. The reactive oxygen species disrupts copper binding to caeruloplasmin thus impairing its antioxidant property and further promoting oxidative pathology. Studies conducted on plasma fibrinogen levels in acute myocardial infarct patients (Harkut et al, 2004; Coppola et al, 2005; Beg et al, 2007; Sivaraman et al, 2004) reported rise in plasma fibrinogen as the present study. Earlier study conducted (Chawla et al, 2006; Auxter, 2003; Bar-Or et al, 2001) in acute myocardial infarct patients also reported higher levels in patients as observed by the present study. Studies on arylesterase activities in acute myocardial infarct patients (Aviram *et al*, 1999; Ayub *et al*, 1999; Richard *et al*, 2000; Jarvik *et al*, 2002; Azizi *et al*, 2002; Singh *et al*, 2007; Sarkar *et al*, 2006) also observed lower activities as concurrent to the current study. Increased C-reactive protein (CRP) concentrations in patients with unstable angina and acute myocardial infarct might induce the production by the monocytes of the tissue factor which initiates the coagulation process. C-reactive protein together with fibrinogen acts as a chemotactic factor. Fibrinogen is responsible for the adhesion of macrophages to the endothelial surface for their migration into the intima. The elevated c-reactive protein levels have been found to be related to the occurrence of cardiovascular complications such as sudden cardiac death or AMI (Pepys and Hirschfield, 2003).

Our study concluded apart from lipid profile, other variables which could be a probable risk for the future myocardial events have to be equally monitored. It is also recommended to increase dietary antioxidant intake in persons who already have known risk factors so that to some extent the myocardial infarction could be delayed. It is also important to check inflammatory markers like c-reactive protein and ischemia-modified albumin in a regular period of time after stepping early forties as they could be a cost effective mode of diagnosis and the subjects can be efficiently monitored and complications of myocardial infarction can be prolonged.

References

1. auxter S. Cardiac Ischemia testing: a new era in chest pain evaluation. *Clin Lab News* 2003; 29, 1-3.
2. Aulinskas TH, Vander Westhuyzen DR. Coetzee GA. Ascorbate increases the number of low density lipoprotein receptors in cultured arterial smooth muscle cells. *Atherosclerosis* 1983; 47: 159-71.
3. Aviram M, Rosenblat M, Billecke S, Eroul J, Sovenson R, Bisaier CL. Human serum paraoxonase (PON1) is in activated by oxidized low density lipoprotein and preserved by antioxidants. *Free Radic Biol Med* 1999; 26:892-904.
4. Awadallah SM, Hamad M, Jbarah I, Salem NM, Mubarak MS. Autoantibodies against oxidized LDL correlate with serum concentrations of caeruloplasmin in patients with cardiovascular disease. *Clin Chim Acta* 2006; 365: 330-336.
5. Ayub A, Mackness MI, Sharon A, Mackness B, Patel J, Durrington PN. Serum Paraoxonase After Myocardial Infarction. Arteriosclerosis, Thrombosis, and Vascular Biology 1999; 19:330-335.
6. Azizi F, Rahmani M, Raiszadeh F, Solati M, Navab M. Associations of lipids, lipoproteins, apolipoproteins and paraoxonase enzyme activity with premature coronary artery disease. *Coronary Artery Dis* 2002; 13(1): 9-16.
7. Balarajan R. Ethnicity and variations in mortality from coronary heart disease. *Health Trends* 1996; 28:45–51.
8. Bar-Or,D, Lau E, Rao N, Bampos N, Winkler JV, Curtis CG. Reduction in the cobalt binding capacity of human albumin with myocardial ischemia. *Ann. Emerg. Med* 1999; 34: 556.
9. Berliner JA, Navab M, Fogelman AM, Frank JS, Demer LL, Edwards PA, et al. Atherosclerosis: basic mechanisms. Oxidation. Inflammarion, and genetics. *Circulation* 1995; 91:2488-96.
10. Bernheim S, Bernheim MLC, Wilbur KM. The reaction between thiobarbituric acid and the oxidant product of certain lipids. *J Biol Chem* 1948; 174: 257-264.
11. Berton G, Cordiano R, Palmieri R, Pianca S, Pagliara V, Palatini P. C-Reactive Protein in Acute Myocardial Infarction: Association With Heart Failure. *Am Heart J* 2003; 145(6):1094-1101.
12. Beutler E. Red Cell Metabolism: *A Manual of Biochemical Methods, 3rd edition. New York, Grune and Stratton* 1984; 105.

13. Beg M, Nizami A, Singhal KC, Mohammed J, Gupta A, Azfar SF. Role of serum fibrinogen in patients of ischemic cerebrovascular disease. *Nepal Med Coll J* 2007; 9: 88-92.
14. Bhagat S, Gaiha M, Sharma VK, Anuradha S A. Comparative Evaluation of C - reactive protein as a Short-Term Prognostic Marker in Severe Unstable Angina- A Preliminary Study. *Journal of Assoc Physicians* 2003; 51:349-354.
15. Bhakuni P, Chandra M, Misra MK. Levels of free radical scavengers and antioxidants in post perfused patients of myocardial infarction. *Current Science* 2005; 89: 168-170.
16. Bhakuni P, Chandra M, Misra MK. Oxidative stress parameters in erythrocytes of post-reperfused patients with myocardial infarction. *J Enzyme Inhib Med Chem* 2005; 20(4):337-81.
17. Boncler M, Luzak B, Watala C. Role of C-reactive protein in atherogenesis. *Postepy Hig Med Dosw* 2006; 60:538-46.
18. Brand FN, Mcgee DL, Kannel WB, Stokes J, Castelli W P. Hyperuricemia as a rsik factor of coronary heart disease: The Framingham Study. *American Journal of Epidemiology* 1985; 121: 11-18.
19. Brown H. *J Clin Chem* 1945; 158:601.
20. Bulatao RAO, Stephens PW. Demographic estimates and projections, by region, 1970-2015. In: Jamison DT, Mosley WH, eds. Disease control priorities in developing countries. *Washington, DC: World Bank,* 1990. (Health sector priorities review no. 13.)
21. Burman A, Jain K, Gulati R, Chopra V, Agrawal DP, Vaisisht S. Lipoprotein (a) as a marker of Coronary Artery Disease and its Association with Dietary Fat. J Assoc Physicians India 2004; 52:99-102.
22. Chawla R, Goyal N, Calton R, Goyal S. Ischemia modified albumin: A novel marker for acute coronary syndrome. *Indian Journal of Clinical Biochemistry* 2006; 21(1):77-82.
23. Chopra V, Wasir H. Implications of lipoprotein abnormalities in Indian patients. *Journal Assoc Physicians of India* 1998; 46:814-8.
24. Coppola G, Rizzo M, Maurizio GA, Corrado E, Alberto DG, Braschi A, Braschi G, Novo S. Fibrinogen as a predictor of mortality after acute myocardial infarction: a forty-two-month follow up study. *Ital Heart J* 2005; 6:315-322.
25. Das S, Yadav D, Narang R, Das N. Interrelationship between lipid peroxidation, ascorbic acid and superoxide dismutase in coronary artery disease. *Current Science* 2002; 83:488-491.
26. Djousse L, Rothman KJ, Cupples LA, Levy D, Ellison RC. Effect of serum albumin and bilirubin as a risk factor for Myocardial infarction. *Am J Cardiol* 2003; 91: 485- 488.
27. El- Badry I, Abon El N, Yehia T K, Zakhari MM. Free radicals activity in Acute Myocardial Infarction. *The Egyptian Heart Journal* 1995; 47: 71-78.
28. Executive Summary of The Third Report of The National Cholesterol Education Program (NCEP) Expert panel on Detection, Evaluation, and treatment of high Blood Cholesterol in Adults (Adult Treatment Panel III). Expert Panel of Detection, Evaluation, and Treatment of High Blood Cholesterol in Adults. *JAMA* 2001; 285(19):2486-97.
29. Frei B, Stocker R, Ames BN. Antioxidant defenses and lipid peroxidation in human blood plasma. *Proc Natl Acad Sci USA* 1988; 85: 9748-9752.
30. Friedewalds, WT, Levy RI, Fredrickson DS. Estimation of the concentration of low density lipoprotein cholesterol in plasma without the use of preparative ultracentrifuge. *Clin. Chem* 1972; 18, 499-502.
31. Ghosh J, Mishra TK, Rao YN, Aggarwal SK. Oxidised LDL, HDL Cholesterol, LDL Cholesterol levels in patients of Coronary Artery Disease. *Indian Journal of Clinical Biochemistry* 2006; 21(1):181-184.
32. Giurgea N, Constantinescu MI, Stanciu R, Suciu S, Muresan A. Caeruloplasmin- acute –phase reactant or endogenous antioxidant? The case of cardiovascular disease. *Med Sci Monit* 2005; 11: RA 48-51.
33. Gomez MA, Anderson JL, Karagounis LA, Muhlestein JB, Mooers FB. An emergency medicine based protocol for rapidly ruling out myocardial ischemia reduces hospital time and expense. Results of randomized study (ROMO). *J. Am. coll. Cardiol* 1996; 28:25-33.
34. Goswami K Bandyopadhyay. Lipid profile in middle class Bengali population of Kolkata. *Ind J of Clin Biochem* 2003; 18:127-130.
35. Gupta M, Chari S. Proxidant and Antioxidant status in patients of type II Diabetes Mellitus with IHD. *Indian Journal of Clinical Biochemistry* 2006; 21(2):118-122.
36. Harkut PV, Sahashrabhojney VS, Salkar RG. Plasma fibrinogen as a marker of major adverse cardiac events in patients of type 2 Diabetes with unstable angina. *Int J Diab Dev Countries* 2004; 24: 69-74.
37. Heitman BL, Frederickson P, Lissner L. Hip Circumference and Cardiovascular Morbidity and Mortality in Men and Women. *Obesity Research* 2004; 12:482-487.
38. Jarvik GP, Tsai NT, Mckinstry LA, Wani R, Victoria HB, Richter RJ, Schellenberg GD, Heagerty PJ, Hatsukami TS, Furlong CE. Vitamin C and E Intake Is Associated With Increased Paraoxonase Activity. *Arteriosclerosis, Thrombosis, and Vascular Biology* 2002; 22:1329.

39. Jendrassik L, Grof B. *Biochem Zeit* 1938; 297:81 9.

188

40. Jing F, Alderman M H. Serum uric acid and cardiovascular mortality. *JAMA* 2000; 283: 2404-2410.

41. Kharb S. Low Glutathione levels in acute myocardial infarction. *Ind J Med Sci* 2003; 57; Issue8: 335-7.

42. Kurl S, Tuomainen TP, Laukkanen JA, Nyyssonen K, Lakka T, Sivenius J, Salonen JT. Plasma Vitamin C Modifies the Association Between Hypertension and Risk of Stroke. *Stroke* 2002; 33:1568.

43. Kulsoom B, Nazrul SH. Association of serum C - reactive protein and LDL: HDL with myocardial infarction. *J Pak Med Assoc* 2006; 56 (7):318-22.

44. Kumar A, Sivakanesan R. Does plasma fibrinogens and C-reactive protein predict the incidence of myocardial infarction in patients with normal lipids profile? *Pak J Med Sci* 2008; 24:336-339.

45. Libby P. Vascular biology of atherosclerosis: Overview and state of art. *Am J Cardiol* 2003; 91(suppl): 3A-6A.

46. Malhotra P, Kumari S, Singh S, Verma S. Isolated Lipid Abnormalities in Rural and Urban Normotensive and Hypertensive North-West Indians. *Journal of Assoc Physicians of India* 2003; 51:459-463.

47. Maritim AC, Sanders RA, Watkins JB. Diabetes, oxidative stress, and antioxidants: a review. *J Biochem Mol Toxicol* 2003; 17: 24-38.

48. Megnien JL, Denarie N, Cocaul M. Predicitve value of Waist-to-hip ratio on Cardiovascular Risk Events. *Int J Obes Relat Metab Disord* 1999; 23:90-97.

49. Mishra A, Luthra K, Vikram NK. Dyspipidemia in Asian Indians: Determmminants and Significance. *Journal Assoc Physicians India* 2005; 52:137-142.

50. Mishra TK, Routray SN, Patnaik UK, Padhi PK, Satapathy C, Behera M. Lipoprotein (a) and Lipid Profile in Young Patients with Angiographically Proven Coronary Artery Disease. *Indian Heart Journal* 2001; 53 :(5) Article No. 60.

51. Nascetti S, D' Addato S, Pascarelli N, Sangiorgi Z, Grippo MC, Gaddi A. Cardiovascular disease and Lp(a) in the adult population and in the elderly: the Brisighella study. *Riv Eur Sci Med Farmacol* 1996; 18(5-6):205-12.

52. Niskanen LK, Laaksonen DE, Nyyssonen K, Alfthan G, Lakka H M, Lakka TA, Salonene JT. Uric acid level as a risk factor for cardiovascular and all- cause moratlity in middle-aged men: a prospective study. *Arch Intern Med* 2004; 164:1546-51.

53. Nyyssonen K, Markku TP, Salonen R, Tuomilehto J, Salonen JT. Vitamin C deficiency and risk of myocardial infarction: prospective population study of men from eastern Finland. *BMJ* 1997; 314:634.

54. Olusi SO, Prabha K, Sugathan TN. Biochemical Risk factors for Myocardial Infarction Among South Asian Immigrants and Arabs. *Annals of Saudi Medicine* 1999; 19: 147-149.

55. Paglia DE, Valentine WN. Studies on quantitative and qualitative characterization of erythrocyte glutathione peroxidase. *J Lab Clin Med* 1967; 70: 158-69.

56. Patil N, Chavan V, Karnik ND. Antioxidant Status in Patients with Acute Myocardial Infarction. *Indian Journal of Clinical Biochemistry* 2007; 22(1):45-51.

57. Pepys MB and Hirschfield G M. C-reactive protein: a critical update. *J Clin Invest* 2003; 111(12): 1805-1812. doi: 10.1172/JCI200318921.

58. Perry BW, Doumas BT. Effect of heparin on albumin determination by use of bromocresol green and bromocresol purple. *Clin Chem* 1979; 25:1520-1522.

59. Rajasekhar D, Srinivasa Rao PV, Latheef SA, Saibaba KS, Subramanyam G. Association of serum antioxidants and risk of coronary heart disease in South Indian population. *Indian J Med Sci* 2004; 58(11):465-71.

60. Rani SH, Madhavi G, Ramachandra RV, Sahay BK, Jyothy A. Risk factors for coronary heart disease in type II diabetes. *Indian Journal of Clinical Biochemistry* 2005; 20(2):75-80.

61. Ravin HA. An improved colorimetric enzymatic assay of caeruloplasmin. *J. Lab. Med* 1961; 58, 161-168.

62. Recknagel RO, Glende EA. Spectrophotometric detection of lipid conjugated dienes. *Methods Enzymol* 1984; 105:331-337.

63. Reddy KS. Cardiovascular disease in India. *World Health Stat Q* 1993; 46:101-7.

64. Reddy KS, Yusuf S. Emerging epidemic of cardiovascular disease in developing countries. *Circulation* 1998; 97:596–601.

65. Richard JW, Leview I, Righetti A. Smoking Is Associated With Reduced Serum Paraoxonase Activity and Concentration in Patients With Coronary Artery Disease. *Circulation* 2000; 101:2252.

66. Roe JH, Kuether CA. *J. Biol Chem* 1943; 147:399.
67. Sarkar PD, TMS Madhusudhan B. Association between paraoxonase activity and lipid levels in patients with premature coronary artery disease. *Clin Chim Acta* 2006; 373:77-81.
68. Senthil S, Veerappan RM, Ramakrishna RM, Pugalendi KV. Oxidative stress and antioxidants in patients with cardiogenic shock complicating acute myocardial infarction. *Clin Chim Acta* 2004; 348 (1-2):131-7.
69. Shrinivas K, Vijaya Bhaskar M, Aruna Kumari M, Nagaraj K, Reddy KK. Antioxidants, lipid peroxidation and lipoproteins in primary hypertension. *Indian Heart J* 2000; 52:285-88.
70. Shinde S, Kumar P, Patil N. Decreased Levels Of Erythrocyte Glutathione In Patients With Myocardial Infarction. *The Internet Journal of Alternative Medicine* 2005; 2:1.
71. Singh S, Venketesh S, Verma JS, Verma M, Lellamma CO, Goel RC. Paraoxonase (PON11) activity in northwest Indian Punjabis with coronary artery disease & type II diabetes mellitus. *Indian J Med Res* 2007; 125:783-7.
72. Sivaraman S K, Zachariah G, Annamalai PT. Evaluation of C - reactive protein and other Inflammatory Markers in Acute Coronary Syndromes. *Kuwait Medical Journal* 2004; 36(1):35-37.
73. Sun Y, Oberly LW, Li Y. A simple method for clinical assay of superoxide dismutase. *Clin Chem* 1988; 34: 497-500.
74. Vasisht S, Narula J, Awtade A, Tandon R, Srivastava LM. Lipids and lipoproteins in normal controls and clinically documented coronary heart disease patients. *Ann Natl Acad Med Sci (India)* 1990; 26:57-66.
75. Yadhav AS, Bhagwat VR, Rathod IM. Relationship of Plasma homocysteine with lipid profile parameters in Ischemic Heart disease. *Indian Journal of Clinical Biochemistry* 2006; 21(1):106-110.

Chapter 18

Oxidative Stress, Endogenous Antioxidant and Ischemia-modified Albumin in Normolipidemic Acute Myocardial Infarction Patients

Abstract

Dyslipidemia appears to be a conventional risk factor for acute myocardial infarction (AMI). Several studies have reported decreased levels of antioxidants and increased levels of ischemia-modified albumin (IscMA) and lipid peroxides in dyslipidemic myocardial infarct patients. However, literature search reveals no reports of normolipidemic AMI patients with reference to antioxidants and IscMA studies. Therefore this study determined the endogenous levels of antioxidants and IscMA in normolipidemic AMI patients so that prospective measures could be taken to avoid acute coronary complications. The serum lipid profile, albumin, uric acid, total bilirubin, malondialdehyde, conjugated dienes and IscMA levels were determined in 165 normolipidemic AMI patients and 165 age/sex-matched controls. In addition, serum lipid concentrations were estimated by enzymatic methods.

Endogenous antioxidants were significantly decreased in AMI patients compared with controls. In parallel with this, serum malondialdehyde and conjugated dienes were significantly increased in AMI patients compared with controls. IscMA levels were significantly increased in AMI patients compared with controls.

As for the serum lipid profile, total cholesterol, cholesterol in low density lipoprotein (LDL) and triglycerides were higher in AMI subjects. High density lipoprotein (HDL)-to-cholesterol and LDL cholesterol-to-HDL cholesterol ratios were also greater in AMI subjects. However, HDL cholesterol was lower in AMI patients than control. AMI is a multifactorial disease that can arise even in normolipidemic subjects. The present study suggests that measuring of serum antioxidants and IscMA in normolipidemic patients would provide an index of oxidative stress and ischemia due to structural modifications of circulating albumin in serum.

Key words: acute myocardial infarction (AMI), normal lipid profile, endogenous antioxidant, ischemia-modified albumin (IscMA)

Introduction

With the explosive rise in the incidence of coronary artery disease (CAD), this entity is predicted to be the leading cause of morbidity and mortality in developing countries by the year 2015. [1] It is a multifactorial disease and predisposing factors suggested so far are hereditary, hyperlipidemia, obesity, hypertension, and environmental factors and life style variables such as stress, smoking and alcohol consumption. [2]

Lipoprotein profile is found to be deranged in the large proportion of CAD patients, especially Asians showing a mixed picture of dyslipidemia. Dyslipidemia is a well-established risk factor as reported in many studies. [3-10] Lowering of high-density lipoprotein (HDL) cholesterol is a common phenomenon observed in myocardial infarction (MI) patients.[3-10] Elevated Low density lipoprotein (LDL) cholesterol is considered the most important risk factor for CAD and its oxidation plays a central role in atherogenesis. Subendothelial accumulation of foam cells initiates the process of atherosclerosis. The generation of foam cells depends on the uptake of oxidized LDL by macrophages via scavenger receptors, leading to accumulation of fatty streaks and more complex fibro fatty or atheromatous plaques. [11] Under oxidative stress, not only LDL but also other serum lipids are exposed to oxidation.

Free radicals play an important role in the pathogenesis of tissue damage in many different clinical disorders. [12] Oxygen free radicals (OFRs) are produced continuously. Normally, OFR is regulated by a balance between tissue oxidant and antioxidant activity. [13] The latter is achieved by the antioxidant scavenger system which includes enzymes (superoxide dismutase, catalase and glutathione peroxidase) and antioxidant vitamins C, A, and E and α-lipoic acid and other carotenoids.[14] The endogenous antioxidant system includes albumin, uric acid, and total bilirubin. Imbalance of this reaction either due to excess free radical formation or insufficient removal by antioxidants leads to oxidative stress. [15]

Most cases of ischemia cause a reduction in oxygen supply to the cells but do not cause cell death. Ideally, one should be able to identify myocardial ischemia before it progresses to irreparable myocardial cell damage. Most of the cardiac markers do not become positive until cell death occurs and provide reliable information when measured in the first 2-6 hours following ischemic events. [16]

Recently, a new parameter, ischemia-modified albumin (IscMA), has been developed and found very useful for the detection of acute myocardial ischemia. While the circulating albumin molecules in the presence of ischemia are modified, this modification does not trigger cell death. [17] However, literature survey reveals that dyslipidemic patients are more prone to MI due to increased free radical generation and ischemic process causing enhanced formation of IscMA. Several studies have reported an increase in IscMA and lipid peroxidation concomitant with lowering of antioxidants.[18] It has been also reported that IscMA is elevated in acute MI (AMI) patients with dyslipidemia. [19,20] In our hospital, we treat a number of normolipidemic myocardial infarct patients. Hence the present study was undertaken to evaluate the levels of IscMA as well as antioxidants and lipid peroxides in normolipidemic AMI patients, as no such study has been conducted so far.

Materials and methods

Setting Design and Patients The study consisted of 165 patients (123 men and 42 women) with AMI, admitted to the Intensive Cardiac Care Unit. The diagnosis of AMI was established according to diagnostic criteria: chest pain lasting for ≤3 hours, electrocardiographic (ECG) changes (ST elevation ≥ 2 mm in at least two leads) and elevation in enzymatic activities of serum creatine phosphokinase and aspartate aminotransferase. The control group consisted of 165 age/sex-matched healthy volunteers (123 men and 42 women). The design of this study was pre-approved by the institutional ethical committee board, and informed consent was obtained from the patients and controls.

Inclusion criteria were patients with a diagnosis of AMI with normal lipid profile. Patients with diabetes mellitus, renal insufficiency, current and past smokers, hepatic disease or taking lipid lowering drugs or antioxidant vitamin supplements were excluded from the study. Normolipidemic status was judged by the following criteria: LDL≤160 mg/dl; HDL, ≥35 mg/dl; total cholesterol (TC), <200 mg/dl; and triglycerides (TG), <150 mg/dl.[21] Ten milliliters of blood was collected after overnight fasting for lipid profile assay. For IscMA analysis, 2 ml of blood was collected from the patients immediately after admission to intensive care unit.

Lipid Profile TC, TG and HDL-cholesterol were analyzed enzymatically using kit obtained from Randox Laboratories Limited, Crumlin, UK. Plasma LDL-cholesterol was determined from the values of total cholesterol and HDL-cholesterol using the following formula:

$$LDL\text{-cholesterol} = TC - \frac{TG}{5} - HDL\text{-cholesterol (mg/dl)}$$

Serum albumin Serum albumin was measured by Bromocresol green binding method. [22]

Other assays All chemicals of analytical grade were obtained from Sigma-Aldrich Company, New Delhi. Serum uric acid was estimated by the method of Brown based on the development of a blue color due to tungsten blue as phosphotungstic acid is reduced by uric acid in alkaline medium. [23] Serum total bilirubin was estimated by the method of Jendrassik and Grof.[24] Malondialdehyde (MDA) derived from lipid peroxides was determined as a thiobarbituric acid (TBA)-reactive substance.[25] Conjugated dienes (CD) were measured according to the method of Recknagel and Glende. [26]

IscMA concentration was determined by addition of a known amount of cobalt (II) to a serum sample and measurement of the unbound cobalt (II) by the intensity of colored complex formed after reacting with dithiothreitol (DTT) by colorimeter.[27] An inverse relationship thus exists between the level of albumin bound cobalt and the intensity of the color formed. The preparations for the Co (II) albumin binding protocol involved the addition of 200 µl of patient serum to 50 µl of a solution of 1g/l cobalt chloride, followed by vigorous mixing and 10-min incubation. Dithiothreitol (50 µl of a 1.5 g/l solution) was then added and mixed. After 2-min. incubation, 1.0 ml of a 9.0 g/l solution of NaCl was added. The absorbance of the assay mixture was read at 470 nm. The blank was prepared similarly with the exclusion of DTT. The values are expressed in U/ml. IMA assay was standardized in the Department of Biochemistry and a standard curve was prepared in the range 6.0-60.0 µg $CoCl_2$/ml. One IMA unit was defined as "µg of free Co (II) in the reaction mixture per ml of serum sample".

Statistical analysis: The data from patients and controls were compared by Student's t-test. Values are expressed as mean ± standard deviation (SD). Microsoft Excel for Windows 2000 was used for statistical analysis. P-value <0.05 was considered to indicate statistical significance.

Results

Serum parameters in AMI patients and control are shown in **Table 1**, and the data in males and females are separately shown in **Tables 2** and **3**, respectively. Total cholesterol, its ratio to HDL-cholesterol (TC/HDL-C) and triglycerides were significantly higher in both sexes of AMI subjects compared with control (**Table 1, 3**). Significant difference for HDL-cholesterol between AMI and control was seen only in female subjects (Table-3). On the other hand, LDL-cholesterol and its ratio to HDL-cholesterol (LDL-C/HDL-C) were higher in male AMI subjects than in control (**Table 2**). The status of endogenous antioxidants (albumin, bilirubin and uric acid) and lipid peroxidation (MDA and CD) are shown in **Tables 1, 3**. All endogenous antioxidants were significantly decreased in AMI patients compared with controls. In agreement with this serum MDA and CD were more abundant in AMI patients compared with controls. IscMA levels were also greater in both male and female AMI patients compared with control (**Tables 1, 3**).

Table 1. Endogenous antioxidants, lipid peroxidation, lipid profile and ischemia-modified albumin in AMI patients and healthy controls (mean ± SD)

Variables	Controls (n=165)	Patients (n=165)	P-value (95%CI)
Age	60.6 ± 4.0	61.8 ± 4.0	0.004(61.26-62.42)
Total Cholesterol (TC) mg%	168.6± 12.2	186.4 ± 14.0	<0.001(184.31-188.56)
HDL-Cholesterol (HDL-C) mg%	50.5 ± 6.8	41.3 ± 4.6	<0.001(40.56-41.97)
TC/ HDL-C ratio	3.4 ± 0.4	4.6 ± 0.6	<0.001(4.48-4.65)
Triglycerides (TG) mg%	107.8 ± 11.5	129.0 ± 12.2	<0.001(127.10-130.82)
LDL-Cholesterol (LDL-C) mg%	83.6 ± 12.0	119.4 ± 14.1	<0.001(17.22-21.51)
LDL-C/HDL-C ratio	1.9 ± 0.3	2.9 ± 0.5	<0.001(2.85-3.00)
TG/ HDL-C ratio	2.2 ± 0.4	3.2 ± 0.5	0.3149(3.086-3.234)
Albumin g%	4.4 ± 0.3	4.2 ± 0.3	<0.001(4.17- 4.28)
Total Bilirubin mg%	0.8 ± 0.2	0.7 ± 0.2	<0.001(0.62 -0.69)
Uric acid mg%	5.8 ± 1.3	4.3 ± 1.0	<0.01(4.18 -4.45)
MDA (nmol/L)	5.7 ± 1.0	14.8 ± 1.7	<0.02 (11.55-15.06)
Conjugated dienes (µmol/L)	31.0 ± 2.7	48.3 ± 5.5	<0.001 (47.44 - 49.11)
Ischemia modified albumin (U/ml)	81.9 ± 3.9	97.5 ± 11.7	<0.001(95.71- 99.28)

Table 2. Endogenous antioxidants, lipid peroxidation, lipid profile and ischemia-modified albumin in male patients and healthy controls (mean ± SD).

Variables	Control Male(n=123)	Male Patients (n=123)	P-value(95%CI)
Age	60.7 ± 4.1	61.5 ± 3.3	0.034 (60.95-62.10)
Total Cholesterol (TC) mg%	168.1 ± 12.1	183.8 ± 13.7	<0.001 (182.41-186.25)
HDL-Cholesterol (HDL-C) mg%	49.9 ± 7.3	41.8 ± 4.9	0.0801(40.91-42.64)
TC/ HDL-C ratio	3.4 ± 0.3	4.5 ± 0.6	<0.001(4.34-4.55)
Triglycerides (TG) mg%	105.0 ± 10.3	126.2 ± 11.7	<0.001(124.14-128.29)

LDL-Cholesterol (LDL-C) mg%	80.0 ± 8.0	116.8 ± 13.8	<0.001(114.38-119.25)
LDL-C/HDL-C ratio	1.9 ± 0.3	2.8 ± 0.5	<0.001(2.74-2.93)
TG/ HDL-C ratio	2.2 ± 0.4	3.1 ± 0.5	0.0123 (2.97-3.14)
Albumin g%	4.5 ± 0.3	4.2 ± 0.4	<0.001(4.14 – 4.27)
Total Bilirubin mg%	0.8 ± 0.2	0.7 ± 0.2	<0.001(0.65 -0.72)
Uric acid mg%	5.4 ± 1.1	4.3 ± 0.9	<0.001(4.18 – 4.49)
MDA (nmol/L)	5.7 ± 1.0	14.8 ± 1.7	<0.001(14.44 – 15.07)
Conjugated dienes (μmol/L)	31.0 ± 2.7	48.3 ± 5.5	<0.001(45.88 – 47.77)
Ischemia modified albumin (U/ml)	81.7 ± 3.9	97.9 ± 12.2	<0.001 (95.71-100.02)

Table 3. Endogenous antioxidants, lipid peroxidation, lipid profile and ischemia-modified albumin in female patients and healthy controls (mean ± SD).

Variables	Control Female (n=42)	Patients Female (n=42)	P value(95%CI)
Age	60.5 ± 2.9	62.7 ± 5.0	0.036(61.22-64.23)
Total Cholesterol (TC) mg%	170.0 ± 12.4	194.0 ± 13.0	<0.001(190.08-197.97)
HDL-Cholesterol (HDL-C) mg%	52.3 ± 4.6	39.8 ± 3.4	<0.001(38.75-40.78)
TC/ HDL-C ratio	3.3 ± 0.5	5.0 ± 0.4	<0.001(4.82-5.09)
Triglycerides (TG) mg%	116.1 ± 11.0	137.0 ± 9.8	<0.001(134.02-139.95)
LDL-Cholesterol (LDL-C) mg%	94.5 ± 14.8	126.9 ± 12.2	0.2044(123.16-130.55)
LDL-C/HDL-C ratio	1.8 ± 0.4	3.2 ± 0.4	0.3066(3.08-3.33)
TG/ HDL-C ratio	2.2 ± 0.3	3.5 ± 0.4	<0.001(3.34-3.59)
Albumin g%	4.4 ± 0.3	3.6 ± 0.2	<0.001(3.53 – 3.66)
Total Bilirubin mg%	0.7 ± 0.2	0.6 ± 0.1	<0.001(0.53 – 0.62)
Uric acid mg%	5.7 ± 1.4	4.3 ± 1.0	<0.001(3.98 -4.53)
MDA (nmol/L)	5.7 ± 1.0	14.8 ± 1.7	<0.001 (14.61 – 15.30)
Conjugated dienes (μmol/L)	31.0 ± 2.7	48.3 ± 5.5	<0.01 (51.36 -53.31)
Ischemia modified albumin (U/ml)	82.4 ± 4.1	96.4 ± 10.2	<0.001(93.33-99.48)

Fig 1. Ischemia-modified albumin (IscMA) in AMI (♦) and control subjects (■).

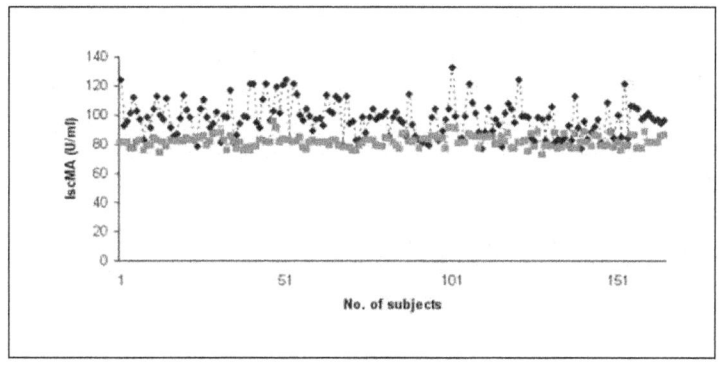

Discussion

Atherosclerosis is one of the major causes of AMI. Contrary to earlier belief, research in the last two decades has shown that atherosclerosis is neither a degenerative disease nor inevitable due to ageing. Atherosclerosis seems to be a chronic inflammatory condition that can be converted to an acute clinical event by the induction of plaque rupture, which in turn leads to thrombosis. Hence inflammation occurs during all phases of atherosclerosis, although it must smolder for decades before resulting in a clinical event such as AMI.[27] Myocardial ischemia is caused due to increased oxygen demand exceeding its supply and, if this condition is not reversed, MI precipitates. During this phase, circulating albumin becomes modified at the N-terminal residues, thus decreasing its affinity to bind to Co (II). Reperfusion of ischemic myocardium not only restores the blood supply but also causes massive production of free radicals, resulting in imbalance between oxidative and anti-oxidative processes. Excess production of reactive oxygen species may initiate lipid peroxidation in cell membranes. These processes reduce the contractile function of the heart and lead to severe myocardial cell damage termed as reperfusion injury.[28] This study suggests that antioxidants depletion has a significant impact on the precipitation of MI and these findings are consistent with the notion that elevated levels of antioxidants are protective against AMI.[29]

The current study observed a significant reduction in albumin, uric acid and total bilirubin and a significant increase in MDA, conjugated dienes and IscMA in AMI patients. The findings of the present study are similar to those of the study conducted by Dubois Rande et al [30] and Mc Murray [31] which reported a significant rise in MDA level and lipid peroxidation, with a concomitant decrease in antioxidants in patients with unstable angina and chronic heart failure. The present study also concurs with studies of Verma et al [32], who demonstrated that there was a significant drop in antioxidant, whereas lipid peroxides were significantly higher in AMI patients, compared with controls. The findings of the present study are also in good agreement with those of the study conducted by Kharb [33] where significantly decreased levels of antioxidants and increased levels of lipid peroxides were reported. This indicates that the antioxidant system combating oxidative stress and inflammation is severely impaired in AMI patients. The findings of the present study indicate that the existence of an abnormal balance between the oxidative and protective mechanisms in patients can be a causative factor for the occurrence of AMI. As has been demonstrated from reperfusion study in ischemic myocardium, [31] increased MDA levels in plasma have been used as an index of free radical-mediated damage, which is significantly elevated in AMI patients.

That the IscMA level in AMI patients was significantly higher than in controls as observed in the present study is similar to previous reports [18, 20, 34] Even though determination of IscMA is promising for the prediction of AMI, its use should be limited until further studies reveal its validity as a biomarker for AMI and usefulness in constructing treatment plans in acute coronary syndrome patients. An extensive study with increased number of patients would be required to compare IscMA with other markers such as troponins and myoglobin. Whether IscMA can be an additional parameter along with troponins to boost the confidence of clinicians in ruling out cardiac ischemia would be of particular interest.

Conclusion

MI is a multifactorial disease that can arise even in normolipidemic subjects. Hence, earlier concepts of maintaining lipid profile within normal limits to prevent MI may be overruled. The present study suggests that measuring serum antioxidants and IscMA in normolipidemic patients will aid better prognosis and management of patients with acute coronary syndromes. Oxidative stress appears an etiological factor for MI as a consequence of free radical scavengers namely antioxidants which tends to be lower in AMI patients.

References

1. Reddy KS. Cardiovascular disease in India. World Health Stat Q 1993; 46:101-7.
2. Chopra V, Wasir H. Implications of lipoprotein abnormalities in Indian patients. J Assoc Physicians India 1998; 46:814-8.
3. Mishra,T.K., Routray, S.N., Patnaik, U.K., Padhi,P.K., Satapathy, C. and Behera, M. Lipoprotein (a) and Lipid Profile in Young Patients with Angiographically Proven Coronary Artery Disease. Indian Heart J 2001; 53 :(5) Article No. 60.
4. Malhotra, P., Kumari, S., Singh, S. and Varma, S. Isolated Lipid Abnormalities in Rural and Urban Normotensive and Hypertensive North-West Indians. J of Assoc Physicians India 2003; 51:459-463.
5. Achari,V. and Thakur, A.K. Association of Major Modifiable Risk factors Among Patients with Coronary Artery Disease –A retrospective Analysis. J Assoc Physicians India 2004; 52:103-108.
6. Mishra, A., Luthra, K. and Vikram, N.K. Dyspipidemia in Asian Indians: Determminants and Significance. J Assoc Physicians India 2005; 52:137-142.
7. Rajasekhar D., Srinivasa Rao P.V., Latheef S.A., Saibaba K.S., and Subramanyam G. Association of serum antioxidants and risk of coronary heart disease in South Indian population. Indian J Med Sci 2004; 58(11):465-71.
8. Rani, S.H., Madhavi, G., Ramachandra Rao, V., Sahay, B.K. and Jyothy, A. Risk factors for coronary heart disease in type II diabetes. Indian J Clin Biochem 2005; 20(2):75-80.
9. Ghosh, J., Mishra, T.K., Rao, Y.N. and Aggarwal, S.K. Oxidised LDL, HDL Cholesterol, LDL Cholesterol levels in patients of Coronary Artery Disease. Indian J Clin Biochem 2006; 21(1):181-184.
10. Patil,N., Chavan,V.and Karnik,N.D.Antioxidant Status in Patients with Acute Myocardial Infarction. Indian J Clin Biochem 2007; 22(1):45-51.
11. Paul H, Johan V, Stefaan J, Frans Van de W, Désiré C. Oxidized LDL and Malondialdehyde-Modified LDL in Patients with Acute Coronary Syndromes and Stable Coronary Artery Disease. Circulation 1998; 98:1487-1494.
12. Halliwell B, Gutteridge GMC, Corss CE. Free radicals and antioxidants and human disease: where we are now? J Lab Clin Invest 1992; 119: 589-620.
13. Frei B, Stocker R, Ames BN. Antioxidant defenses and lipid peroxidation in human blood plasma. Proc Natl Acad Sci USA 1988; 85: 9748-9752.
14. Shrinivas K, Vijaya Bhaskar M, Aruna Kumari M, Nagaraj K, Reddy KK. Antioxidants, lipid peroxidation and lipoproteins in primary hypertension. Indian Heart J 2000; 52:285-88.
15. Maritim AC, Sanders RA, Watkins JB. Diabetes, oxidative stress, and antioxidants: a review. J Biochem Mol Toxicol 2003; 17: 24-38.
16. Gomez, M.A., Anderson, J.L., Karagounis L.A., Muhlestein, J.B. and Mooers, F.B. An emergency medicine based protocol for rapidly ruling out myocardial ischemia reduces hospital time and expense. Results of randomized study (ROMO). J Am Coll Cardiol 1996; 28:25-33.
17. Christenson, R.L., Duh SH, Sanhai WR, et al. Characteristics of an Albumin Cobalt Binding Test for Assessment of Acute Coronary Syndrome Patients: A Multicenter Study. Clin Chem 2001; 47: 464-470.
18. Sinha, M.K., Roy, D., Gaze, D.C. Collinson, P.O., Kaski,J.C. Role of Ischemia Modified Albumin", a new biochemical marker of myocardial Ischaemia, in the early diagnosis of acute coronary syndromes. Emerg Med J 2004; 21:29-34.

19. Robert, H. C., Show, H. D., Wendy, R. S., Alan, H.B.W., Verena, H.,Pennell, P., Elizabeth, B., Fred, S. A., MaryAnn, M. and Deborah, L. M. Characteristics of an Albumin Cobalt Binding Test for Assessment of Acute Coronary Syndrome Patients: A Multicenter Study. Clin Chem 2001; 47:464-470.

20. Collinson,P.O., Gaze,D.C., Bainbridge, K., Morris, F., Morris,B., Price,A. and Goodacre, S. Utility of admission cardiac troponin and "Ischemia Modified Albumin" measurements for rapid evaluation and rule out of suspected acute myocardial infarction in the emergency department. Emerg Med J 2006; 23: 256-261.

21. Executive Summary of The Third Report of The National Cholesterol Education Program (NCEP) Expert Panel on Detection, Evaluation, and Treatment of High Blood Cholesterol in Adults (Adult Treatment Panel III). Expert Panel of Detection, Evaluation, and Treatment of High Blood Cholesterol in Adults. JAMA 2001; 285(19):2486-97.

22. Perry,B.W., Doumas,B.T. Effect of heparin on albumin determination by use of bromocresol green and bromocresol purple. Clin Chem 1979; 25:1520-1522.

23. Brown, H. J Clin Chem 1945; 158:601.

24. Jendrassik L, Grof B. Biochem Zeit 1938; 297:81 9.

25. Bernheim S, Bernheim MLC, Wilbur KM. The reaction between thiobarbituric acid and the oxidant product of certain lipids. J Biol Chem 1948; 174: 257-264.

26. Recknagel RO, Glende EA. Spectrophotometric detection of lipid conjugated dienes. Methods Enzymol 1984; 105:331-337.

27. Libby P. Vascular biology of atherosclerosis: Overview and state of art. Am J Cardiol 2003; 91(suppl): 3A-6A.

28. Jacobson, M. D., Reactive oxygen species and programmed cell death. Trends Biochem Sci 1996, 243, 81–119.

29. Tomoda, H. et al., SOD activity as a predictor of myocardial reperfusion and salvage in acute myocardial infarction. Am Heart J 1996, 131, 849–856.

30. Dubois-Rande JL, Artigou JY, Darmon JY, Habbal R, Manuel C, Tayarani I, et al. Oxidative stress in patients with unstable angina. Eur Heart J 1994; 15(2): 179-83.

31. McMurray J. Evidence of oxidative stress in chronic heart failure in humans. Eur Heart J 1993; 14 (11): 1493-7.

32. Verma V.K., Ramesh, V., Tewari,S., Gupta, R.K., Sinha,N.& Pandey,C.M. Role of Bilirubin, Vitamin C and Ceruloplasmin as antioxidants I Coronary Artery Disease (CAD). Indian J Clin Biochem 2005 20(2): 68-74.

33. Kharb S. Low blood glutathione levels in acute myocardial infarction. Indian J Med Sci 2003; 57 (8): 335-7.

34. Bar-Or, D., Lau, E., Rao, N., Bampos, N., Winkler, J.V. and Curtis, C.G. Reduction in the cobalt binding capacity of human albumin with myocardial ischemia. Ann Emerg Med 1999; 34:556.

Chapter 19

Is Waist to Hip Ratio a better index than BMI in determining the risk of Myocardial Infarction in Normolipidemics?

Abstract

Objectives: To observe the changes in anthropometric variables in normolipidemic AMI patients and determine the significance of waist-hip ratio and basal metabolic index in assessment of risk of myocardial infarction compare to normal healthy control.

Materials and Methods

The study was conducted at Department of Biochemistry, Hindustan Institute of Medical Sciences and Research, Sharda Hospital, India and Faculty of Medicine, University of Peradeniya, Sri Lanka. The study subjects were categorized into two groups – one being control and the other being normolipidemic AMI patients. The study consisted of 165 normolipidemic AMI patients from India (87 males; 22 females) and Sri Lanka (36 males; 20 females) and 165 age-sex matched normal healthy control from India and Sri Lanka. The physical examination emphasized measurement of height (H), weight (W), waist circumference (WC), hip circumference(Hp), waist-hip ratio (W/H ratio), mid arm circumference (MAC), biceps skin fold thickness (BSFT)and triceps skin fold thickness (TSFT) was measured using standardized techniques.

Results: The present study observed highly significant changes (p<0.001) in weight, waist circumference, hip circumference, biceps and triceps skin fold thickness in cases compared to healthy age-sex matched control. The relative risk of MI was increased by 2.6 folds in subjects whose waist /hip ratio was ≥0.95 compared to those with normal waist/hip ratio.

Conclusion: Waist-to-hip ratio is a marker for determining the patients of myocardial infarction. The importance of anthropometric measurement should be implemented in ruling out the patients of high risk groups apart from considering the conventional risk factors.

Key words: Normolipidemia, Acute myocardial infarction, Waist - Hip ratio, BMI.

Introduction

Coronary artery disease (CAD) is a major cause of mortality and morbidity in the industrialized world which develops through the chain of events. The presence of certain risk factors elicits changes in the heart and vascular, some of which may initially be beneficial but may be maladaptive or become pathogenic when they progress. Cardiac biochemistry- hyperlipidemia is a subject of rapidly growing importance among Indian and Sri Lankan population. In fact, on account of neglect and ignorance, this area has not received any attention at all [1]. Recent studies on focused on waist-to-hip ratio, irrespective of other heart disease risk factors. Until now, body mass index (BMI) was used to judge overweight, but a global study found waist –to-hip ratio would more accurately predict the risk of myocardial infarction. A ratio of ≥ 0.85 for women and ≥ 0.9 for men is considered for the prediction of risk. [2] This is because fat stored around the waist is more likely to affect lipids in the blood and clog up arteries than fat stored around the thighs and hips. Myocardial infarct patients had "strikingly higher" waist-to-hip ratios, irrespective of other heart disease risk-factors. This observation was also found to be consistent in men and women across all ages, and in all regions of the world. A larger waist size was found to be harmful, whereas larger hip size - possibly indicating lower-body muscle mass - was protective.[3] With a view of the above studies, the current study was undertaken to assess the anthropometric variables in normolipidemic MI patients.

Setting Design and Patients The study consisted of 165 normolipidemic AMI patients from India (87 males; 22 females) and Sri Lanka (36 males; 20 females) and 165 age-sex matched normal healthy control. The diagnosis of AMI was established according to diagnostic criteria: chest pain lasting for up to 3 hours, electrocardiographic (ECG) changes (ST elevation of 2 mm or more in at least two leads) and elevation in the enzymatic activities of serum creatine phosphokinase and aspartate aminotransferase. The design of this study was pre-approved by the institutional ethical committee board of Chaudhary Charan Singh University, and informed consent was taken from the patients and controls.

An inclusion criterion was set to be patients with the diagnosis of AMI with normal lipid profile. Patients with diabetes mellitus, renal insufficiency, current and past smokers, hepatic disease or taking lipid lowering drugs or antioxidant vitamin supplements were excluded from the study. Normolipidemic status was judged by the following criteria: LDL<160mg/dl; HDL, ≥ 35 mg/dl; total cholesterol (TC), <200 mg/dl and triglycerides (TG), <150 mg/dl. [4] Ten ml of blood was collected after overnight fasting for lipid profile assay.

Lipid Profile TC, TG and HDL-cholesterol were analyzed enzymatically using kit obtained from Randox Laboratories Limited, Crumlin, UK. Plasma LDL-cholesterol was determined from the values of total cholesterol and HDL-cholesterol using the following formulae:

$$LDL\text{-cholesterol} = TC - \frac{TG}{5} - HDL\text{-cholesterol (mg/dl)}$$

Anthropometric examination: The anthropometric examination measurement of height (H), weight (W), waist circumference(WC), hip circumference (Hp), waist-hip ratio(W/H ratio), mid arm circumference (MAC), biceps skin fold thickness (BSFT)and triceps skin fold thickness (TSFT) was done by standardized procedure.

Height was measured in centimeters and weight in kilograms using calibrated spring balance. Supine waist girth was measured at the level of umbilicus with a person breathing silently and standing hip girth was measured at inter-trochanteric level.

Mid arm circumference was measured half way between the acromion process of the scapula and the tip of the elbow. Triceps skin fold thickness (TSFT) measurements were made at a point over the triceps muscle mid way the acromion and olecranon process on the posterior aspect of the arm.

Statistical Analysis: For statistical analysis two-sample t-test was performed and the results were expressed as mean ± SD, P≤0.05 was considered significant.

Results: The findings of the present study are shown in **Table 1** and **2.** The present study observed highly significant changes in W, WC, Hp, BSFT and TSFT when controls and cases were compared. The relative risk of MI was increased by 2.6 folds in subjects whose waist /hip ratio was ≥0.95 compared to those with normal waist/hip ratio.

Table 1. Lipid Profile in Control and AMI Patients.

Variables	Control(n=165)	Patient (n=165)	P value (95%CI)
Age (Mean ± SD)	60.55 ± 3.98	61.84 ± 3.80	0.0037(61.26-62.42)
Total Cholesterol (mg/dl)	168.58 ± 12.16	186.44 ± 13.95	<0.001(184.31-188.56)
HDL-Cholesterol (mg/dl)	50.51 ± 6.78	41.27 ± 4.62	<0.001(40.56-41.97)
TC: HDL-C ratio	3.39 ± 0.36	4.57 ± 0.58	<0.001(4.48-4.65)
Triglycerides (mg/dl)	107.84 ± 11.51	128.96 ± 12.19	<0.001(127.10-130.82)
LDL-Cholesterol (mg/dl)	83.59 ± 11.95	119.37 ± 14.05	<0.001(17.22-21.51)
LDL:HDL-C ratio	1.90 ± 0.31	2.93 ± 0.51	<0.001(2.85-3.00)
TG: HDL-C ratio	2.17 ± 0.35	3.16 ± 0.49	0.3149(3.086-3.234)

Table 2. Anthropometric variables in Control and AMI patients.

Variables	Control(n=165)	Patient (n=165)	P value (95%CI)
Height (cm)	1.63 ± 0.04	1.64 ± 0.05	>0.1 (1.63-1.64)
Weight (kg)	68.34 ± 3.97	72.01 ± 5.37	<0.001(71.19-72.82)
BMI (kg/m^2)	25.40 ± 1.20	26.16 ± 1.45	<0.01 (25.93-26.38)
Waist Circumference(cm)	93.70 ± 3.63	100.77 ± 6.06	<0.001(99.84-101.69)
Hip Circumference (cm)	100.01 ± 3.16	105.72 ± 5.23	<0.001(104.92-106.51)
Waist: Hip ratio	0.93 ± 0.01	0.95 ± 0.01	<0.02(0.94-0.95)
Mid Arm Circumference(cm)	29.70 ± 1.47	30.63 ± 1.87	<0.05(30.34-30.91)
Biceps skin fold thickness (mm)	6.95 ± 1.05	7.5 ± 1.38	<0.001(7.29-7.70)
Triceps skin fold thickness (mm)	11.97 ± 1.27	12.89 ± 1.69	<0.001(13.63-14.14)

Discussions

The anthropometric data of control and myocardial infarct patients are shown in **Table 1** and **2**. The body weight (W), waist circumference (WC), mid arm circumference (MAC), hip circumference (Hp), waist to hip ratio (W/H ratio) were significantly (p<0.0001) higher in MI patients compared to controls. Study reported that waist to hip ratio is a dominant, independent and predictive variable of CVD and CHD deaths in Australian men and women.[2] They stressed that the assessment of obesity by waist-hip ratio would be a better predictor of CVD and CHD mortality than waist circumference, which in turn, is a better predictor than BMI. The recognition of central obesity is clinically important, as life style intervention is likely to provide significant health benefits. Another study reported that high hip circumference, relative to body size and waist circumference predicts low incidence of CVD and CHD and total deaths in women and BMI and WC were the strongest independent predictors of CVD. [5] The present study is in good agreement with the observations of the above studies.

The clinical usefulness of waist-to-hip ratio (W/H ratio) for predicting the risk of cardiovascular events, was assessed with models based on the data from Framingham and Prospective Cardiovascular Munster (PROCAM) studies. [6] In this study abdominal fat was found to be the strongest predictor of cardiovascular complications in subjects whose W/H ratio was in the top quartile (>0.98 for men and >0.091 for women). The estimated percentage rate of coronary heart disease (CHD, p<0.01) and death (p<0.01), myocardial infarction (p<0.01), stroke (p<0.01), total CVD (p<0.01) increased with increasing quartile of W/H ratio in both men and women. In the highest W/H ratio, the number of subjects exceeding a 15% risk of developing a coronary event over the next 10 years was more than two-fold greater than in the lowest W/H ratio quartile. Their study concluded that abdominal deposition of fat assessed by W/H ratio is a strong predictor of cardiovascular events.

Cardiovascular risk factors have been reported in Asian Indians even though the prevalence of obesity is not high. [7] In a cross-sectional study, that involved subjects from low socioeconomic stratum residing in urban slums of New Delhi, approximately 68% of men and 88% of women had at least one risk factor for CVD. They concluded that Asian Indians have higher cardiovascular risk even at BMI and WC values within normal range and suggested that the definitions of "normal" ranges of BMI and WC need to be revised for Asian Indians.

Another reported [8] the prevalence of overweight to be 13.6% and obesity to be 2.2% in myocardial infarct subjects; 45.5% of them had normal weight and 38.4% were underweight. A higher W/H ratio (≥ 0.92) was observed in 11.4%. They found positive correlation between BMI and W/H ratio. In the present study the mean BMI and W/H ratio of all the subjects was 26.56 and 0.96 respectively, tending towards overweight and higher W/H ratio, with a significantly higher BMI and W/H ratio in study group compared to control subjects.

Based on the observations of the aforementioned studies it could be concluded that waist-hip ratio is a better predictor of CVD than BMI and same is observed in the present study. The significantly higher triceps skin fold thickness observed in MI patients in the present study has not been reported previously.

Conclusion: Apart from conventional risk factors for myocardial infarction, it is important for clinicians and researchers to go for non-invasive anthropometric measurement to rule out the risk for myocardial infarction.

References

1. Mendis, S. and Wissler, R. A Nutritional experiment to study short term effects of coconut in diet on serum cholesterol and platelet factor 4 in man. International Congress on Coronary Heart Disease 18th to 21st February 1988, Bombay, India.
2. Welborn,T.A., Dhaliwal, S.S. and Bennett, S.A.Waist-hip ratio is the dominant risk factor predicting cardiovascular death in Australia. Med J Aust; 2003; 179:580–5.
3. Barclay, L. Waist-to-Hip-Ratio May Predict Mortality Risk Better Than BMI in Elderly. Am J Clin Nutr. 2006; 84:449-460.
4. National Cholesterol Education Programme. Third report of the expert panel on detection, evaluation and treatment of high blood cholesterol in adults (Adult Panel III). (2001).
5. Heitman, B.L., Frederickson, P. and Lissner, L. Hip Circumference and Cardiovascular Morbidity and Mortality in Men and Women. Obesity Research 2004; 12:482-487.
6. Megnien J.L., Denarie N., and Cocaul M. Predicitve value of Waist-to-hip ratio on Cardiovascular Risk Events. Int J Obes Relat Metab Disord 1999; 23:90-97.
7. Vikram N.K., Pandey R.M., Misra A., Sharma R., Devi J.R and Khanna N. Non-Obese (body mass index<25kg/m2) Asians Indians with normal waist circumference have high cardiovascular risk. Nutrition 2003; 19(6):503-9.
8. Shahbazpour, N. Prevalence of Overweight and Obesity and Their Relation to Hypertension in Adult Male University Students in Kerman, Iran. Int J Endocrinol Metab 2003; 2:55-60.

Chapter 20

Thyroid Stimulating Hormone and its Correlation with Lipid Profile in the Obese Nepalese Population

Abstract

Background and Objectives: Obesity is an epidemic problem across the globe including developing countries. Obesity is associated with derangements in lipid profile, which further increases the risk of coronary heart disease, diabetes mellitus, stroke and certain cancers like endometrial, colon, esophageal and uterine. However, the association of obesity and thyroid stimulating hormone (TSH) is equivocal. The current study was undertaken

1. To establish the correlation between serum TSH level and varying degree of obesity depending on the body mass index (BMI).
2. To evaluate the relationship with BMI and lipid profile.

Materials and Methods: Two hundred and thirty seven (183 obese and 54 control) subjects were recruited for this study with age ranging from 30-65 y attending Western Regional Hospital, a government referral centre in Western region of Nepal. Subjects with history of familial hypercholesterolemia, hyperthyroidism, diabetes, hypertension, renal disease, cardiovascular disease and cancer were excluded from the study. Anthropometric variables, lipid profiles and TSH levels were determined in control and obese subjects. Blood glucose, serum urea, serum creatinine, SGPT levels were also determined in the participants.

Result: Significant difference in Systolic blood pressure (SBP) and diastolic blood pressure (DBP) was observed between obese and non-obese subjects (SBP; $p < 0.05$; DBP; $p < 0.05$). Weight, WC and W/H ratio significantly was positively correlated with increasing BMI ($p < 0.001$). Higher TC, TG, LDL-C and VLDL-C were observed in obese compared with control, except HDL-C which was significantly lower in obese subjects.

Significant difference ($p < 0.05$) was observed in TSH levels in control compared with obese. When the TSH levels were correlated among the obese subjects with grade I and grade II obesity according to BMI values, a significant differences ($p < 0.05$) in TSH levels were observed highlighting the variation in TSH levels depending on the extent of obesity.

Conclusion: With the current understanding of patients with thyroid disorders, the lipid profile, BMI and TSH should be well correlated among the subjects presenting with obesity. As lipid profile is deranged with higher BMI which impairs resistant to TSH in peripheral tissue further aggravating the thyroid problem. A closer examination of TSH is required in obese subjects, as these subjects are prone for cardiovascular diseases.

Key words: Thyroid Stimulating hormone, Lipid Profile, Obesity, BMI, Nepal.

Introduction

Obesity is noticed among all strata of population in developing countries (1). It is one of the conventional risk factor for cardiovascular disease (CVD) apart from hypertension, diabetes, hyperlipidemia and various endocrine disorders (2). Obesity is defined when a body mass index value exceeds the cut-off values of $\geq$ 24.9. Obesity is associated with lipoprotein metabolism abnormalities, and its assessment is extremely important in obese subjects as they are more likely to develop CVD (3). In context to Asians, the criteria of defining obesity are different from Western countries (4). Among Asian adults, a BMI value of $\geq$ 23.0 is considered as Obese, as per WHO Experts (5).Hypothyroidism is linked to obesity and so there must be any link with thyroid profile with lipid profile as derangements of lipid profile is observed in obesity. Even though numerous studies has been conducted earlier to link the thyroid profile parameters namely thyroid stimulating hormone (TSH) to those with lipid profile, a clear cut relationship between TSH and lipid profiles has not been established so far (6,7). Latest researches in this area tried to link with thyroid abnormalities with respect to body weight, the result seems to be normal in euthyroid subjects. Studies showed positive correlation between TSH levels and BMI $(kg/m^2) \geq$ 40 kg/m^2 (8). In European population a positive correlation is established between obesity (BMI > 30 kg/m^2) and TSH levels (9). However, recent study reported from United Kingdom failed to link between these two variables in euthyroid subjects (10). In context to Nepal, till today no literature is reported focusing between TSH levels and its relation to BMI in Nepalese population. The present study was aimed with hypothesis of increased TSH levels in obese subjects compared to control.

Thus the current study was undertaken to:

1. To establish the correlation between serum TSH level and varying degree of obesity depending on the body mass index (BMI).
2. To evaluate the relationship with BMI and lipid profile.

Material and methods

Two hundred and thirty seven subjects including both obese and control subjects with age ranging from 30 to 65 years, mean ($\pm$SD) 40.56 $\pm$ 0.93 were recruited from Western Regional Hospital, Pokhara, Nepal. Obesity was defined by a BMI values $\geq$ 23 kg/m^2 as obese and BMI values $\leq$ 23 kg/m^2 as controls. Among obese, it was further classified into two groups, Obese I (23- 26 kg/m^2) and Obese II ($\geq$ 26 kg/m^2).

Following the above criteria, 183 obese subjects (102 males; 81 females) and 54 controls (29 males; 25 females) were recruited for the study. An informed consent was obtained from the subjects before participating in the study and the study design was pre-approved by the institutional ethical committee board of Pokhara University, Nepal.

Exclusion criteria: Subjects with known hypercholesterolemia, hyperthyroidism, diabetes, hypertension, renal failure, cardiovascular disease, cancer and other known diseases.

A pre-tested questionnaire was used to record the age, height, weight, waist circumference (WC), Hip circumference (Hp) and waist-to-hip ratio (W/H) was calculated. Height was measured in centimeters and weight in kilograms using calibrated spring balance. Supine waist girth was measured at the level of umbilicus with a person breathing silently and standing hip girth was measured at inter-trochanteric level.

The BMI was calculated by weight (kg) divided by height (m²).

Blood pressure and pulse rate was also recorded from the participants. The blood pressure was measured using standard mercury manometer. At least two readings at 5 minutes intervals as per World Health Organization guidelines were recorded. If high blood pressure (≥140/90 mmHg) was noted a third reading was taken after 30 minutes. The lowest of the three readings was taken as blood pressure. The measurement of pulse rate was done by feeling palpitation on the wrist for one minute.

Lipid Profile Total Cholesterol (TC), Triglyceride (TG) and High-density lipoprotein cholesterol (HDL-C) were analyzed enzymatically using kit obtained from Randox Laboratories Limited, Crumlin, UK. Plasma LDL-cholesterol (LDL-C) was determined from the values of total cholesterol and HDL-cholesterol using the following formulae:

$$\text{LDL-cholesterol} = TC - \frac{TG}{5} - \text{HDL-cholesterol (mg/dl)}$$

Other assays The blood sugar was determined using enzymatic glucose oxidase peroxidase (GOD-POD) method with deproteinisation using Human Diagnostic kit obtained from Germany.

The Serum Creatinine was determined by Jaffes' method using Human kit.

The Serum Urea was determined by Berthelot reaction based on the hydrolysis of urea to ammonia and carbondioxide, further the ammonium ions reacts with hypochlorite and salicylate to form a green dye and the absorbance was proportional to the concentration of urea.

The serum SGPT was determined using enzymatic method based on the formation of glutamate and oxaloacetate from α-ketoglutarate and aspartate. The oxaloacetate formed further in the presence of malonate dehydrogenase converted to malate. The absorbance was based on formation of NAD⁺ at 340 nm. TSH was determined by enzyme linked immunosorbent assay (ELISA) using kit obtained from Ranbaxy Laboratories.

Statistical analysis

All statistical analysis was performed using SPSS version 11.0. Data were presented as mean ± Standard error mean. Correlations between measured parameters were assessed using the analytical method of Pearson co-efficient. Comparison of parameters between obese and non-obese subjects was performed with Mann-Whitney test and Kruskal-Walis test. $P < 0.05$ was considered to be statistically significant.

Result

The mean and standard error mean (SEM) of age, weight, height, WC, W/H ratio, Systolic blood pressure (SBP) and Diastolic blood pressure (DBP) are presented in **Table 1.** Significant difference in Systolic blood pressure (SBP) and diastolic blood pressure (DBP) was observed between obese and non-obese subjects (SBP; p<0.05; DBP; p<0.05). Weight, WC and W/H ratio significantly was positively correlated with increasing BMI (*p*<0.001). Systolic and diastolic blood pressure, weight, WC and W/H ratio also positively correlated with BMI (data not shown).

The biochemical parameters of the participants are presented in **Table 2.** The study observed significantly higher TC, TG, LDL-C and VLDL-C compared with control, except HDL-C which was significantly lower in obese subjects (**Table 2**).

The mean TSH level in control and obese is presented in **Table 3.** Significant difference (p<0.05) was observed in TSH levels in control compared with obese. When the TSH levels were correlated among the obese subjects with grade I and grade II obesity, BMI values significantly increased (p<0.05) (**Table 4**), highlighting the variation in TSH levels depending on the extent of obesity.

Table 1. Anthropometric variable in Obese and Non- Obese subjects.

Parameters	Control (n=54)	Obese (n=183)	P value (95% CI)
Age (years)	40.63 ± 1.33	40.77 ± 0.78	0.087 (40.65-40.80)
Height (mt)	1.56 ± 0.01	1.58 ± 0.09	0.0456 (1.56-1.59)
Weight (kg)	52.21 ± 0.98	69.36 ± 0.87	<0.001 (69.23-69.48)
WC (cms)	75.28 ± 1.48	91.30 ± 0.86	<0.001(91.17-91.42)
Hip circumference (cms)	88.56 ± 0.78	103.75 ± 0.73	<0.001(101.34- 104.21)
W/H ratio	0.85 ± 0.01	0.88 ± 0.01	<0.001(0.87-0.88)
SBP(mmHg)	118.39 ± 2.72	124.29 ± 1.39	<0.05(124.09-124.48)
DBP(mmHg)	78.50 ± 1.65	83.76 ± 1.04	<0.05(83.21-83.90)

Values are in mean (± SEM)

Table 2. Lipid profile and biochemical variable in Control and Obese subjects.

Parameters	Control (n=54)	Obese (n=183)	P Value (95% CI)
Total cholesterol (mg/dl)	160.73 ± 4.75	173.97 ± 3.19	<0.01(173.51-174.42)
Triglycerides (mg/dl)	108.59 ± 7.82	162.44 ± 11.94	<0.001(160.75-164.12)
HDL (mg/dl)	41.02 ± 1.52	39.08 ± 1.36	0.0864 (38.88-39.27)
LDL (mg/dl)	95.43 ± 5.18	104.38 ± 4.27	<0.05(103.77-104.98)
VLDL (mg/dl)	22.28 ± 1.56	31.91 ± 2.37	<0.05(31.57-32.24)
Fasting Glucose (mg/dl)	77.71 ± 1.94	80.12 ± 1.67	0.134 (79.88-80.35)
Serum Urea (mg/dl)	26.89 ± 1.19	28.18 ± 1.24	0. 245 (28.00-28.35)
Serum Creatinine (mg/dl)	0.97 ± 0.41	1.02 ± 0.37	0. 324 (0.96-1.07)
SGPT (U/L)	27.45 ± 1.09	30.71 ± 2.45	0. 068 (30.36-31.05)

Values quoted as mean ± SEM

Table 3. TSH level in Obese and Control subjects.

Parameter	Control (n = 54)	Obese (n = 183)	P value (95% CI)
Mean TSH(µIU/mL)	2.32 ± 0.23	2.64 ± 0.11	<0.05 (2.62-2.65)

Table 4. TSH level in Grade I and II Obesity

Parameter	Obese I (n = 79)	Obese II (n = 104)	P value (95% CI)
TSH(µIU/mL)	2.62 ± 0.23	2.68 ± 0.13	<0.05 (2.66-2.69)

Discussion

Obesity is a conventional risk factor for cardiovascular disease and is emerging as a major health problem in developing countries. The relationship between obesity, lipid profile and thyroid dysfunction is a concern for researchers and are carried out to link up these three aspects. Lipid and thyroid profiles are the most common investigations called for obese subjects by clinicians even though data linking obesity and thyroid function fail to prove its significant relationship (11, 12). Lipid abnormalities have been reported in obese individuals especially in central obesity (8, 9, 13). The present study was aimed to examine the relationship between obesity and lipid profile in context to Nepalese population inhabitant of Pokhara Valley, where there is higher trends of obesity among the locals in recent years. International Obesity Task Force stated that the approach to obesity should be considered on the basis of regional variations. Among Asians the cut-off value for BMI is 23 kg/m^2 to define obesity and the classification of obesity is based on BMI values ranges from 22-26 kg/m^2, however, clear cut demarcation of obesity is on BMI values more than 26 kg/m^2(14,15,16).

In the present study, dyslipidemia was observed among obese subjects and significantly higher levels of TC, TG, VLDL-C and LDL-C was observed in obese compared to non-obese which concurs with the reports of the previous studies (3, 17). The current study observed only TG levels to be positively correlated with BMI. Study conducted else where reported an increase in BMI was associated with increase in TG and decrease in HDL-C levels (5, 6, 7).

In the current study, a positive correlation was observed between TSH levels and obesity. In addition, TSH level was significantly higher, with high borderline value of BMI compared to the lower BMI values. Similar findings were reported (9) where a positive correlation between varying degree of obesity with varying TSH levels. Earlier study conducted also observed an association of BMI and TSH levels, showing varying TSH levels depending on the degree of obesity from mild to severe (8). The mechanism of elevated TSH levels in obese subjects still remains unclear (11) but increased TSH levels is suggestive of non responding receptors of target cells to TSH, a phenomenon similar to insulin resistant observed in diabetes (18,19). This theory has some merit, since T$_3$ receptors are decreased in obesity, resulting in a relative pituitary resistance to thyroid hormones (20, 21). A TRH stimulation test (TRH-t) could rule out whether pituitary response is altered in obese population (22, 23). It is also postulated that the production of TSH is also regulated by transmitters and hormones that regulate body weight satiation such as neuropeptide Y (alpha), melanocyte stimulating hormones and the agouti-related peptide innervating TRH synthesizing neurons (24,25). The other possible mediator of increased TSH secretion could be Leptin as suggested by earlier reports (11). The study has its limitations, as we did not measure serum fT_4 and fT_3 in our subjects, which could have added more information on status of thyroid function.

The current study did not observe any significant difference between TSH levels and lipid profile pattern, as reported in earlier studies (3, 4). In obese sub clinical hypothyroid patients higher energy expenditure is observed with higher TSH levels but does not alter body composition and lipid profile (26).

The study did not observe significant differences in BMI, body weight, WC, W/H ratio and dyslipidemia in elevated TSH levels compared with normal TSH levels, but significant difference in BMI was observed within normal TSH levels.

Furthermore, the study observed elevated TG and lower HDL-C associated with higher BMI showing the higher risk of cardiovascular diseases in obesity. A large scale study involving more health personnel and researchers are required to further carry out this work to validate the findings of the current study.

Conclusion

With the current understanding of patients with thyroid disorders, the lipid profile, BMI and TSH should be well correlated among the subjects presenting with obesity. As lipid profile is deranged with higher BMI which impairs resistant to TSH in peripheral tissue further aggravating the thyroid problem. A closer examination of TSH is required in obese subjects, as these subjects are prone for cardiovascular diseases.

Acknowledgements

The authors express their gratitude towards Pokhara University, for granting funds for this project. The authors are also thankful to Mr. Niranjan Shrestha, Lecturer, Biostatistics, School of Pharmaceutical and Biomedical Sciences Pokhara University for data analysis.

References

1. Jafar TH, Chaturvedi N, Pappas G. Prevalence of overweight and obesity and their association with hypertension and diabetes mellitus in an Indo-Asian population. *Canadian Medical Association Journal* 2006; 24:1071-1077.
2. Murray RK, Granner DK, Mayes PA, Rodwell VW. Harper's Illustrated Biochemistry (26th ed.). *Appleton-Lange, New York* 2003.
3. Hu D, Gray RS, Jablonski KA *et al.* Effects of obesity and body fat distribution on lipids and lipoproteins in nondiabetic American Indians: the Strong Heart Study. *Obesity Research* 2000; 8: 411-421.
4. Seidell J C, Kahn HS, Williamson DF, Lissner L and Valdez R. Report from a centers for disease and prevention workshop on use of Adult Anthropometry for Public Health and Primary Health Care. *Am J Clin Nutr* 2001; 73:123-126.
5. WHO Expert Consultation: Appropriate body mass index for Asian Populations and its implications for Policy and intervention strategies. *Lancet* 2001; 363:157-163.

6. Canaris GJ, Manowitz NR, Mayor G, Ridgway EC. The Colorado thyroid disease prevalence study. *Arch Intern Med* 2000; 160: 526-534.
7. Caraccio N, Ferannini E, Monzani F. Lipoprotein profile in subclinical hypothyroidism: response to levothyroxine replacement, a randomized placebo-controlled study. *J Clin Endocrinol Metab* 2002; 37: 1533-1538.
8. Iacobellis G, Ribaudo MC, Zappattereno A, Iannucci CV, Leonetti F. Relationship of thyroid hormone with body mass index, leptin, insulin sensitivity and adiponectin in euthyroid obese women. *Clinical Endocrinology* 2005; 62: 487-491.
9. Knudsen N, Laurberg P, Rasmussen LV *et al*. Small differences in thyroid function may be important for body mass index and the occurrence of obesity in the population. *Journal of Clinical Endocrinology and Metabolism* 2005; 90: 4019-4024.
10. Manji N, Boelaert K, Sheppard MC, Holdert RL, Gough SC, Franklyn JA. Lack of association between serum TSH or free T4 and body mass index in euthyroid subjects. *Clinical Endocrinology* 2006; 64: 125-128.
11. Bhowmick SK, Dasari G, Levens KL, Rettig KR. The prevalence of elevated serum thyroid-stimulating hormone in childhood/adolescent obesity and of autoimmune thyroid diseases in a subgroup. *Journal of the National Medical Association* 2007; 99: 773-776.
12. Terry RB, Wood PD, Haskell WL, stefanick ML, Kruss RM. Regional adiposity patterns in relation to lipid, lipoprotein cholesterol, and lipoprotein subfraction mass in men. *J Clin Endocrinol Metab* 1989; 68: 191-199.
13. Howard BB, Lee ET, Yeh JL, Go O, Fabsitz RR, Devereux RB, Welky TK. Hypertension in adult American Indians. *The Strong Heart study Hypertension* 1996; 28: 256-264.
14. WHO expert Consultation. Appropriate body mass index for Asian Populations and its implications for policy and intervention strategies. *Lancet* 2004; 363: 157-163.
15. Asia Pacific cohort studies collaboration. The Burden of over weight and obesity in the Asia pacific region. *Obesity Reviews* 2006; 8: 191-196.
16. Freedman DS, Jacobsen SJ, Barboriak JJ *et al*. Body fat distribution and male/female differences in lipids and lipoproteins. *Circulation* 1990; 81: 1498-1506.
17. Srinivasan SR, Myers L, Berenson GS. Temporal association between obesity and hyperinsulinemia in children, adolescents and young adults: the Bogalusa Heart Study. *Metabolism* 1999; 48: 928-934.
18. Reinher T, Andler W. Thyroid hormones before and after weight loss in obesity. *Arch Dis Child* 2002; 87: 320-323.
19. Burman KD, Latham KR, Djuh YY *et al*. Solubilized nuclear thyroid hormone receptors in circulating human mononuclear cells. *J Clin Endocrinol Metab* 1980; 51: 106-116.
20. Kvtny J. Nuclear thyroxine receptors and cellular metabolism of thyroxine in obese subjects before and after fasting. *Horm Res* 1985; 21: 60-65.
21. Glass AR, Kushner J. Obesity, nutrition and thyroid. *Endocrinologist* 1996; 6: 392-403.
22. Wilcox RG. Triiodothyronine, TSH and prolactin in obese women. *Lancet* 1997; 1: 1027-1029.
23. Stichel H, Allemand D, Gruter A. Thyroid function and obesity in children and adolescents. *Horm Res* 2000; 54: 14-9.
24. Mihaly E, Fekete C, Tatro JB *et al*. Hypophysiotropic thyrotropin releasing hormone synthesizing neurons in the human hypothalamus are innervated neuropeptide Y, agouti-related protein and alpha melanocyte-stimulating hormone. *J Clin Endocrinol Metab* 2000; 85: 2596-603.
25. Tagliaferri M, Berselli ME, Calo G *et al*. Subclinical hypothyroidism in obese patients: relation to resting energy expenditure, serum leptin, body composition, and lipid profile. *Obesity Research* 2001; 9: 196-200.

Chapter 21

Does plasma fibrinogens and c-reactive protein predict the incidence of myocardial infraction in patients with normal lipids profile?

Abstract

Objectives: To evaluate plasma fibrinogen and C-reactive proteins in patients with acute myocardial infarction (AMI) and compare it with normal lipid profile in healthy controls.

Methodology: Plasma fibrinogen and C-reactive proteins were determined in 165 patients and 165 age –sex matched control. The plasma fibrinogen was determined using kit, which was obtained from TECO GmbH, Dieselstr. 1, 84088 Neufahrn NB. The C-reactive protein were determined using high sensitivity enzyme Immunoassay kit manufactured by Life Diagnostics, inc. Also lipid profile was analysed enzymatically in these subjects. The values were expressed as means ± standard deviation (SD) and data from patients and controls was compared using student "t" test.

Results: Serum CRP and Plasma Fibrinogen were increased significantly (p<0.001) in AMI subjects compared to controls. High fibrinogen concentration and C-Reactive proteins seem to be important contributory risk factor in Indian CAD patients.

Conclusions: Thrombotic and inflammatory markers in combination may contribute to AMI with increased severity of the disease. Further larger studies on a nationwide basis recruiting a large number of AMI patients should be done to substantiate these findings.

Key words: Normal lipid profile, Plasma Fibrinogen, C-Reactive proteins and AMI.

Introduction

Although studies have demonstrated the role of fibrinogen and C-reactive protein as a coronary risk factor, there are controversial data on the correlation between plasma fibrinogen and c-reactive proteins and the ischemia process. Data regarding the role of fibrinogen and C-reactive proteins in patients of acute myocardial infarction with normal lipid profile is scanty. With the current understanding of the role of fibrinogen and C-reactive protein the present study was undertaken in normolipaedemic patients of acute myocardial infarction. Coronary Heart Disease (CHD) is associated with the greatest morbidity and mortality in industrialized countries.[1] The cost of management of CHD is a significant economic burden and so early detection and management is crucial. In the last decades a number of studies showed effective cost-benefit ratio of interventional approaches on the so-called "traditional" risk factors for coronary artery disease, with significant reductions in both cardiovascular morbidity and mortality.[2,3] The advancement in the understanding of pathophysiology of atherosclerotic vascular disease has given new insights regarding potential indicators of underlying atherosclerosis and cardiovascular risk. Thus, it has been recently tried world-wide to identify "new" possible atherosclerosis risk factors, including biochemical factors and genetic polymorphisms.[4] Several studies have suggested that high concentrations of fibrinogen may represent a strong risk factor for cardiovascular diseases[5-7] particularly Acute Myocardial Infarction.[8-10] Some of the newly emerged risk factors are called 'novel risk factors' which includes Lp(a), homocysteine, and hs CRP. Therefore, the aim of the present study was to evaluate, in a group of patients of AMI with normal lipid profile, the possible predictive role of plasma fibrinogen and C - reactive protein levels compared to normal healthy control. This study was undertaken due to lacunae of data on plasma fibrinogen and C-Reactive proteins in AMI patients with normal lipid profile.

Patients and methods

Setting Design and patients: The study consisted of 165 patients (123 men and 42 women) with AMI, admitted to the Intensive Cardiac Care Unit. The diagnosis of AMI was established according to diagnostic criteria: chest pain, which lasted for up to three hours, ECG changes (ST elevation of 2mm or more in at least two leads) and elevation of serum creatine phosphokinase (CPK-MB) and aspartate aminotransferase enzyme elevation. The study was conducted for a period of four and half years from April 2002 to September 2006. Informed consent was taken.

Inclusion criteria: Patients with diagnosis of AMI with normal lipid profile.

Exclusion criteria: Patients with diabetes mellitus, renal insufficiency, current and past smokers, hepatic disease or taking lipid lowering drugs or antioxidant vitamin supplements.

Selection of Controls: Age-, sex-matched subjects healthy volunteers consisting of 165 subjects, 123 men and 42 women were studied as control.

Collection of Samples: Blood collection and biochemical methods used: 10ml of blood was collected after overnight fasting in different containers.

1. EDTA vial: 5.0ml of blood was taken which was used for Plasma Fibrinogen assay.

2. Plain vial: Remaining blood was taken and serum was separated. Serum was used for determination of lipid profile, C-reactive proteins.

Lipid profile: Total cholesterol, triglycerides, and HDL-cholesterol) were analyzed enzymatically using kit obtained from (Randox Laboratories Limited, Crumlin, UK). Plasma LDL-cholesterol was determined from the values of total cholesterol and HDL-cholesterol using the following formulae:

$$LDL = TC - \frac{TG}{5} - HDL \text{ (mg/dl)}$$

C-reactive protein: The C-reactive protein were determined using high sensitivity enzyme Immunoassay kit11 manufactured by Life Diagnostics,inc., Catalog Number: 2210. The principle of the assay was based on a solid phase enzyme-linked immunosorbent assay.

Plasma Fibrinogen: The plasma fibrinogen was determined using kit12 which was obtained from TEClot Fib Kit 10 Catalog No: 050-500, manufactured by TECO GmbH, Dieselstr. 1, 84088 Neufahrn NB Germany.

Statistical Analysis: The data from patients and controls were compared using Student's 't'-test. Values were expressed as mean ± standard deviation (SD). Microft excel for windows 2000 was used for statistical analysis. 'P' value of less than 0.05 was considered to indicate statistical significance.

Results and observations

Baseline variable of control and AMI patients are shown in **Table 1.** The differences in age, height and body mass index (BMI) in control and AMI patient are insignificant. The weight, waist circumference, mid arm circumference, biceps and triceps skin fold thickness were higher in AMI subjects as compared to control (p<0.001) **(Table 1)** and **(Table 2)**. Systolic and diastolic blood pressure was significantly higher in AMI patient compared with controls (p<0.05) **(Table 1)**.

Table 1. Baseline Variables in Controls and AMI Patients (mean ±SD).

Variable	Control (n =165)	Patients (n = 165)
Age	60.6 ± 4.0	61.8 ± 3.8†
Height (cm)	1.6 ± 0.1	1.6 ± 0.1 ‡
Weight (kg)	68.3 ± 4.0	72.0 ± 5.4 §
BMI (kg/m2)	25.4 ± 1.2	26.2 ± 1.5||
Waist circumference(cm)	93.7 ± 3.6	100.8 ± 6.1 §
Hip circumference (cm)	100.0 ± 3.2	105.7 ± 5.2 §
Waist : Hip*	0.9	1.0 ¶
Systolic blood pressure(mm Hg)	113 ± 8	136 ± 2 **
Diastolic blood pressure(mm Hg)	85 ± 7	95 ± 10 **

*Ratio † (p = 0.0037) ; ‡ (p = 0.2919); § (p < 0.001); \|\|(p < 0.01); ¶ (p < 0.02);** (p < 0.05)

Table 2. Lipid Profile, plasma fibrinogen and C-reactive protein in Control and AMI Patient (mean ± SD)

Variable	Controls (n=165)	Patients (n=165)
Total cholesterol §	168.6 ± 12.2	186.4 ± 14.0 †
HDL-cholesterol §	50.5 ± 6.8	41.3 ± 4.6 †
TC : HDL-C*	3.4 ± 0.4	4.6 ± 0.6 †
Triglycerides §	107.8 ± 11.5	129.0 ± 12.2 †
LDL-cholesterol §	83.6 ± 11.9	119.4 ± 14.1 †
LDL:HDL-C*	1.9 ± 0.3	2.9 ± 0.5 †
TG:HDL-C*	2.2 ± 0.4	3.2 ± 0.5 ‡
C-Reactive protein §§	1.12 ± 0.33	2.97 ± 1.11 ††
Plasma fibrinogen§	237.55 ± 17.40	357.88 ± 23.18†

* Ratio † p<0.001; ‡ p= 1.0008; ††p<0.05; § mg/dl. §§ mg/l

The lipid profile are shown in **Table 2** Total cholesterol, TC: HDL-C ratio, triglycerides, LDL-cholesterol, LDL: HDL-C ratio were higher in AMI subjects as compared to control (**Table 2**) (p<0.001). Also, significant differences were seen in HDL-C levels between AMI and controls (p<0.001). LDL-cholesterol, LDL: HDL-C ratio were higher in male AMI subjects compared to control (**Table 4**) (p<0.001).

The C-reactive protein and plasma fibrinogen concentrations are shown in **Table 2**. Both parameters were significantly increased (p<0.001) in AMI patients compared to controls.

Discussion

The present study investigated fibrinogen and C-reactive protein in acute myocardial infarct patients since there is a paucity of data in Indian patients. There have also been reports which show that cardiovascular disease has reached alarming proportions in India and it cannot be neglected.13,14 The present study found higher levels of plasma fibrinogen and C-reactive protein (CRP) in patients with AMI compared to control (p<0.001). Fibrinogen levels were significantly elevated in MI patients in agreement with previous Indian studies.15-17

Various studies have18 suggested that the genesis of atherosclerotic plaque is dependent on the interplay of cellular components of the immune system like cytokines, adhesion molecules, lipids, platelets and endothelial cells, and the role of inflammatory markers like C-reactive protein cannot be ignored.19 It is an acute phase reactant considered as a classical marker for inflammation. Acute inflammation, infection, or tissue injury induces a marked increase in CRP. As atherosclerosis involves inflammation of the vascular endothelium, CRP levels tend to be raised.20 The notion that fibrinogen is strongly, consistently, and independently related to coronary risk has been widely accepted. The evidence is based on numerous prospective epidemiological studies and clinical observations. However, the reasons why fibrinogen is elevated in coronary disease and in atherosclerosis are not fully understood. All cells involved in the atherogenetic process are able to produce cytokines which induce an acute phase reaction. The potential pathophysiologic mechanisms by which elevated fibrinogen levels mediate coronary risk are manifold: It forms the substrate for thrombin and represents the final step in the coagulation cascade; it is essential for platelet aggregation; it modulates endothelial function; it promotes smooth muscle cell proliferation and migration; it interacts with the binding of plasminogen with its receptor; and finally it represents a major acute phase protein. Whether or not fibrinogen is causally involved in atherothrombogenesis still remains to be determined and even though other unsolved issues await conclusive answers, fibrinogen has emerged as an important additional marker of coronary risk.

Conclusions

High fibrinogen concentration and C-Reactive proteins seem to be important in Indian CAD patients. Thus, it can be said that thrombotic and inflammatory markers in combination may contribute to AMI with increased severity of the disease. Further larger studies on a nationwide basis recruiting a large number of AMI patients should be done to substantiate these findings.

References

1. Mendis S, Wissler R. A Nutritional experiment to study short term effects of coconut in diet on serum cholesterol and platelet factor 4 in man. Scientific Proceedings of the International Congress on Coronary Heart Disease Conference; 1988;18-21; Bombay, India.
2. Neaton JD, Wentworth D. Multiple Risk Factor Intervention Trial Research Group.Serum cholesterol, blood pressure, cigarette smoking, and Death from coronary heart disease. Overall findings and differences by age for 316099 white men. Arch Intern Med 1992;152:56-64.
3. Gould AL, Roussouw JE, Santanello NC, Heyse JF, Furberg CD. Cholesterol reduction yields clinical benefit. Impact of statin trials. Circulation 1998;97:946-52.
4. Ridker PM. Evaluating novel cardiovascular risk cfactors: Can we better predict heart attack? Ann Intern Med 1999;130:933-7.
5. Gil M, Zarebinski M, Adamus J. Plasma fibrinogen and troponin I in acute coronary syndrome and stable angina. Int J Cardiol 2002;83:43-6.
6. Ridker PM, Stamper MJ, Rifai N. Novel risk factors for systemic atherosclerosis: a comparison of C-reactive protein, fibrinogen, homocysteine, lipoprotein(a) and standard cholesterol screening predictors of peripheral arterial disease. JAMA 2001;285:2481-5.
7. Smith EB, Crospbie L. Fibrinogen and fibrin in atherogenesis. In: Ernst E, Koeing W, Lowe GD, Meade TW, eds, Fibrinogen: a new cardiovascular risk factor. Wein: Blackwell, 1992;4-10.
8. Seifried E, Oethinger M, Tansewell P, Hoegee-de Nobel E, Nieuwenhuizen W. Influence of acute myocardial infarction and rt-PA therapy on circulating fibrinogen. Thromb Haemost 1993;69:321-7.
9. Wilhelmsen L, Svardsudd K, Korsan-Bengsten K, Larson B, Welin L, Tibblin G. Fibrinogen as a risk factor for stroke and myocardial infarction. N Engl J Med 1984;311:501-5.
10. Tataru MC, Schulte H, von Eckardstein A, Heinrich J, Assmann G, Koehler E. Plasma fibrinogen inrelation to the severity of arteriosclerosis in patients with stable angina pectoris after myocardial infarction. Coron Artery Dis 2001;12:157-65.
11. Kindmark CO. The concentration of C-reactive protein in Sera from Healthy Individuals. Scand J Clin Lab Invest 1972;29:407-11.

12. Stefan Wagener. National Committee for Clinical Laboratory Standards: Guidelines for the Standardized Collection, Transport and Preparation of Blood Specimens for Coagulation Testing and Performance of Coagulation Assays. American Biological Safety Association (April 5, 2004), http://www.absa.org/0404nccls.html

13. Reddy KS. Neglecting cardiovascular disease is unaffordable. Bulletin of WHO 2001;79:984-5.

14. Reddy KS. Cardiovascular diseases in the developing countries: dimensions, determinants, dynamics and directions for public health. Public Health Nutr 2002;51:231-7.

15. Gheye S, Lakshmi AV, Krishna TP, Krishnaswamy K. Fibrinogen and Homocysteine levels in coronary artery disease. Ind Heart J 1999;51:499-502.

16. Deepa R, Velmurugan K, Saravanan G, Dwarkanath V, Agarwal S, Mohan V. Relationship of tissue plasminogen activator, plasminogen activator inhibitor-1 and fibrinogen with coronary artery disease in South Indian male subjects. J Assoc Physicians Ind 2002;50:901-6.

17. Chambers JC, Obeid OA, Refsum H, Ueland P, Hackett D, Hooper J, et al. EORTC Breast cancer group and EORTC radiotherapy group. Plasma homocysteine concentrations and risk of coronary heart disease in UK Indian Asian and European men. Lancet 2000;355:523-7.

18. Ridker PM. High-sensitivity C-reactive protein: Potential adjunct for global risk assessment in the primary prevention of cardiovascular disease. Circulation 2001;103:1813-18.

19. Berton G, Cordiano R, Palmieri R, Pianca S, Pagliara V, Palatini P. C-Reactive Protein in Acute Myocardial Infarction: Association with Heart Failure. Am Heart J 2003;145:1094-1101.

20. Rosenson RS, Koenig W. Utility of inflammatory markers in the management of coronary artery disease. Am J Cardiol 2003;92(Suppl):10i-18i.

Chapter 22

Hypertriglyceridemia: A Case Report from Diagnostic Laboratory, Barasat, West Bengal, India

Introduction

Hypertriglyceridemia is defined as an abnormal concentration of triglyceride in the blood and has been associated with atherosclerosis, even in the absence of hypercholesterolemia [1]. It can also lead to pancreatitis in excessive concentrations [2]. According to National Commission on Macroeconomics and Health (NCMH), a government of India undertaking, there would be around 62 million patients with CAD by 2015 in India and of these, 23 million would be patients younger than 40 years of age [3]. As per the National Cholesterol Education Program Adult Treatment Panel (NCEP ATP III) guidelines, a normal triglyceride level is 150 mg/dl [4]. In India, the prevalence of hypertriglyceridemia defined as a triglyceride level >150 mg/dl is 3.4% [5]. Hypertriglyceridemia could be of primary or secondary in nature. The primary hypertriglyceridemia arises from various genetic defects leading to disordered triglyceride metabolism. Secondary causes are acquired ones, could be due to high dietary fat, obesity, diabetes, hypothyroidism, and certain medications. Hypertriglyceridemia is a risk factor for pancreatitis and it accounts for 1 to 4% of cases of acute pancreatitis. Although a few patients can develop pancreatitis with triglyceride levels 500 mg/dl, the risk for pancreatitis does not become clinically significant until levels are 1000 mg/dl [6]. More importantly however, hypertriglyceridemia is typically not an isolated abnormality. It is frequently associated with other lipid abnormalities and the metabolic syndrome (abdominal obesity, insulin resistance, low high-density lipoprotein (HDL), high triglyceride, and hypertension), which are linked to coronary artery disease. Considering the current status of cardiovascular diseases among Indians, a drastic rise in the incidence of the metabolic syndrome is foreseen. Thus, primary care physicians would come across hypertriglyceridemia more frequently and should be familiar with the evaluation and management of this common disorder.

Case Report

A healthy 40-year-old man who came for a routine screening in our diagnostic laboratory at Barasat, Medicave Diagnostic Laboratory was detected to have hypertriglyceridemia. On interrogation, he was found to be a nonsmoker, has a reasonable diet with abundant fruits and vegetables, non-alcoholic, and exercises regularly. He has not been taking any lipid lowering medications. He works in a private sector in Barasat. His father died at the age of 57 years in an accident; but his mother is healthy and now almost 62 years of age, and he has two brothers one elder and another younger to him. His blood pressure was normal, his body-mass index was 27, and his waist circumference is 96 cm.

For lipid profile analysis twelve hours fasting blood samples were collected from the subject in our laboratory at Barasat. Five ml of blood samples was collected in a sterile test tube, allowed to clot and then carefully centrifuged at 3000 r.p.m for 10 minutes. Clear serum was used for analysis of lipid profile. The total cholesterol, triglyceride and high-density lipoprotein were analyzed enzymatically using kit obtained from Randox Laboratories Limited, Crumlin, UK. Plasma LDL-cholesterol was determined from the values of total cholesterol and HDL-cholesterol using the following formula [7]:

$$LDL\text{-cholesterol} = TC - \frac{TG}{5} - HDL\text{-cholesterol (mg/dl)}$$

One examination his fasting triglyceride level was 780 mg/dl.

The lipid profile was repeated in the subject after one week and the values almost remained the same.

Discussion

This study reveals hypertriglyceridemia with normal total cholesterol and very low LDL-C and HDL-C levels. Increased prevalence hypertriglyceridemia are more prominent in 31- 40 years age group as observed earlier studies [8], conforms with the current report. Enas et al. in their study on coronary artery disease in Indians (CADI) study reports the prevalence of diabetes to be three to six times higher among south Asian's than Europeans, Americans and other Asians [9] but in this subject we observed normal blood glucose levels with hypertriglyceridemia. We Indians have relatively higher risk of predisposition to coronary artery disease even at relatively lower level of cholesterol [10]. Further hospital based study also observed lower levels (<200 mg/dl) of cholesterol in 75% of patients with myocardial infarction which is indicative of the fact that we have lower threshold for the total cholesterol levels compared to western population adding to further risk of CAD [11]. The overall prevalence of hypertriglyceridemia differs between the age groups and it is higher in men than in women [12]. The contributing factor for hypertriglyceridemia in our report might be due to genetic predisposition as the subject is on a well balanced diet devoid of rich carbohydrates. High triglycerides levels have been associated with increased levels of small dense LDL which are considered to be highly atherogenic [13] which is not a risk in our report as the patients LDL cholesterol is also within normal reference range as per NCEP-ATP-III. Increased prevalence of low HDL has been reported earlier by Enas et al. who found that only 4% of Asian Indian men and 5% Asian Indian women had optimal HDL levels [9]. Low HDL-C levels are stronger predictor of occurrence and reoccurrence of MI and stroke and are also associated with premature and severe CAD [8]. Oxidative modification of LDL-C is a key process of atherosclerosis and elevated LDL-C has been recognized as primary risk factor for CAD [14] by NCEP – ATPIII but our report didn't observe any significant increase in LDL-C. So the current report suggests, hypertriglyceridemia could be presented in a patient without blood glucose elevation and not necessarily be accompanied by dyslipidaemia.

Conclusion

This study revealed the increased prevalence of dyslipidemia to be more prevalent in 31-40 year males, suggesting that this group is at increased risk of developing CAD leading to young infarcts. Combination lifestyle therapies i.e., enhanced physical activity and dietary modification and therapeutic intervention would help us in treatment and management of dyslipidemia.

References

1. http://www.news-medical.net/tag/feed/Hypertriglyceridemia.aspx
2. S Ian Gan, Alun L Edwards, Christopher J Symonds, Paul L Beck. Hypertriglyceridemia-induced pancreatitis: A case-based review World J Gastroenterol 2006; 12(44): 7197-7202.
3. Report of the National Commission on Macroeconomics and Health. Ministry of Health and Family Welfare, Government of India, 2005.
4. Executive Summary of The Third Report of The National Cholesterol Education Program (NCEP) Expert panel on Detection, Evaluation, and treatment of high Blood Cholesterol in Adults (Adult Treatment Panel III). Expert Panel of Detection, Evaluation, and Treatment of High Blood Cholesterol in Adults. JAMA 2001; 285(19):2486-97.
5. Rajmohan L, Deepa R, Mohan A, Mohan V. Association between isolated hypercholesterolemia, isolated hypertriglyceridemia and coronary artery disease in south Indian type 2 diabetic patients. Indian Heart J. 2000 Jul-Aug; 52(4):400-6.
6. Rade N. Pejic, Daniel T. Lee. Hypertriglyceridemia. J Am Board Fam Med. 2006; 19(3):310-316.
7. Friedewalds, W.T., Levy, R.I. and Fredrickson, D.S. Estimation of the concentration of low density lipoprotein cholesterol in plasma without the use of preparative ultracentrifuge. Clin. Chem 1972; 18: 499-502.
8. Sawant AM, Shetty D, Mankeshwar R, Ashavaid TF. Prevalence of dyslipidemia in young adult Indian population. J Assoc Physicians India. 2008 Feb; 56:99-102.
9. E. A. Enas & A. Senthilkumar : Coronary Artery Disease In Asian Indians: An Update And Review. The Internet Journal of Cardiology. 2001 Volume 1 Number 2.
10. Leea J, Hengb D, Chiaa KS, Chewc SK, Tanc BY, Hughesa K. Risk factors and incident coronary heart disease in Chinese, Malay and Asian Indian males: the Singapore Cardiovascular Cohort Study. International Journal of Epidemiology 2001; 30(5): 983-988.
11. Kumar A, Sivakanesan R. Behavioral pattern, life style and socio economic status in elderly Normolipidemic Acute Myocardial Infarct Subjects - A case control study from South Asia. The Internet Journal of Cardiovascular Research. 2009 Volume 6 Number 2.
12. Gomez-Huelgas R, Bernal-López M R, Villalobos A, Mancera-Romero J, Baca-Osorio A J, Jansen S, Guijarro R, Salgado F, Tinahones F J & Serrano-Ríos M. Hypertriglyceridemic waist: an alternative to the metabolic syndrome? Results of the IMAP Study (multidisciplinary intervention in primary care) International Journal of Obesity, 15 June 2010 doi:10.1038/ijo.2010.127.
13. Gupta R, Rastogi S, Panwar RB, Soangra MR, Gupta VP, Gupta KD. Major coronary risk factors and coronary heart disease epidemic in India. South Asian J Prev Cardiol 2003; 7:11-40.
14. Antonio M. Gotto J. Antioxidants, statins, and atherosclerosis.Am Coll Cardiol, 2003; 41:1205-1210, doi: 10.1016/S0735-1097(03)00082-2.

Other titles by iMedPub:

- *Social Medicine in the 21st Century* by Samuel Barrack.

- *World Health Report 2012: No Health Without Research* by Samuel Barrack.

- *Quality design in Anatomical Pathology* by Anil Malleshi Betigeri.

- *Escherichia coli infections* by Viroj Wiwanitkit.

- *Atlas of Biomarkers for Alzheimer's disease* by Manuel Menendez.

- *Advances in Research and Treatment for Alzheimer's disease by* Samuel Barrack.

www.ingramcontent.com/pod-product-compliance
Lightning Source LLC
Chambersburg PA
CBHW081439170526
45166CB00008B/2250